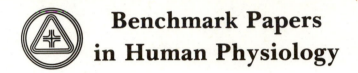

Benchmark Papers
in Human Physiology

Series Editor: L. L. Langley
University of Missouri School of Medicine

Published Volumes and Volumes in Preparation

HOMEOSTASIS: Origins of the Concept
    L. L. Langley
CONTRACEPTION
    L. L. Langley
MICROCIRCULATION
    Mary P. Wiedeman
THE PHYSIOLOGY OF RESPIRATION
    Julius H. Comroe, Jr.
ELECTROPHYSIOLOGY
    Hebbel E. Hoff
HUMAN CARDIOVASCULAR PHYSIOLOGY
    James V. Warren
THERMAL HOMEOSTASIS
    T. H. Benzinger
INFANT NUTRITION
    Doris Merritt
OVULATION INDUCTION
    S. M. Husain

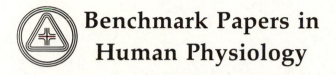

Benchmark Papers in
Human Physiology

─── A *BENCHMARK* ® Books Series ───

MICROCIRCULATION

Edited by
MARY P. WIEDEMAN, Ph.D.
Temple University, School of Medicine

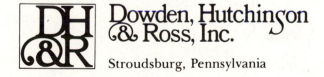

Dowden, Hutchinson
& Ross, Inc.
Stroudsburg, Pennsylvania

Manufactured in the United States of America.

Exclusive distributor outside the United States and
Canada: John Wiley & Sons, Inc.

74 75 76   5 4 3 2 1

Library of Congress Cataloging in Publication Data

Wiedeman, Mary P
    Microcirculation.

    (Benchmark papers in human physiology, v. 3)
    1. Microcirculation--Addresses, essays, lectures.
I. Title. [DNLM: 1. Microcirculation--Collected
works. WG103 W644m 1974]
QP106.6.W53   599'.01'1   73-22327
ISBN 0-87933-066-X

Permissions

The following papers have been reprinted with the permission of the authors and the copyright holders.

Academic Press, Inc.—*Microcirculation as Related to Shock*
   "Rheological Aspects of Low Flow States"

Angiology Research Foundation, Inc.—*Angiology*
   "Vascular Patterns and Active Vasomotion as Determiners of Flow Through Minute Vessels"

Blackwell Scientific Publications Ltd.—*Movement of the Heart and Blood in Animals*

The Heymans Institute of Pharmacology—*Archives Internationales de Pharmacodynamie et de Thérapie*
   "Transmural Pressure and Vascular Tone—Some Aspects of an Old Controversy"

The Rockefeller University Press
   Journal of Biophysical and Biochemical Cytology
      "Studies on Inflammation: II. The Site of Action of Histamine and Serotonin Along the Vascular
         Tree: A Topographic Study"
   Journal of General Physiology
      "Dynamics of Transcapillary Fluid Exchange"

Charles C Thomas, Publisher—*Selected Readings in the History of Physiology*
   De pulmonibus: Observationes anatomicae

The Wistar Institute Press
   American Journal of Anatomy
      "Microscopic Observations on the Extra-endothelial Cells of Living Mammalian Blood Vessels"
      "Observations on Living Preformed Blood Vessels As Seen in a Transparent Chamber Inserted into
         the Rabbit's Ear"
      "A Quantitative Study of the Hemodynamics in the Living Microvascular System"
   Anatomical Record
      "The Character and Distribution of the Blood Capillaries"
      "Contraction of Blood Vessels and Observations on the Circulation in the Transparent Chamber in
         the Rabbit's Ear"
      "Spleen Studies: I. Microscopic Observations of the Circulatory System of Living Unstimulated Mam-
         malian Spleens"
      "The Use of the Hamster Cheek Pouch for the Study of Vascular Changes at the Microscopic Level"
   Circulation Research
      "Dimensions of Blood Vessels from Distributing Artery to Collecting Vein"

Yale University Press—*The Anatomy and Physiology of Capillaries*

Series Editor's Preface

The Benchmark Books Publishing Program is a new and unique concept, a concept that has rapidly spread to myriad fields and which has already won wide acceptance. In essence, each volume contains reproductions of the original articles vital to the development of a particular field, or to a major concept within a field. When the publisher asked me to be Series Editor for the "Benchmark Papers in Human Physiology," I decided that I should not only encourage leaders in various subdisciplines of human physiology to prepare volumes but that I should undertake two myself. The two, *Homeostasis: Origins of the Concept,* and *Contraception,* were both published in 1973. The present volume, by Dr. Mary Wiedeman, will soon be followed by others, edited for example, by Hebbel Hoff, James Warren, Julius Comroe, T. H. Benzinger, Doris Merritt, and S. M. Husain. In due time, then, this series will contain a collection of the most important original publications in the major areas of human physiology.

Dr. Mary Wiedeman has long been recognized as a leader in the field of microcirculation. She is also a superb writer. Recently she undertook to revise the classic textbook "Physiology and Anatomy," by Esther Greisheimer. In view of the fact that I authored a competing text, I know all too well how successful Dr. Wiedeman's revision is!

Microcirculation, in current jargon, is what it's all about. The rest of the circulatory system, and indeed the respiratory system too, are designed to deliver blood with an adequate oxygen load to the microcirculation, that is, to the capillaries, where blood–tissue fluid exchange occurs. This is where the action is, and therefore, knowledge of microcirculation is essential. In this volume, the classic, early papers are presented, beginning, quite logically, with William Harvey. The giant in the field, August Krogh, is accorded a separate section, and the volume concludes with the landmark papers that followed. Characteristically modest, Dr. Wiedeman includes but one of her own publications, a crisp, meaty article that provides essential data on the dimensions of these microvessels.

Microcirculation is a rapidly expanding field. A second volume will be needed in a few years.

L. L. Langley

Contents

V.   IN THE LAST DECADE

Contents by Author

Introduction

At present, the term "microcirculation" is used to designate blood flow through small vessels at the capillary level. The microcirculatory bed is that portion of the cardiovascular system involved in the transfer of nutrients and the removal of metabolic waste products. Minute precapillary arterioles and postcapillary venules are included with the capillaries as the major components of the microcirculatory system.

Although the term microcirculation is relatively new, the study of the flow of blood through very small blood vessels dates back to Malpighi, who used magnifying lenses to look at blood vessels in frog lung and mesentery 300 years ago. During the 300 years since those observations were first recorded, an untold number of investigators have been exploring vascular beds in practically every tissue of a large variety of amphibians and mammals. The ingenuity that has been shown in the design of techniques for microscopic observations of the circulation of blood through arterial and venous vessels is breathtaking. It is difficult to understand why our knowledge of the structure and functional behavior of capillary networks is not complete, if one considers the talent, the vigor, and the excellence of the investigators who have devoted themselves to the study. The fact remains that there are still areas of disagreement regarding the nomenclature, architecture, and control mechanisms of this special area of the circulatory system.

It is of interest that the structural organization of all of the microcirculatory networks that have been studied reveal more similarities than dissimilarities. Although minor differences in vascular patterns (between, for example, skin and skeletal muscle) seem to be associated with the structure of the tissue in which the vessels lie, the basic pattern remains the same.

A consideration of the entire vascular system leads one to the conclusion that the heart and the macrocirculation are present for the sole purpose of supplying blood to the microcirculation, where the delivery of life-sustaining nutrients to tissue cells and the removal of their metabolic waste takes place. It is therefore appropriate that

1

a great deal of study has been devoted to the design and regulation of these minute vessels.

The results of investigations using *in vivo* microscopy have been, until recently, primarily descriptive. To some extent, the anatomical structure and physiological functions of the terminal vascular bed have been clarified. The concept of a preferential, or thoroughfare, channel has been presented, challenged, and is now partially dispelled.

Vasomotion, the spontaneous contraction and relaxation of both arterial and venous vessels (independent of innervation), has been described and assigned a function in the regulation of blood flow into and out of capillary networks. The concept of the Rouget cell as a major contractile element has been abandoned, and capillary contractility has been disproved.

The phenomenon of vasomotion (the word first appeared in the literature in 1944) may be seen wherever smooth muscle exists—in arteries, arterioles, precapillary sphincters, venules, and veins. Such activity in venous vessels, especially if intravascular pressure serves as the mechanism that controls its frequency and intensity, may serve as an effective aid to venous return of blood from postcapillary vessels. Vasomotion may also serve as the regulator of arterial blood flow through capillary nets and as a mechanism whereby capillary vessels could be protected against sudden or prolonged increases in pressure that might rupture their thin walls.

The concept that intraluminal pressure change activates vascular smooth muscle and that the resultant vasoconstriction controls the flow of blood into capillaries has recently been expanded to explain autoregulation of blood flow in terminal beds. "Autoregulation" is defined as the capability of an organ to regulate its blood supply in accordance with its needs, or, in a more restricted sense, as the tendency of an organ to maintain constant blood flow despite changes in arterial perfusion pressure. Thus far, autoregulation has been noted and described in the kidney, skeletal muscle, brain, intestine, myocardium, and liver of experimental animals, including dogs, cats, rats, bats, and calves. There is evidence that it also occurs in the brain and kidney of humans.

The entrance to a capillary network is guarded by the precapillary sphincter, whose contractile activity is regulated by its local intravascular and extravascular environment. Once whole blood or plasma has entered the capillaries, its flow path is determined by the various resistances occurring within the nets. These resistances result from pressure changes in the venous vessels that may temporarily curtail outflow from the capillaries or from alternation in arterial pressures that vary according to the activity of the precapillary sphincter. Thus blood flow within the capillary network changes from moment to moment, frequently reversing direction and often bypassing one route to follow another. The primary control of the flow lies in the spontaneous contractile activity of the precapillary sphincter, a smooth muscle cell that is independent of control by the central nervous system, but one that is influenced by local changes in intraluminal pressure and by the accumulation or washout of metabolic by-products and humoral agents (metabolic autoregulation).

2

A brief description of the structural organization of the large vessels that deliver blood to the exchange vessels is in order here. From the large artery to the terminal arteriole, each arterial vessel is accompanied by a vein. A major artery gives rise to numerous smaller arteries that have a diameter about one-half that of their parent vessel and which branch off at right angles. These branches occur at irregular intervals along the length of the artery, which actually terminates by forming an arterial anastomosis or arcade with another artery of the same type that lies parallel some distance away. The branches, called small arteries, are approximately one-fifth the length of their parent vessel, but they give rise to a relatively large number of arterioles with a small diameter (about one-third that of the small artery). The arterioles continue to become terminal arterioles, from which the capillaries originate. Arterial arcades are formed at all levels, and it is therefore almost impossible for a capillary network to be isolated from the main blood supply unless an extensive obstruction occurs.

On the venous side of the system, postcapillary venules are formed as capillary nets begin to converge. In diameter, they are almost twice as large as the arterioles that they accompany. Venules converge to form twice as many small veins as there are small arteries. Venules have a diameter three times as large as the arterioles; small veins are three times larger than small arteries.

The next step after this rather cursory survey of the current state of our knowledge of the structural and functional aspects of the microvasculature is to review some of the outstanding papers that have led to this understanding.

This book is divided into five parts: I. Early Investigators; II. From van Leeuwenhoek to Krogh; III. The Era of Krogh; IV. The Renaissance After Krogh; and V. In the Last Decade.

Part I necessarily begins with the work of William Harvey, who first postulated the existence of small hair-like vessels to connect the arterial and venous systems, a mandatory condition if blood truly did circulate from the heart to tissues and lungs and back again to the heart. Also included in this section are papers that prove the existence of the postulated vessels, which could not be seen or accurately described until the development of magnifying lenses—an event that took place some 50 years after Harvey had made his original speculations. Space restrictions permit the inclusion of only a few of the most innovative papers, but a survey of a number of informative works is presented. There are some seemingly fallow periods that account for extended periods of time between the investigations that are reported in this section (as well as between Parts I and II). The primary reason for this is the repetitive nature of some of the earlier works, presumably due to a lack of communication—the result of the sparcity of circulated journals and of geographical distances. "Early Investigators" covers the period from 1628 to 1688.

Part II provides a survey of the work done between 1733 and 1852 on microcirculation. Because much of the work is available only in book form, it would be difficult to do justice to the ideas and conclusions of the investigators by including only small excerpts from their publications. Instead, a short summary of their work is presented, along with a reference list designed to help interested readers locate the original publication.

Part III is devoted entirely to the work of August Krogh, with excerpts from his book *The Anatomy and Physiology of Capillaries*. The book was compiled from Krogh's lectures at Harvard in 1922 and acts as a survey of prevailing concepts. Krogh draws heavily on workers immediately preceding him and on his contemporaries and thus gives us a clear picture of the progress made from the middle of the 1800s to his time. Only a small portion of Krogh's extensive work is reproduced here.

Part IV contains works dealing with fresh, new ideas and techniques. I apologize for the omission of interesting and relevant papers by proven investigators in the field, but it was necessary to conserve space. Selection was made on the basis of a desire to present work that was the most influential in promoting subsequent research. Pioneers in the establishment of a group that was later to be identified as microcirculatory anatomists and physiologists, such as Bloch, Knisely, Irwin, Zweifach, Fulton, Webb, and Nicoll, are well known, and the works of some of them are presented here. Many current investigators are former students or followers of these men.

This part is called "The Renaissance After Krogh" because it is undeniable that Krogh's book was the stimulus for an explosive effort to confirm, expand, or refute his stated concepts. It became fashionable to study microcirculation, and much emphasis was placed on actually looking at small blood vessels directly rather than attempting to deduce peripheral vascular changes from indirect parameters. The latter approach was referred to as working around the "little black box," which contained hitherto unseen and unknown regulatory responses and adjustments of the microcirculation to variations in the macrocirculation. Part IV includes papers from 1932 through 1955.

Part V consists of papers published between 1961 and 1968 that contain several new approaches to the study of microvascular beds, a reiteration and clarification of some older concepts, and some corrections, refinements, and applications of previously collected data.

More information is available each year, and new applications of *in vivo* microscopy are apparent in the current literature as technical advances permitting more accurate quantitative measurements of variations in blood pressure and blood flow are made. Intravascular phenomena, such as platelet aggregation, red and white blood cell behavior, and vascular responses to toxic materials introduced into the system, are now being observed through the microscope. The potential for advances is limitless.

I

Early Investigators

Editor's Comments on Papers 1, 2, and 3

1   **Harvey:** Excerpts from *Movement of the Heart and Blood in Animals*
    K. J. Franklin, trans., Blackwell Scientific Publications Ltd., Oxford, 1957, pp. 70, 87

2   **Harvey:** Excerpts from "An Anatomical Disquisition on the Motion of the Heart and Blood in Animals"
    The Works of William Harvey, Robert Willis, ed., The Sydenham Society, London, 1847, pp. 54–55, 68

3   **Harvey:** The First Anatomical Disquisition on the Circulation of the Blood, Addressed to Jo. Riolan.
    The Works of William Harvey, Robert Willis, ed., The Sydenham Society, London, 1847, pp. 89–92

    The three papers presented first represent the very beginning of the idea of microcirculation. William Harvey's essay on the movement of the heart and blood is well known, but his letter to John Riolan, written in 1649, has had less exposure.

    The length of Harvey's initial paper (72 pages) and of his subsequent letter (16 pages) to Riolan, who sought to refute the Harverian theory of blood circulation, precludes inclusion in their entirety, but excerpts from these writings must be included if we are to visualize the entire history of the study of microcirculation. The passages that follow are selected to show that logical reasoning demanded the existence of microvessels to connect the arterial and the venous circulation, as stated in *De motu cordis*. The rebuttal to criticism from a colleague 21 years later shows how vigorously Harvey was forced to defend his revolutionary idea.

    Excerpts from the 1957 translation of *De motu cordis* by K. J. Franklin appear first. For comparison, they are followed by a translation of the same passages by Robert Willis, who compiled the works of Harvey in 1847.

1

Copyright © 1957 by Blackwell Scientific Publications Ltd.

Reprinted from *Movement of the Heart and Blood in Animals,* by William Harvey, K. J. Franklin, trans., Blackwell Scientific Publications Ltd., Oxford, 1957, pp. 70, 87

Movement of the Heart and Blood in Animals

WILLIAM HARVEY

CHAPTER ELEVEN

The second supposition is confirmed

IN order that the second supposition which I have to confirm may be better appreciated by my readers, I must refer to certain experiments which make it clear that the blood goes into each member through the arteries and flows out of it through the veins; that the arteries are the vessels which carry blood away from the heart, and the veins the vessels and pathways for the return of the blood to the same heart; that in the members and extremities the blood passes from the arteries into the veins either directly by anastomosis, or indirectly through the porosities of the flesh, or in both ways, just as it passes (see earlier) from the veins into the arteries in its cardio-pulmonary course. Hence it is manifest that it moves from one region to a second and back again, that is to say, from the centre to the farthest parts and thence back to the centre. If after that premise you make a calculation as before, it will at that very point be manifest that such an amount of blood cannot be supplied from the food intake or necessarily be required for nutrition.

* * * * * * *

Editor's Note: A row of asterisks indicates material that has been omitted from the original article.

CHAPTER FOURTEEN

Conclusion of my description of the circuit of the blood

MAY I now be permitted to summarize my view about the circuit of the blood, and to make it generally known!

Since calculations and visual demonstrations have confirmed all my suppositions, to wit, that the blood is passed through the lungs and the heart by the pulsation of the ventricles, is forcibly ejected to all parts of the body, therein steals into the veins and the porosities of the flesh, flows back everywhere through those very veins from the circumference to the centre, from small veins into larger ones, and thence comes at last into the vena cava and to the auricle of the heart; all this, too, in such amount and with so large a flux and reflux— from the heart out to the periphery, and back from the periphery to the heart—that it cannot be supplied from the ingesta, and is also in much greater bulk than would suffice for nutrition.

* * * * * * *

2

Reprinted from *The Works of William Harvey*, Robert Willis, ed., The Sydenham Society, London, 1847, pp. 54–55, 68

An Anatomical Disquisition on the Motion of the Heart and Blood in Animals

WILLIAM HARVEY

CHAPTER XI.

THE SECOND POSITION IS DEMONSTRATED.

THAT this may the more clearly appear to every one, I have here to cite certain experiments, from which it seems obvious that the blood enters a limb by the arteries, and returns from it by the veins; that the arteries are the vessels carrying the blood from the heart, and the veins the returning channels of the blood to the heart; that in the limbs and extreme parts of the body the blood passes either immediately by anastomosis from the arteries into the veins, or mediately by the pores of the flesh, or in both ways, as has already been said in speaking of the passage of the blood through the lungs; whence it appears manifest that in the circuit the blood moves from thence hither, and from hence thither; from the centre to the extremities, to wit; and from the extreme parts back again to the centre. Finally, upon grounds of calculation, with the same elements as before, it will be obvious that the quantity can neither be accounted for by the ingesta, nor yet be held necessary to nutrition.

* * * * * *

CHAPTER XIV.

CONCLUSION OF THE DEMONSTRATION OF THE CIRCULATION.

AND now I may be allowed to give in brief my view of the circulation of the blood, and to propose it for general adoption.

Since all things, both argument and ocular demonstration, show that the blood passes through the lungs and heart by the action of the [auricles and] ventricles, and is sent for distribution to all parts of the body, where it makes its way into the veins and pores of the flesh, and then flows by the veins from the circumference on every side to the centre, from the lesser to the greater veins, and is by them finally discharged into the vena cava and right auricle of the heart, and this in such a quantity or in such a flux and reflux thither by the arteries, hither by the veins, as cannot possibly be supplied by the ingesta, and is much greater than can be required for mere purposes of nutrition; it is absolutely necessary to conclude that the blood in the animal body is impelled in a circle, and is in a state of ceaseless motion; that this is the act or function which the heart performs by means of its pulse; and that it is the sole and only end of the motion and contraction of the heart.

* * * * * *

9

3

Reprinted from *The Works of William Harvey*, Robert Willis, ed., The Sydenham Society, London, 1847, pp. 89–92

THE FIRST ANATOMICAL DISQUISITION ON THE CIRCULATION OF THE BLOOD, ADDRESSED TO JO. RIOLAN.

WILLIAM HARVEY

SOME few months ago there appeared a small anatomical and pathological work from the pen of the celebrated Riolanus, for which, as sent to me by the author himself, I return him my grateful thanks.[1] I also congratulate this author on the highly laudable undertaking in which he has engaged. To demonstrate the seats of all diseases is a task that can only be achieved under favour of the highest abilities; for surely he enters on a difficult province who proposes to bring under the cognizance of the eyes those diseases which almost escape the keenest understanding. But such efforts become the prince of anatomists; for there is no science which does not spring from preexisting knowledge, and no certain and definite idea which has not derived its origin from the senses. Induced therefore by the subject itself, and the example of so distinguished an individual, which makes me think lightly of the labour, I also intend putting to press my Medical Anatomy, or Anatomy in its Application to Medicine. Not with the purpose, like Riolanus, of indicating the seats of diseases from the bodies of healthy subjects, and discussing the several diseases that make their appearance there, according to the views which others have entertained of them; but that I may relate from the many dissections I have made of the bodies of persons diseased, worn out by serious and strange affections, how and in what way the internal organs were changed in their situation, size, structure, figure, consistency, and other sensible qualities, from their natural forms and appearances, such as they are usually described by anatomists; and in what various and remarkable ways they were affected. For even as the dissection

Encheiridium Anatomicum et Pathologicum. 12mo, Parisiis, 1648.

of healthy and well-constituted bodies contributes essentially to the advancement of philosophy and sound physiology, so does the inspection of diseased and cachectic subjects powerfully assist philosophical pathology. And, indeed, the physiological consideration of the things which are according to nature is to be first undertaken by medical men; since that which is in conformity with nature is right, and serves as a rule both to itself and to that which is amiss; by the light it sheds, too, aberrations and affections against nature are defined; pathology then stands out more clearly; and from pathology the use and art of healing, as well as occasions for the discovery of many new remedies, are perceived. Nor could any one readily imagine how extensively internal organs are altered in diseases, especially chronic diseases, and what monstrosities among internal parts these diseases engender. So that I venture to say, that the examination of a single body of one who has died of tabes or some other disease of long standing, or poisonous nature, is of more service to medicine than the dissection of the bodies of ten men who have been hanged.

I would not have it supposed by this that I in any way disapprove of the purpose of Riolanus, that learned and skilful anatomist; on the contrary, I think it deserving of the highest praise, as likely to be extremely useful to medicine, inasmuch as it illustrates the physiological branch of this science; but I have thought that it would scarcely turn out less profitable to the art of healing, did I place before the eyes of my readers not only the places, but the affections of these places, illustrating them as I proceed with observations, and recording the results of my experience derived from my numerous dissections.

But it is imperative on me first to dispose of those observations contained in the work referred to, which bear upon the circulation of the blood as discovered by me, and which seem to require especial notice at my hands. For the judgment of such a man, who is indeed the prince and leader of all the anatomists of the present age, in such a matter, is not to be lightly esteemed, but is rather to be held of greater weight and authority, either for praise or blame, than the commendations or censure of all the world besides.

Riolanus, then, admits our motion of the blood in animals,[1]

[1] Enchiridion, lib. iii, cap. 8.

and falls in with our conclusions in regard to the circulation; yet not entirely and avowedly; for he says[1] that the blood contained in the vena portæ does not circulate like that in the vena cava; and again he states[2] that there is some blood which circulates, and that the circulatory vessels are the aorta and vena cava; but then he denies that the continuations of these trunks have any circulation, "because the blood is effused into all the parts of the second and third regions, where it remains for purposes of nutrition; nor does it return to any greater vessels, unless forcibly drawn back when there is a great lack of blood in the main channels, or driven by a fit of passion when it flows to the greater circulatory vessels;" and shortly afterwards: "thus, as the blood of the veins naturally ascends incessantly or returns to the heart, so the blood of the arteries descends or departs from the heart; still, if the smaller veins of the arms and legs be empty, the blood filling the empty channels in succession, may descend in the veins, as I have clearly shown," he says, "against Harvey and Walæus." And as the authority of Galen and daily experience confirm the anastomoses of the arteries and veins, and the necessity of the circulation of the blood, "you perceive," he continues, "how the circulation is effected, without any perturbation or confusion of fluids and the destruction of the ancient system of medicine."

These words explain the motives by which this illustrious anatomist was actuated when he was led partly to admit, partly to deny the circulation of the blood; and why he only ventures on an undecided and inconclusive opinion of the subject; his fear is lest it destroy the ancient medicine. Not yielding implicitly to the truth, which it appears he could not help seeing, but rather guided by caution, he fears speaking plainly out, lest he offend the ancient physic, or perhaps seem to retract the physiological doctrines he supports in his Anthropology. The circulation of the blood does not shake, but much rather confirms the ancient medicine; though it runs counter to the physiology of physicians, and their speculations upon natural subjects, and opposes the anatomical doctrine of the use and action of the heart and lungs, and rest of the viscera. That this is so shall readily be made to appear, both from his own words and avowal, and partly also from what I shall supply;

[1] Enchiridion, lib. ii, cap. 21.   [2] Ib. lib. iii, cap. 8.

viz., that the whole of the blood, wherever it be in the living body, moves and changes its place, not merely that which is in the larger vessels and their continuations, but that also which is in their minute subdivisions, and which is contained in the pores or interstices of every part; that it flows from and back to the heart ceaselessly and without pause, and could not pause for ever so short a time without detriment, although I admit that occasionally, and in some places, its motion is quicker or slower.[1]

[1] Vide Chapter III.

Editor's Comments on Papers 4 and 5

4 **Malpighi:** Excerpts from *De pulmonibus: Observationes anatomicae*
Selected Readings in the History of Physiology, J. F. Fulton, ed., Charles C Thomas, Publisher, Springfield, Ill., 1966, pp. 68–71

5 **van Leeuwenhoek:** 65th Missive
Opuscula selecta Neerlandicorum de arte medica (int. ed.), **1**, 37, 51–81 (1907)

The next two articles, the first written by Malpighi in 1661 and the second written by van Leeuwenhoek in 1688, contain reports of the first microscopic observations of blood vessels and blood flow in living animals. Here, again, the extraordinary length and diversity of the articles make it impractical to include the entire texts. Important passages have been excerpted, however, and should be read in order to appreciate the stimulating influence of Harvey's treatise and of the subsequent results of the first use of a magnifying lens that confirmed Harvey's speculations about connections between arteries and veins.

Malpighi studied the lungs and mesentery in frogs and observed small channels connecting arteries and veins, the reports of which are accepted as being the first descriptions of capillaries. Van Leeuwenhoek, who studied small vessels in frog feet, bat wings, and tadpole tails, began to describe his findings in 1673, but the edition of his collected works did not appear until 1688. He saw and described pulsatile blood flow in relation to heart beat, red and white blood cells, and continuous flow between arteries and veins. He noted that blood cells were flat and oval and that they became "long ovals" in a narrow vessel. He remarked that one could be misled about the pattern of circulation if one did not see blood flowing through the vessels, and he observed that pulsation died out in the smallest vessels, vessels so small that only one blood cell could pass through at a time. He was impressed by the fact that the cells that gave the blood its red color were so small that ten hundred thousand were not as large as a grain of coarse sand. His observations proved a continuity between arterial vessels and venous vessels in many sites other than the lung, which had been shown by Malpighi. Thus began a series of investigations describing capillaries and their behavior by Hales, Whytt, Haller, Philip, and Black between 1733 and 1825 (see the introductory essay to Part II).

4

Reprinted from *Selected Readings in the History of Physiology*, J. F. Fulton, ed., Charles C Thomas, Publisher, Springfield, Ill., 1966, pp. 68–71. Courtesy of the publisher.

De pulmonibus: Observationes anatomicae

MARCELLO MALPIGHI

EPISTLE II TO BORELLI—ABOUT THE LUNGS

So now, most distinguished Sir, I shall deal more closely with two matters which in my letter containing observations on the lungs I left in doubt as requiring more exact study. The first was what might be that network I have described by which the single vesicles and spaces are somehow bound together in the lungs. The second was whether the vessels of the lungs are joined together by mutual anastomosis or whether on the other hand they open into the common substance and spaces of the lungs. The solution of any problem prepares the way for solving greater ones and places the operations of nature more clearly before the eyes. Toward the disentangling of these matters I have sacrificed nearly the whole genus of frogs which did not occur even in that wild *batrachomyomachia* of Homer. For in the anatomy of frogs which I have studied through the courtesy of my excellent colleague Master Carolo Fracassati in order that I might determine with greater certainty the nature of the membranous substance of the lungs it occurred to me that I might not improperly better apply to the present problem that saying of Homer—"With my eyes I see a great and true work. . . ."

Microscopic observation detects in these terminal vessels something more wonderful than mere structure and connection, for, with the heart still beating, there may be observed in the vessels, although with difficulty, an opposite movement of the blood [i.e., in opposite directions in arteries and veins] so that here is clearly revealed the circulation of the blood which may also be observed more satisfactorily in the mesentery and in the other larger veins contained in the abdomen. Therefore, the blood is impelled by this force into each cellule through the arteries and thereby distributes its current in very small amounts through branches either passing through the cellule or ending therein. When the blood is thus much divided, its red color disappears and winding sinuously it is distributed everywhere, even to the walls and corners and to the branches of the veins one calls the resorbing ones.

The power of the eye could not be extended further in the opened living animal, hence I had believed that the mass of the blood broke out into empty spaces and was re-collected by an open-mouthed vessel and by the structure of its walls. To this problem the diverse, tortuous, and diffuse movements of the blood and its reunion at a fixed place offered a clue. However, my doubts were resolved by the dried lung of a frog which accidentally preserved its blood redness even in the smallest portions (as it had been detached later from its vessels). There, with a more perfect glass the points forming the skin which is called *Sagrino* no longer were seen to occur but rather interwoven looped vessels. So great is the branching of these vessels as they extend out hither and thither from the vein and artery that no further order is maintained by the vessels, but a network appears formed from the offshoots of the two vessels and this network occupies not only the whole floor [of the vesicle] but extends also to the walls and afterwards connects with the outgoing vessel as I was able to observe more abundantly, though with greater difficulty, in the oblong lung of a tortoise which is likewise membranous and translucent. Hence, it lay revealed to observation that the blood passes out through these twisting divided vessels and is not poured out into spaces but is always conveyed through tubules and is distributed by the many windings of the vessels. Nor is it a new caprice of Nature that the ultimate openings of the vessels join together since the same thing occurs in the intestines and other parts. Nay it will certainly seem more marvellous that the upper ends of the veins connect to the lower by visible anastomoses as the very learned Fallopio has so well observed.

But in order that you may be able to grasp more easily what I have proposed and follow it with your own sight, tie off, by the

thread with which it is joined to the heart, the bulging and swollen
lung of a dissected frog while it is abundantly nourished with blood
in every part, for this when dried will keep the vessels swollen with
blood which you will then see very well if you examine it with a
microscope, consisting of one flea lens, exposed against the horizontal sun. Or you can use another method in seeing these things.
You may place the lung on a plate of crystal illuminated from below
by the light of a lamp through a tube and bring to it a microscope
of two lenses. The vessels, proliferated in loops, will then be revealed to you. By the same arrangement of instruments and light
you will observe the movement of the blood through the vessels
mentioned and you will yourself be able, with different degrees
of light, to contrive to see other things which escape description by
the pen. In fact one matter concerning the movement of the blood
promises to be worthy of your speculation for when both auricle
and heart have been tied off so that the movement and impulse
which might have been transmitted from the heart into the attached vessels has been removed, the blood is still moved through
the veins to the heart. Thus it distends the vessels with its own
force and abundant flow, and this continues for several hours. Yet
in the end, especially if it be exposed to the rays of the sun, it is
not excited with the same continued movement but advances and
recedes, fluctuating at the same time as if impelled by alternating
forces. This also occurs when the heart and auricle have been excised.

Therefore, to resolve the primary problems, from these facts
and from the analogy and simplicity which Nature uses in her works,
it can be concluded that the network, which elsewhere I thought
consisted of nerves mixed in among vesicles and spaces, is a vessel
carrying away the mass of blood or conducting it out, and although
in the lungs of perfect animals a vessel may sometimes seem to end
and open in the middle of the loops of the network, it is nevertheless probable that just as occurs in the *cellulae* of frogs and tortoises
that very small vessel has further vessels arising from it in the form
of a network, which on account of its exquisite smallness also escapes observation.

The problem of the mutual junctions and anastomoses of the
vessels can in all likelihood also be solved from these facts. For if
in one case Nature turns about the blood within vessels and joins
the ends of the vessels together in a network, it is also probable
that in other cases they are joined by anastomosis. This may be

clearly perceived in a frog's bladder swollen with urine in which may be observed the rapid movement of the blood through transparent vessels joined together by mutual anastomosis. Nay rather those vessels receive that connection and order which the veins or fibres in the leaves of nearly all trees invariably display.

But to what end are these things made—beyond that which in my preceding letter I touched upon concerning pulmonary mixture— you yourself seem particularly to have perceived; nor is it my intention to defraud you of this your discovery which in your kindness you have committed to me in your elegant letters in which you philosophized subtly in observing the wonderful manifestations of nature in vegetables. We marvel that an apple hangs from a trunk not its own and that the grafting of plants has produced a happy mixture of bastard and legitimate parts. For we see that one and the same tree has taken on different habits in its branches; while on one the hanging fruits gratify the taste of some with their pleasant sharpness, all desire the nectar-like sweetness of those on another. You give confidence to truth when at Rome you marvelled that both the vine and the jasmine were produced from the trunk of a Massilian apple. He who made these ingenious things nurtured his plantations with a small scion grafted on larger branches and trained the not unwilling trees to bring forth a variety of things. In this connection Virgil in the Georgics aptly sang:

> *From an alien tree the sprout they ingraft*
> *And teach it to shoot from the moist inner bark. . . .*

I have included these few trifles in a letter in order that I might now add to the things discovered concerning the lungs. If I have brought forward any new point I owe the whole of my observations to the frog. By your authority and ingenuity you may gain value and dignity for these matters. In the meantime, may you philosophize felicitously and continue to make me perfectly happy in the knowledge that these very trifling thoughts of mine may contribute in some small way to your writings on the movement of animals. Farewell. (Malpighi, M. *De pulmonibus. Observationes anatomicae.* Bologna, Baptista Ferronius, 1661. 14, 9 pp., 2 pl. [Epistola altera, pp. 1-9. Translated by L.G.W.])[1]

Reprinted from *Opuscula selecta Neerlandicorum de arte medica* (int. ed.), **1**, 37, 51–81 (1907)

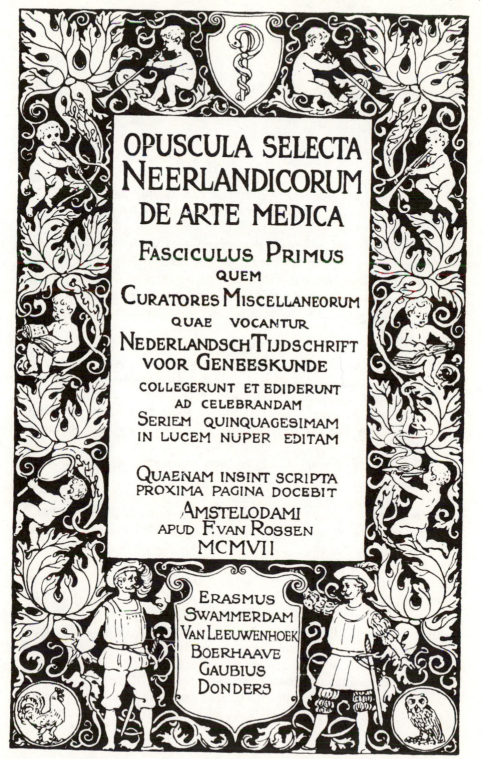

OPUSCULA SELECTA
NEERLANDICORUM
DE ARTE MEDICA

FASCICULUS PRIMUS
QUEM
CURATORES MISCELLANEORUM
QUAE VOCANTUR
NEDERLANDSCH TIJDSCHRIFT
VOOR GENEESKUNDE

COLLEGERUNT ET EDIDERUNT
AD CELEBRANDAM
SERIEM QUINQUAGESIMAM
IN LUCEM NUPER EDITAM

QUAENAM INSINT SCRIPTA
PROXIMA PAGINA DOCEBIT
AMSTELODAMI
APUD F. VAN ROSSEN
MCMVII

ERASMUS
SWAMMERDAM
VAN LEEUWENHOEK
BOERHAAVE
GAUBIUS
DONDERS

65th Missile

ANTONY VAN LEEUWENHOEK

Then I placed a frog-worm, as it lives in the water and adheres to glass, under a magnifying-glass and gave it to the draughtsman to make a picture of it.

Fig. 4. G H I K L M N O P Q R S. shows the frog-worm as it had fastened itself, when alive, to the glass, and with the belly turned towards the beholder. This worm had only a few hours before swum out of the slime in which it had lain.

L M N O P. indicates the head, H I R S. the belly and G H S. the tail. On the head of this animal is seen a part of the skin, thicker than the skin around it, so that I asked myself whether this might not be a part of the new skin with which the whole body was going to be covered. It is indicated by M N O.

T. denotes the mouth, which, so far as I could see, the animal, when so young, did not move. V V. are two brown spots on the head. In this specimen these spots were quite round (this being not nearly the case in others), and in some they might be taken for eyes. But the eyes cannot be seen in this position, because they are turned away from us. I K L. and P Q R. are six transparent projecting parts, of which there are three on either side of the head.

These parts only have caused me to have the frog-worm drawn: or in each of these parts I was greatly pleased to see very distinctly the circulation of the blood, which was driven on from the parts that were nearest to the body to those on the outside, thus causing an uninterrupted, very rapid circulation. This circulation was not regular in its movement, but at very short intervals it was continually brought about anew with sudden impulses, and before there was an other sudden impulse we might (in case we had not observed a continual increase in the rapidity) have thought that a stoppage in the circulation would follow. But scarcely had the blood begun to move more slowly, when there was again a sudden impulse of the blood, so that there was an uninterrupted current; and trying accurately to measure the very short time in

4*

which each impulse took place, I found that in the time wanted to count rapidly to a hundred, there were as many as a hundred sudden impulses. From this I concluded that as often as these sudden impulses occurred, the blood was driven from the heart. Indeed, I saw this current (the impulse of the blood from the heart and its passing from the arteries, where these meet together, into the veins) as clearly as I or anybody else could possibly imagine.

Having seen this many times to my great satisfaction, I would not keep the knowledge to myself, but I showed it to five distinguished gentlemen, who told me they had never seen anything deserving so much to be seen. I must add that, if the blood had been an even thin liquid, we could not possibly have distinguished it; but as the blood consisted of a very clear liquid, mixed as it appeared to the eye, with larger and smaller globules, which though they had no colour, yet were plainly visible, so the observation of the circulation was the more distinct.

When these frog-worms were a few days old, I could no longer see all these six projecting parts (in each of which the circulation of the blood took place), but it seemed to me that they were covered with a skin.

Then I also noticed on either side of the head a sudden impulse (as described above), but I did not perceive any circulation of the blood. Neither could I distinguish the head from the body, for they seemed to form one whole. When these worm-frogs were about eight or ten days old, and had grown to twice their size, I saw their mouths open and shut with a sudden movement such as I described before of the current of the blood; and then the teeth in the mouth in both jaws had become so large that I could see them quite well. These teeth were as numerous and were placed in the same order

as the rows of teeth in the mouth of a fish which we call shark.

I have not confined myself to these observations, but I have exerted myself to the utmost to know more about the said circulation of the blood. I have observed these worm-frogs, eight or ten days old, in all imaginable ways, and I have seen inside the body something small that moved, and that I imagined to be the heart, and then the liquid which was in it and driven out of it began to assume a red colour. This part, taken by me for the heart, showed the same sudden movements as I said before that took place in the blood-vessels. Then, as often as I saw this supposed heart move, also the eyes of the animal were slightly moved, so that I imagined that the movement of the eyes depended only on the movement of the heart and the mouth. These eyes, in their projecting roundness, as well as in their blackness in the middle, appeared to my sight as clearly as the eyes of any small animal can be visible to our naked eyes.

When I opened the belly of such an animal, I found that the entrails were filled with a brownish substance, and that they were arranged in a circular order.

When I came to examine the tail of this little worm, I saw something so amusing that it surpassed anything I had ever seen in my life, for here I discovered more than fifty circulations of the blood in particular places, whenever I could place the animal as it was living in the water and lying still, under the magnifying-glass. For I not only saw that the blood was driven in many places through very thin vessels from the middle of the tail to the outside of it, but also that each such vessel was bent in a curve and carried the blood back to the interior or thickest part of the tail, in order to convey it back to the heart. So that it appeared to me that the blood-vessels, observed in this animal and called arteries and veins, are exactly alike; only they can be called arteries when they carry the blood to the utmost extremities of the small blood-vessels, and veins when they carry the same blood back to the heart. For example I saw many blood-vessels in the tail of the frog-worm, which have their course as in Fig. 5. A B C. of which A. and C. extend in the direction of the tail-bone, and B. in that of extremity of the tail. A B. carries the blood away from the heart and B C. carries the blood back to the heart; and so we may say that the blood-vessel A B C. is an artery and a vein, for we only call the said blood-vessel an artery in so far as it carries the blood away or sends it to its farthest end, that is here from A to B, and we can or must call B C. a vein, because the blood is carried back to the heart from B to C. And so it has been proved here that arteries and veins are one and the same continued blood-vessels.

When I thus observed the circulation of the blood through the veins, the veins were just wide enough for a single blood corpuscle (which seemed a globule to the sight, but which, as has been said before, is nevertheless a flat oval substance) to pass through without any difficulty. But another time I saw that these corpuscles, owing to the narrowness of the vein, changed into long ovals; and when I took the animal out of the water, and it began to die, I saw that the blood in the thinnest arteries sometimes stopped; and when in the same artery the blood was pushed on again, I saw that then several corpuscles of blood became twice as long as they were broad, and that the two ends seemed to be pointed. In another place I saw that a thicker artery divided itself into two branches, as in E., and that each of these branches continued in a curve as is indicated by E F. and E G. If now we assume D E F. and D E G. to be arteries, because they carry the blood away from the heart, it follows that F H. and G I K. are veins, because both of them carry the blood back to the heart.

At the same time I saw that at a short distance from K. there was a smaller or thinner artery, indicated by M L. The last named artery ran into the vein I K, so that the arteries D E G. and M L. were joined in the vein I K. Therefore H F. in Fig. 6 A., is a vein, D E F. and D E G. are arteries; G I K. and K I L. are veins and M L. is an artery, and yet we may say that it is one continued blood-vessel.

In another place I saw that three of the thinnest arteries, each running in a curve, all met together in one point and there formed a blood-vessel or vein, and consequently this blood-vessel was as wide as the three arteries mentioned. These three distinct vessels with their somewhat circular course, in which the circulation took place, were so small that a grain of sand could have covered them.

I also observed several times that an artery crossed a vein, and unless it had been possible to distinguish the particular course of each of them, many persons would have thought that the circulation originated there, and this I saw not only in the smallest vessels, but also in vessels ten times wider than those in which the circulation took place.

Such blood-vessels running across each other I often noticed before when I tried to discover the junction of arteries and veins in other animals, but I was quite certain that the circulation of the blood does not take place in the large vessels, but in the smallest or thinnest, for if it were otherwise, I conclude that all the parts of the body could not be fed. And as these discoveries seemed inscrutable to me, I gave up my investigations on this head for some years. If now we see clearly with our eyes that the passing of the blood from the arteries into the veins, in the frog-worm, only takes place in such blood-vessels as are so thin that only one corpuscle can be driven through at one time, we may conclude that the same thing takes place in the same way in our bodies as well as in that of all animals. And this being so, it is impossible for us to discover the passing of the blood from the arteries into the veins in our bodies or that of other animals, first because a single globule of blood being in a vein, has no colour; secondly because the blood does not move in the blood-vessels when we make this investigation.

I have said before that the corpuscles or globules that make the blood red, are so small that ten hundred thousand of them are not so big as a grain of coarse sand, and so we can easily imagine how very small the blood-vessels are in which the circulation of the blood takes place.

The observations told here have not been made once, but they have been resumed repeatedly, giving me much pleasure, and every time on different worms, and the result has almost always been the same. But it is remarkable that in the very small vessels mentioned above and placed furthest from the heart, as here at the end of the tail, the impulse was not by far so sudden and strong as in the vessels nearest to the heart. And though the un-interrupted current could be clearly observed, it could be distinctly seen that at each impulse from the heart the current was a little quicker.

When I looked along the length of the tail and at the thickest part of it, I could clearly see that on either side of the bone there was a large artery, through which the blood was carried to the extremity of the tail, and which on its way sent out several small branches.

When I looked at the part of the tail beside these arteries on the outside, I discovered there two large veins, which carried the blood back again to the heart, and moreover I saw that blood was driven into this large vein from several small veins. In short, I saw here the circulation of the blood to my perfect satisfaction, because there was nothing, though ever so slight, that caused me any doubt. I even saw that in the small part of the tail the blood circulated in more than five-and-twenty distinct veins. Besides the above-mentioned veins I discovered in the tail an immense number of other veins with their branches, which ultimately divided into such small branches that they became invisible to the eye. These veins also sprung from the thickest part of the tail, and however closely I looked, I could not discover any the least circulation in them, though these vessels were much thicker than those in which I saw the circulation of the blood. This suggested to me the idea that all these vessels might be nerves.

I did not wish to keep the sight of this to myself, but I showed it to two scholars of distinction. Not only did I show them that the blood was carried from the big artery to the end of the tail, and that by the side of it there lay a large vein conveying the blood continually back to the heart, but I also showed them in various places how the blood was driven into the smallest vessels on the outside of the tail and thence came back through the said veins and was conveyed to the inside of the tail.

Also I observed the young frogs when they had changed from worms into frogs and I also discovered in them a very large number of small blood-vessels which, continually running in curves, formed the vessels called arteries and veins, from which it was perfectly clear to me that the arteries and veins are one and the same continuous blood-vessels. But I saw them clearest of all and most of all at the end of the projecting parts of the legs, which we may call fingers, and of which the frog has four on each fore-leg and five on each hind-leg.

These blood-vessels, called arteries and veins (being nevertheless identical) were exceedingly numerous at the ends of these fingers, and each ran in a curve, which made it impossible to follow the particular course of each vessel. All these vessels were so small or thin that no more than one corpuscle could pass through it at a time. But when I examined these fingers about the first or second joint, I found the blood-vessels there, which we call arteries and veins, bigger, so big even that the blood in these vessels had a red colour.

These young frogs I have not examined in parts, but I have placed them before the magnifying-glass whole, and the said blood-vessels have been noticed by me as I have described above. This current or circulation I have shown to two distinguished gentlemen, who beheld it with great wonder. This was especially the case when they saw the parts of the blood by which this is made red, move through such thin vessels (with great rapidity) that only a few blood corpuscles could pass through one after another.

I had also some of the biggest frogs, called "Works" by us, caught. These I also left whole, and holding them with their fingers before the magnifying-glass, I could see the circulation of the blood in then too, but only with great difficulty: if I had not discovered it first in the young frog, it would have been impossible for me to see the circulation of the blood in the smallest vessels.

But when I examined these big frogs in other parts of their bodies, I could quite distinctly see the circulation of the blood.

Amongst other things I saw once that the blood in an artery (which was so wide that three corpuscles of blood could pass through it at a time) ran back or contrary to its first course, but this contrary current did not last longer than one can count four, and after that the blood resumed its ordinary first course.

For example I saw the blood go through a big artery as in Fig. 6 B., N R O P, running from N to O, and from this artery issued a branch or small artery, as has been said above. Now it happened while I was looking on, that the blood in artery P Q. not only ceased moving all at once, but also came running back from Q. to P, and poured into artery N R O P. The cause of this, I imagine, may have been either that the blood in the small artery P Q. or in the smaller branches into which P Q. is divided, was stopped by some slight obstruction, or that the muscle or nerve lying by the side of these small vessels, pressed or squeezed them so much that the circulation was prevented by it, which caused not only a stopping of the current, but also a going back of the blood in the big artery close by. For after the said short time was past, the blood resumed its previous quick course.

In an other place I saw that the current of the blood in such an artery became much slower in a short time and that then again

5

it was followed in the same artery by a sudden impulse; but shortly after this impulse there was again a slower current, and sometimes also a very short stopping. This impulse and this slackening of the current alternated as many as five or six times in succession, and then there followed again a continuous quick progress, and all this happened in such a short time that one could not have spoken ten words.

Several times I have had frog-worms caught in the canal, and found among them three or four very small fishes, a little longer than the frog-worm, when it has grown into a worm after leaving the egg. The skin of these fishes was covered with black spots, some of which looked like stars.

I thought that these fishes would not grow bigger, because I had never seen with my naked eye such creatures as they appeared to me through the microscope. At first I observed one of these fishes, but then I could not see anything remarkable in it.

These fishes I observed again after they had been a fortnight in my study alive among the frog-worms (and had grown during that time), that I might, if possible, also in them discover the circulation of the blood and its passage from the arteries into the veins, and at last I saw in the tail close to the farthest tail-fin, a large blood-vessel, which was an artery, that carried the blood to the end of the tail, and near to that blood-vessel was also a large vein, through which the blood was conveyed back to the heart. Both blood-vessels extended lengthwise through the tail.

When I looked at the tail-fin forming the end of the tail, I could see very clearly that on each side of the bones (that make the tail-fin stiff) there ran very thin arteries and veins, for I could very clearly distinguish the course of each of them, but not so clearly as in the frog-worm: partly because this little fish rarely did not move its tail, partly because the particles of blood (which during these observations I could not but take for globules) were much smaller than in the frog-worm. The last mentioned blood-vessels were also so small that only a single particle of blood

5*

could pass through them, and if these said particles of blood did not appear distinctly in the thin liquid in which they float (which some call the serous part of the blood), it would be altogether impossible to discover the circulation of the blood.

Although I could distinctly see the course of the blood both in the arteries and in the veins, yet it was impossible for me, however closely I looked, to see the ends of the arteries and the beginning of the veins. But when afterwards I made my observations on the only and last fish I had kept alive, in a manner different from that mentioned before, I saw to my very great satisfaction the circulation of the blood very clearly not only in one place, but as a rule in several places, for on either side of the above-mentioned bones (that give strength to the fins) each artery ran in a smal curve and there formed the beginning the vein.

When I looked at the tail of the fish, where the tail-fin begins, I saw with great wonder how the big artery spread there into the said very thin vessels or arteries, and how many of the thin veins of the tail-fin close by united again in the large vein. In short there was such a quick current of the blood flowing or driven from the thick artery to the farthest end of the tail and the tail-fin, and coming back from the many small veins to the large vein, that it was incomprehensible.

When I observed the two outer edges of the tail, where the short bones of the tail-fin have their beginning, I saw that many of the smallest veins met or united, and thus formed a large vein there. But this very agreeable sight did not last long, for I had taken the fish out of the water and quickly placed before my eye, and in such a case the current of the blood in the extremities of the body slackened in less than a minute.

After that I often went to catch this kind of fish myself, because I was not satisfied with this fine sight of one fish, and generally I came to the same result.

Further I observed that the large artery (from which many small arteries take their origin) and the large vein (into which the blood flows from many small veins) were placed close to or beside each other lengthwise in the fish, near to the spine, that is to say not to the side of the back, but to the lower side of the spine, and on the side of the back I could not at all discover any large blood-vessel. In the said large artery I could generally distinguish again the impulse or the increase of rapidity that the blood receives from the heart, but in the thinnest arteries I did not notice any change in the current of the blood, for there the current was quite regular. As I said before, there was no colour in the thinnest vessels; but I could clearly discover that the blood was red in the large artery and vein (very near to the end of the tail.)

In order to show the size of the said fish, in which I have also discovered the circulation of the blood, I have had a drawing made of it of the same size as it appears to the naked eye, as in Fig. 7.

Fig. 8 also shows the size of an other fish I had caught, but most of them were smaller, and among eight or ten I had only one that was somewhat larger.

I placed a fish before the magnifying-glass and gave orders that everything that was visible in the fish should be drawn, as is here indicated in Fig. 9 by A B C D E F G H I K L M N.

B C. indicates the eye of the fish. This generally appeared to me as large and perfect as the eye of a haddock seen with the naked eye. But as the fish had been dead more than a whole day and in that time the head and the eye had become drier than the other parts of the body, the draughtsman could not see it better.

Between C. and D. there were several short projecting parts on the back.

D E. is a fin near the tail.

F G H I K. is the tail-fin, which contains seventeen small bones, three of which are indicated by G, H and I. These bones make the tail-fin stiff and strong and consist of joints, and I also saw that these were composed of long parts, apparently hollow.

At the same time I could see that the membrane or skin covering these bones and forming the greater part of the tail-fin, also consisted of long parts, but the draughtsman was unable to see all these parts, because they had become invisible, owing to the dying of the fish.

L M. is also a fin near to the tail on the lower part of the body.

N A. is the mouth, which, when the fish was being dried, remained very wide open, whereas the fish otherwise when it is alive, opens and closes its mouth very quickly but not much, in rapid succession.

I said before how I could see very distinctly the circulation of the blood on either side of the bone that for the greater part forms the tail-fin, there being two distinct circulations between each two bones. So there were in the tail-fin thirty-four separate circulations, that is, there were in the tail-fin of such a small fish sixty-eight blood-vessels, namely thirty-four arteries and an equal number of veins, not reckoning the blood-vessels that may be found in the shortest part of the same fin in F. or K, to which I have not paid any attention.

In order to show the circulation in the fail-fin the better, I have had a part of the fin-bone drawn on a larger scale, as in Fig. 10 O P Q R.

On each side of this bone and very near to it runs an artery, both indicated here by ST. and WX. In these blood-vessels those globules of blood are drawn that appear to be round.

When this blood had completed its quick course from S. to T, it returned with the same speed from T. to V, so that S T. is an artery and TV. a vein, and nevertheless it is a continuous and uninterrupted blood-vessel. This was also the case with the blood-vessels on the other side of the bone, indicated by WXY. But this artery and vein were not so far apart as seems to be the case in the drawing, but they were in many places so close together that the artery and the vein touched each other.

In other places and even in the fins DE. and LM. I saw not only the blood run in the same way both in the arteries and in the veins, but in them I could also distinguish the circulation of the blood as described in the tail-fin.

The said circulation of the blood in this little fish I made known to two distinguished scholars, who were allowed to see it, having expressed a desire to that effect. Several fishes I then placed before the magnifying-glass in such a way that they could observe very distinctly with great wonder and attention the circulation of the blood in several separate blood-vessels at the same time.

If now in the tail-fin of such a small fish, as is indicated by Fig. 7 or Fig. 8 we see thirty-four separate circulations of the blood, how immense must not then be the number of circulations in our own body. This being so, we need not wonder any longer that blood appears when we prick ourselves with a needle or other small instrument.

Nay, after my observations described, I feel sure that in a space the size of a nail, there are on our fore-finger, or I may say, all over our skin, generally more than a thousand separate circulations of the blood.

After my previous observations I have also thought of our common river fish, namely the roach and the bream, that possibly I might also see in them the circulation of the blood. So I took a young roach and a young bream, two years old as I thought, and held them with their heads down in the water and their tails sticking out of the water, that the fishes might move their heads or jaws and the circulation of the blood might not be hindered, but might continue uninterrupted for some time.

As it is impossible to observe the circulation of the blood in any other parts of these fishes than the fins, because their bodies are covered with scales, I only examined the tail-fin as being most convenient, and in it I saw very distinctly a great many blood-vessels, so thin that only a single particle of blood could pass through at the same time, and besides these I saw vessels in which the blood was driven to the extremities of the tail-fin, and others through which the blood came back, without, however, being able to distinguish the extreme parts of the arteries and veins, for when I wanted to follow them with my eyes to the extremity of the tail-fin, I lost sight both of the arteries and of the veins.

It seemed to me more than once that an artery so wide that only one single particle of blood could get through at a time, happened to get stopped up, which came to pass in this way: the blood, after having been forcibly propelled through the artery a few times, suddenly came back a little way and was checked in its first and regular course. After this the blood sometimes took another direction (not far from the original vessel) and then continued unimpeded, with this difference only that it did not flow so fast. Seeing this, I concluded that the new course taken here by the blood was not through a blood-vessel with a membrane, but that the blood had forcibly made a new channel.

As I said before, all the particles that make the blood of fishes as well as of birds red, consist of flat oval corpuscles that in the aforesaid observations seemed round to me, because in these investigations I had not at my disposal such magnifying-glasses as were required to see these particles distinctly.

But in the last mentioned new course of the blood I could see that the particles that make the blood red, were flat. Nay, I not only saw that they were flat, but besides this I also saw that they were more long than broad.

The reason why these particles appeared to me in such different shapes is that they turn round so often in their course, so that what offered its narrow side to the eye one moment, presented its broad side the next; another particle again was turned over lengthwise after it had gone on the distance of a hair-breadth. In short, I saw here as many turnings-over of the flat particles of blood as

I could possibly imagine. This view was so clear first, because the space in which the current of the blood took place was so transparent that the particles of blood seemed to move in a glass tube; and secondly I could judge about the particles of blood the better as it was known to me that the particles which make the blood red in fish, were flat and oval.

If now we have been fortunate enough (for which we have longed so much and diligently looked in vain for many years) to expose so clearly the circulation of the blood and its passing from the arteries into the veins in the foresaid frogs and fishes, we shall not be satisfied with it, but we shall do our best to examine it also in other animals and if possible to discover it there also.

Before I stop I find it necessary to add that some time ago telling a certain medical Professor about my discoveries regarding the circulation of the blood, this gentleman said that when people chanced to speak about my observations and made use of them to confirm something or other, they were often met with the question, Must we believe it, because Leeuwenhoek tells us? What security does he give? For this reason that gentleman advised me to enable myself to produce attestations from some persons of distinction who had been eye-witnesses of these my discoveries, that I might be less liable to contradiction.

It is true that for some special reason I have hitherto mentioned by name none of those who with myself saw some of the most remarkable things with their own eyes with the aid of my microscope, but I have only said in general that some gentlemen of learning and judgment, lovers of physical science, have seen them.

But now that I hear that more credit will be given to my words when I mention the names of those who have partly seen the aforesaid circulation of the blood, about which I write to your honourable society, and which I have discovered, I have no objection to mentioning instead of many, such as I trust will deserve most belief, as for example *Mr. Cornelius 's-Gravesande, M. D. and ordinary professor of anatomy and surgery, and also councillor and late sheriff of this town; Mr. Cornelius Valensis, also councillor and late sheriff; Mr. Antoni Heinsius, L. L. D., councillor and "Pensionaris" of this town, late Envoy Extraordinary to His Majesty the King of France, and not long ago Ambassador of this state to the court of his Royal Majesty of England.* To these gentlemen, to whom I usually communicate many of my discoveries, I have also shown the true circulation of the blood, as distinctly as we see the current of the water in a running river with our naked eyes.

Here, Most Honourable Gentlemen, you have my observations concerning the circulation of the blood as I have from time to time noted them down; and after completing this, I have made several more observations about the circulation of the blood, and to my great satisfaction I have seen the same circulation in four particular living creatures, and these being large bodies in comparison to the foregoing, I have been thinking about means to demonstrate the circulation of the blood in one of these large creatures clearly afterwards to other people, details of which later on.
Meanwhile I am

Most Honourable Gentlemen, etc.

ANTONI VAN LEEUWENHOEK.

II

From van Leeuwenhoek to Krogh

It is not feasible to include here all the observations and theories of the early investigators who followed van Leeuwenhoek; but it is necessary for reasons of continuity to describe briefly their findings and to indicate how slow was the progress in collecting new information about microcirculation until a renaissance of interest followed the publication of August Krogh's book in the 1920s. Two excellent sources of more detailed information regarding the scientists mentioned here are Fulton (1966) and Fishman and Richards (1964).

Stephen Hales (1733) is best known for his experiment to determine blood pressure by the direct method. He tied a horse to a gate, connected its carotid artery to glass tubing by means of a goose trachea, and recorded the height to which blood rose in the tubing.

He also made numerous observations on flow through the smallest blood vessels and described the diameter of a blood globule as being 1/3240 inch. He supposed that capillary vessels must be a "small size" larger than the globules and gave them a diameter approximately double that of a globule, or 1/1620 inch. Hales described certain features of peripheral circulation, such as contraction and relaxation of small blood vessels. He calculated cardiac output in the horse, vessel resistance to blood flow, and the number of capillary arteries. Hales was undoubtedly the first man to observe, during his numerous perfusion experiments, the effects of alcohol on small blood vessels. He noted that brandy contracted the fine capillary arteries of the gut and that relaxation followed rinsing them out with water.

Robert Whytt (1755), who published his *Physiological Essays* in 1755, was concerned about the force that aided circulation of blood through the smallest vessels, having shown, by calculation, that the force exerted by a contraction of the heart was not strong enough to move blood through the capillary arteries. He knew that pulsation of the arteries did not extend to the small arterial vessels, but he thought it "highly probable" that the vessels were undergoing small alternate contractions to promote circulation of blood through them. His speculation has since been proved to be correct by the observation of spontaneous contractile activity of the arterioles, terminal arterioles, and precapillary sphincters.

Albrect von Haller (1756) disagreed with the concept of contractility of small arterial vessels because of his observations of frog arteries and veins. He saw blood corpuscles move in the arteries even though the arteries did not contract, and he believed that the effect of the contracting heart was diminished beyond this point and had no effect on flow in the small vessels. Perhaps he was not justified in speaking of the absence of capillary contractility because there was still no definitive delineation between the small arteriolar vessels and the capillaries, but Haller's writings were interpreted to mean that there was no contractile activity in capillaries.

A. P. W. Philip (1826) studied circulation in the webbed feet of frogs after decapitation of the frog and injury to its "spinal marrow" and tried to establish that the central nervous system had some influence on blood flow.

James Black (1825) continued the controversy regarding contraction and relaxation of small blood vessels. He concluded that blood flow in the capillary circulation was independent of both the heart and the brain.

In the 1830s, two investigators who pursued the study of capillary vessels avidly were still describing vascular beds and searching for definitions of the components. Marshall Hall (1831) described precapillary, capillary, and postcapillary vessels in the most reasonable way. He stated that small vessels should be considered as arterial vessels as long as they continued to divide and subdivide into smaller and smaller vessels; venous vessels would, conversely, become larger as vessels joined one another. Although he did not mention the direction of blood flow, it seems apparent that the dividing vessels would distribute blood while the coalescing vessels would collect it. This is still the best means of identifying the arterial and venous components in the microcirculation. Hall also recognized the fact that capillary vessels differed from the vessels that supplied them and collected from them. He referred to true capillary vessels as those that "do not become smaller by subdivision, nor larger by conjunction" and noted that they had a nearly uniform diameter. When he compared the anatomical pattern of capillary beds in various tissues of fish, frogs, toads, and salamanders, he was impressed with the architecture of the vessels. He noted that the design seemed to fit the function, that only a few vessels were necessary if their only function was to provide nutrition, and that more vessels were present in more complex tissues. He also described an arterial vessel in the tail of a small fish that ran its course and then looped around to become a venous vessel. This is very similar to the pathway that would later be described in the rat cecal mesentery.

In 1838, Johannes Müller expanded the current store of information by recording the diameters of capillary vessels in skin, brain, and intestine, and noting the absence of capillaries in the cornea. He actually described terminal arterioles, stating that certain minute arteries had no termination other than communication with veins through the capillaries, which he accepted as being uniform in diameter, as described by Hall. With regard to the passage of materials through capillary walls, Müller postulated that there were invisible pores that permitted the escape of fluid but not of particles.

It was much later, however, before any other significant advances in the knowledge about capillary circulation and its control were forthcoming, especially until there was some agreement about the definition of a capillary. As we proceed through the nineteenth-century and into the twentieth-century literature, the reader will notice a certain repetition of van Leeuwenhoek's observations.

References

Black, J. *A Short Inquiry into the Capillary Circulation of the Blood.* Longman, Hurst, Rees, Orme, Brown and Green, London, 1825.

Fishman, A. P., and Richards, D. W. *Circulation of the Blood: Men and Ideas.* Oxford University Press, New York, 1964.

Fulton, J. F. *Selected Readings in the History of Physiology,* 2nd ed. Charles C Thomas, Publisher, Springfield, Ill., 1966.

Hales, S. *Statical Essays: Containing Haemastaticks; or, An Account of Some Hydraulick and Hydrostatical Experiments Made on the Blood and Blood Vessels of Animals,* Vol. II. W. Innys and R. Manby, London, 1733.

Hall, M. *A Critical and Experimental Essay on the Circulation of the Blood.* R. B. Seely and W. Burnside, London, 1831.

Haller, A. von *Deux mémoires sur le mouvement du sang, et sur les effets de la saignée; fondés sur des expériences faites sur des animaux.* M. M. Bousquet and Co., Lausanne, 1756.

Müller, J. *Elements of Physiology,* translated by W. Baly. Taylor and Walton, London, 1838–1842.

Philip, A. P. W. *An Experimental Inquiry into the Laws of the Vital Functions,* 3rd ed. T. and G. Underwood, London, 1826.

Whytt, R. *Physiological Essays.* Hamilton, Balfour, and Neill, Edinburgh, 1755.

Editor's Comments on Paper 6

6 Jones: Discovery That the Veins of the Bat's Wing (Which Are Furnished with Valves) Are Endowed with Rhythmical Contractility, and That the Onward Flow of Blood Is Accelerated by Each Contraction
Phil. Trans. Roy. Soc. Lond., Pt. 1, **142**, 131–136 (1852)

An interesting report forthcoming in 1852, from the laboratory of T. Wharton Jones concerned microscopic observations made on blood vessels in the transparent membrane of bat wing.

Jones describes certain features of vascular behavior that had not previously been clearly stated, including spontaneous contractile activity of both arterial and venous vessels, and he was aware of changes in wall thickness of blood vessels during contraction and relaxation. He also observed the action of venous valves in preventing backflow and discussed the backward eddy of blood cells behind venous valves. In addition, he accurately described capillaries, noting their origin, their termination, and the fact that they are noncontractile.

Finally, Jones produced platelet aggregates mechanically by compressing vessels for a short period of time. Although unaware of the existence of platelets at that time, he described the response to mechanical compressions as producing a "viscid-looking grayish granular lymph," and he observed that portions of the deposit became detached and were carried away in the flowing blood.

6

Reprinted from *Phil. Trans. Roy. Soc. Lond.*, Pt. 1, **142**, 131–136 (1852)

X. *Discovery that the Veins of the Bat's Wing (which are furnished with valves) are endowed with rythmical contractility, and that the onward flow of blood is accelerated by each contraction.* By T. WHARTON JONES, *F.R.S., Fullerian Professor of Physiology in the Royal Institution of Great Britain, Ophthalmic Surgeon to University College Hospital, and Corresponding Member of the Society of Biology of Paris, &c. &c.*

Received November 20, 1851.—Read February 5, 1852.

IN entering on the investigation of the state of the blood and the blood-vessels in inflammation excited in the web of the Bat's wing, I applied myself, in the first place, to the study of the distribution, structure and endowments of the arteries, capillaries and veins of the part, and of the phenomena of the circulation in them.

I had not observed the circulation under the microscope long, before I was struck with something peculiar in the flow of blood in the veins; I therefore directed my attention to them, and discovered that they contracted and dilated rythmically. Following the veins for some extent in their course, I further discovered them to be provided with valves, some of which completely opposed regurgitation of blood, others only partially.

The cause of the peculiarity in the flow of blood in the veins was thus no longer doubtful, but some continued observation was required before I was able to make out exactly its mode of operation.

The act of contraction of the vein is manifested by progressive constriction of its caliber and increasing thickness of its wall; the relaxation of the vessel, by a return to the former width of caliber and thickness of wall.

The rythmical contractions and dilatations of the veins are, in the natural state, continually going on; but sometimes with greater, sometimes with less rapidity, and sometimes to a greater, sometimes to a less extent. The average number of contractions in a minute, I have found to be ten. I have on some occasions counted only seven or eight, and on other occasions as many as twelve or thirteen. Most usually, the numbers were nine and eleven. The supervening dilatations take place rather more quickly than the contractions. The amount of constriction of one of the larger veins—one about $\frac{1}{300}$dth or $\frac{1}{400}$dth of an inch in width when dilated—at each contraction of its walls, may be put down at a fourth or fifth of its whole width when in a state of dilatation; I have sometimes estimated it at nearly a third, sometimes at not more than a sixth.

s 2

The contractions *centrad* and *distad* of a valve appeared to be simultaneous, as did also the dilatations.

The smaller veins, those of the first and second order, proceeding from the radicles, contract, but not in a very marked manner, and are destitute of valves.

During contraction, the flow of blood in the vein is accelerated. On the cessation of the contraction, the flow is checked, and a tendency to regurgitation of the blood takes place, which brings the valves into play. Where the valves are perfect, the backward movement of the blood is at once stopped by their closure ; but where the valves are not complete, the blood regurgitates more or less freely *. But this check to the onward flow of the blood is usually only for a moment or two. Already, even while the vein is in the act of again becoming dilated, the onward flow of blood recommences and goes on, though comparatively slowly, until dilatation is completed and contraction supervenes ; whereupon acceleration of the flow takes place as before.

It is to be observed, that in determining the flow of blood in the veins (the phenomena of which I have now described), the action of the heart is concerned as well as the contractions of the veins themselves. It appears to be the heart's action which maintains the onward flow of blood during the dilatation of the vein, whilst it is the contraction of the vein, coming in aid of the heart's action, which causes the acceleration. Sometimes the *vis a tergo* is sufficient to keep up a pretty steady flow in the veins, this being only accelerated at each contraction of these vessels.

The check to the flow of blood in the veins takes place at the completion of the contraction or commencement of the dilatation. The number of checks observable in a minute, therefore, corresponds with the number of contractions. In one case, while an assistant marked the time by a seconds' watch, I observed that a complete valve checked the tendency to regurgitation nine times in a minute ; and on counting the number of contractions of the same vessel, I found them also nine in a minute. In another case, eleven checks and eleven contractions were counted ; and so on repeatedly. Though I quote these little experiments, I would remark that, after some practice in the observation, the eye is quite able to take in at one glance the succession and relations of the two phenomena.

The valves of the veins are composed sometimes of but a single flap, sometimes of two. In the situation of a valve, and *centrad* of the insertion of its flaps, the veins present the usual dilatations or sinuses corresponding to the sinuses of Valsalva at the origin of the pulmonary artery and aorta. These sinuses are best seen when the valve happens to present its flaps edgeways to the observer.

Valves are found close to the entrance of a large branch, but distad of it (Plate IV. fig. 2). They are also found at intermediate parts of the veins (fig. 1). Tracing the

---

* Sometimes, as for example, into a venous branch with an incomplete valve, a retrograde flow of blood takes place from a large vein, at the moment this latter is contracting and propelling its blood onwards.— May 7, 1852.

veins from radicles to trunks, the first valves I have noticed were at the junction of the second order of veins to form the third.

In watching the circulation, it is interesting to observe the backward eddy of blood-corpuscles into the sinuses of the valves, when the blood issues from the narrow valvular opening into the wide part of the vein beyond (fig. 1).

In structure, the valves are seen to be a reduplication of the clear innermost coat of the vein, with sometimes a pretty evident layer of fibrous tissue intervening.

Each vein is closely accompanied by an artery, a nerve only intervening. The average diameter of a vein is to that of its accompanying artery as about 3 to 2.

The contractility of the arteries is altogether different in its nature from that of the veins. It is *tonic contractility, not rythmical.* On the application of pressure over an artery, this vessel may be seen to become constricted, sometimes even to temporary obliteration of its caliber, and that uniformly throughout some extent of its course, both above and below the point where the pressure was applied; or, the constriction is greater or less at intervals, so that the vessel presents a varicose appearance. This tonic contraction of the arteries of the Bat's wing does not take place quite so quickly as the same phenomenon in the Frog's web, and, ordinarily, continues a longer time*.

The pulsation of a vein so affects its accompanying artery as to push the latter, as a whole, to and fro. That the movement of the artery referred to is really owing to this cause, and not to any pulsation or rythmical contraction and dilatation of its own walls, is evident from this, that the movements are synchronous with the contractions and dilatations of the vein, and that *both sides of the artery move in the same direction*, not approximating and receding from each other, so as to constrict or dilate the caliber, as in the case of the vein.

I have not been able to observe unequivocal evidences of tonic contractility of veins in addition to their rythmical contractility. When pressure is, at the same time, applied over the vein as well as the artery, the vein is not found to become tonically constricted in the same manner as the artery, upward and downward. At the place where the vein was pressed on, a mechanical indentation of its wall may perhaps be seen. And in addition to this, there may often be observed an appearance of great and abrupt constriction. This appearance, however, is not owing to contraction of the walls of the vein, but to a deposit of a viscid-looking grayish granular lymph within the vessel at the place, obstructing its channel and narrowing the stream of blood (figs. 3 and 4). On watching, I have seen portions of this deposit detached and carried away by the stream of blood, with corresponding enlargement of the channel, and again an additional deposit with renewed narrowing of the stream. When the pressure has been considerable, I have seen the vein become for a time wholly obstructed by the deposit. A similar deposit of lymph takes place in the artery. In one case, I observed that the artery, at the place pressed on, was

* When a frog under examination struggles, the arteries of the web are seen to become constricted. I have observed the same thing in the web of the Bat's wing and the ear of a white rabbit.

actually not so much constricted as above and below, though, on account of the narrowness of the stream of blood from the presence of the lymphy deposit, it appeared as much so at first sight (fig. 4).

Having subjected the web to the galvanic influence from a single pair of plates, I found all the smaller arteries of the part in a state of considerable tonic constriction, but the larger arteries constricted in a less degree. The effect of galvanism on the veins appeared to be to render their rythmical contractions somewhat more brisk, they having been previously rather languid. On cutting a vein across, I did not observe tonic constriction of it, any more than in the Frog.

After the application of a drop of Vinum opii to the web, the veins were found dilated as well as the arteries, and their rythmical contractions appeared to be suspended.

It has been stated by an authority not liable to err, that, on mechanical irritation, both artery and vein of the Bat's web gradually contract and close, and, by and by, dilate wider than before. And, again, that in Bats, contraction of veins is quite as well marked as that of arteries.

These statements, it will be observed, imply tonic contractility of the veins.

Notwithstanding my attention has been repeatedly directed to the point, I have not, as previously stated, been able to observe unequivocal evidences of tonic contractility of veins, in addition to their rythmical contractility. For this reason, I cannot help venturing on the supposition that Mr. PAGET* must have made his statements either from a hasty and imperfect observation of the proper rythmical contractions of the veins; or, seeing that in rythmical contraction of the veins the constriction is never to closure, like that of the arteries, under some such misapprehension as to the nature of the vessel observed, as he certainly must have laboured under when he supposed that arteries and veins of the second and third order open directly into each other without any intermedium of capillaries.

The arteries and their subdivisions anastomose freely with each other, forming a network all through the web, the meshes of which go on to diminish towards the free margin. Each artery and each subdivision of an artery is closely accompanied by a vein; and these veins, like the arteries they accompany, anastomose with each other. But it is to be remarked that nowhere do the arteries and veins directly communicate. The only communication is the usual one through the medium of capillaries. The capillaries, the walls of which are destitute of contractility, receive the blood from small arterial twigs which arise from the arterial network, and return it to the venous radicles which open into corresponding veins. These arterial twigs, capillaries and venous radicles, form networks within the meshes of the great vascular network, and a looped network at the margin of the web† (Plate V.).

The observations recorded in the preceding pages were made principally with

---

* Lectures on Inflammation at the Royal College of Surgeons in 1850.

† I shall have occasion to treat of this point more in detail in a paper on the state of the blood and the blood-vessels in inflammation of the web of the Bat's wing.

one-eighth of an inch object-glass, and the two lowest eyepieces, affording magnifying powers of 370 and 550 diameters.

The web of the wing was stretched out on the object plate, wetted on both sides with water, and covered with a thin plate of glass at the spot to be examined.

Appendix to the Foregoing Paper.

Received December 11, 1851,—Read February 5, 1852.

In consequence of the dark pigment in the cells of the epidermis of the web of the Bat's wing, the structure of the vessels cannot be well made out except by dissection.

A small piece of the web containing vessels being detached and disposed in a drop of water, under the simple microscope, the two layers of skin may be readily torn from each other with needles, and the artery and vein with their accompanying nerve, which lies between the two, separated in one bundle.

In pieces cut out of a web which had been dried, the bundle of vessels and nerve was, after tearing away the skin, left surrounded by a sheath of cellular and elastic fibres disposed longitudinally; but in pieces cut out from the living web and directly examined, this sheath was always detached along with the skin, and the vessels with their accompanying nerve at once laid bare (see Plate IV. fig. 5.).

Both artery and vein are seen to have a middle coat of circularly disposed muscular fibres; but the appearance of the fibres is different in the two vessels.

The fibres of the vein are about $\frac{1}{3600}$ths of an inch broad, pale, grayish, semitransparent and granular-looking. In general aspect they very much resemble the muscular fibres of the lymphatic hearts of the frog. In none of the muscular fibres of the vein, however, did I detect an unequivocal appearance of transverse marking.

The fibres of the middle coat of the artery are not so pale-looking as those of the middle coat of the vein, are clearer, and exhibit a more strongly marked contour.

Second Appendix.

Received May 10,—Read May 13, 1852.

From a microscopical examination of the blood-vessels and circulation in the ears of the Long-eared Bat, I have ascertained that, different from what I discovered to be the case in the wings, the veins of the ears are unfurnished with valves, and are not endowed with rythmical contractility, and that the onward flow of blood in them is consequently uniform. I ought, perhaps, to qualify the statement that the veins of the ear are not endowed with rythmical contractility, by saying, that I think I noticed a very slight tendency to it, here and there in a vein, but so slight as not to have the smallest effect on the flow of blood.

This observation regarding the ear of the Bat illustrates how that the heart's action is sufficient of itself for the circulation of the blood in the body generally; but that being sufficient for that only, the supplementary force of rythmical contractility of veins, supported by the presence of valves, is called forth to promote the flow of blood in the wings, which, on account of their extent, are, as regards their circulation, in a considerable degree, though not entirely, beyond the sphere of the heart's influence.

I may take this opportunity to mention that I have also found the veins of the mesentery of the Mouse destitute of rythmical contractility.

EXPLANATION OF THE PLATES.

PLATE IV.

Fig. 1. A vein with a complete valve. In this figure an attempt has been made to represent the backward eddy of blood-corpuscles into the sinuses of the valve, at the time the blood issues from the narrow valvular opening into the wide part of the vein beyond.

Fig. 2. A vein with a valve close to the entrance of a large branch.

Fig. 3. An artery and vein over which pressure had been applied. The artery is seen constricted at intervals, above and below the place of pressure *a*. The vein is not constricted, but there is seen, at the place where the pressure was applied, a grayish granular deposit of lymph within the vessel, giving rise to the appearance of constriction by narrowing the stream of blood.

Fig. 4. Representation of the case in which the artery, at the place pressed on, was actually not so much constricted as above and below; though, on account of the narrowness of the stream of blood from the presence of the lymphy deposit, it appeared as much so at first sight.

In this case the channel of the vein was much narrowed by a deposit of lymphy matter on either side within the vessel.

Fig. 5. This represents an artery (*a*) and a vein (*v*), with an accompanying nerve (*n*) lying between the two, as seen with a magnifying power of about 370 diameters; immediately after being separated, by dissection under the simple microscope, from a small piece cut out of the living web. The cellular sheath was detached along with the two layers of skin.

The artery is at one place tonically constricted, and there the middle coat is seen to be thicker.

The difference in the general aspect of the fibres of the middle coats of the two vessels may be recognised.

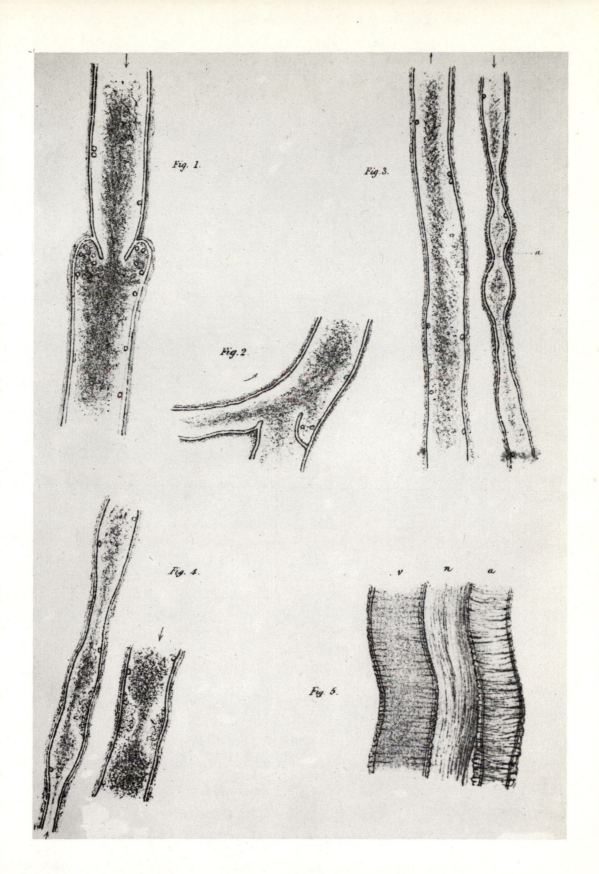

Fig. 1.

Fig. 3.

Fig. 2.

Fig. 4.

Fig. 5.

47

III
The Era of Krogh

Editor's Comments on Paper 7

7 **Krogh:** Excerpts from *The Anatomy and Physiology of Capillaries*
   Yale University Press, New Haven, Conn., 1929, pp. 1–18, 25–31, 47–48, 61–80, 100–105

Important contributions to the field of microcirculation between 1852 and 1922 are discussed by August Krogh in *The Anatomy and Physiology of Capillaries*. Krogh's book, which can only be regarded as a classic, was a review of his own studies and of those of other scientists who were interested in capillaries. The information was presented in lectures at Yale University in 1922, and these were published as a book in 1929. Needless to say, the book's impact was tremendous, and it became not only a reference source but a mediator and touchstone for all other work in the field.

Many aspects of Krogh's work have been confirmed, but many others were hotly contested and have since been refuted. Excerpts of material that is considered to be of particular importance are included here, but the interested reader is encouraged to read the book in its entirety.

In the opening lecture, Krogh points out that the heart and blood vessels are designed to serve the capillaries, the area where exchange of materials takes place, and that "capillaries constitute the most important part of the whole circulatory system." He proposes, in these lectures, to review the current information without conducting an exhaustive literature search and to permit his own views to dominate.

He discusses axial flow in small vessels and "plasma skimming," a term that he introduced in 1921. He describes the deformation of red blood cells passing through capillaries that are 4–5 microns in diameter, the irregularity of rate of flow and direction in single capillaries, and stasis, in which corpuscles lose their identity. They resume their normal size and shape when they are swept into flowing blood. He also describes the behavior of white blood cells that can be seen rolling slowly along the walls of small venous vessels and suggests that some slight adhesion between the cells and the endothelium accounts for their peculiar movement along the vessel wall, outside the rapidly flowing blood steam.

Krogh's description of the blood vessels of muscles, the measurements of which are still in use today, is interesting to review. His interest in the functional aspects of those vessels is apparent as he discusses the relationship between the number of capillaries that are present and the supply of oxygen to muscular tissue.

Lecture III is concerned with the independent contractility of capillaries. The opening paragraph of this lecture, has been reproduced, but the following 14 pages, dealing with the older experiments on capillary contractility, have been deleted to save space. Before proceeding with Krogh's own experiments and views, we should note some comments by E. M. Landis. Landis wrote, regarding the Krogh lectures:

> Most controversy has focused on the phrase "independent contractility of capillaries" and on the role of the "Rouget cell." If, however, we simply substitute the phrase "independent variations of capillary blood flow" and substitute for Rouget cells "certain scattered smooth muscle cells of metarterioles and arteriocapillary sphincters," then even this criticism becomes

merely a matter of new classifications, changing definitions, and, in part, semantics. The basic concept remains unchanged.

In a sense, this is true, although Krogh does state on page 81 that "the whole length of a capillary from an arteriole to a venule can be contractile." We must assume either that the frog tongue has vessels unlike those seen in mammalian beds or that the optical resolution and magnification of his microscope were not good enough to permit the necessary accuracy of visualization. It took many years to refute the idea of capillary contractility.

Lecture IV, the last lecture included in these excerpts, is concerned with the structure of the capillary wall. Krogh begins with the question of how a capillary, an endothelial tube, can contract. He then proceeds to tell of Rouget's 1873 observations, which were forgotten for 30 years until Mayer, in 1902, reported cells similar to those seen by Rouget. This work was continued by Steinach and Kahn in 1903, but histological evidence was still lacking. To solve the problem, Krogh, in 1922, assigned the task of investigating the presence of capillary cells to Dr. Vimtrup, who reached definite conclusions about the existence of muscle cells in the capillary wall. Vimtrup elected to name them after the man who had first discovered them; thus the term "Rouget cell" came into the literature.

The remaining lectures deal with innervation of capillaries and their reflexes (which today we recognize as being inaccurate), with capillary reactions to stimulation, and, finally, with the exchange of substances through capillary walls, a discussion that is not relevant here.

Reprinted from *The Anatomy and Physiology of Capillaries*, Yale University Press, New Haven, Conn., 1929, pp. 1–18, 25–31, 47–48, 61–80, 100–105

The Anatomy and Physiology of Capillaries

AUGUST KROGH

LECTURE I

INTRODUCTORY—THE FLOW OF BLOOD IN THE MICROSCOPIC VESSELS

THE circulatory system of man and the vertebrate animals can be considered as made up of a small number of organs or subordinate systems, which are easy to recognize anatomically, and the functions of which are on the whole quite distinct. We have a propulsive organ: the heart; a distributing organ: the system of arteries; an organ for interchange of substances between the blood and the tissues: the capillaries; an organ for collecting the blood and carrying it back to the heart: the venous system. It is evident that the organs of propulsion, distribution, and carrying back are all subservient to the functions of exchange carried out in the capillaries, and though, of course, each of the great organs is absolutely necessary for the functioning of the whole, it will be difficult to challenge the proposition that the capillaries constitute the most essential part of the whole circulatory system. It is a little strange, therefore, to find that, far from being a favorite subject for anatomical and physiological research, the capillaries have been neglected in an extraordinary degree. Though about two hundred years have passed since the capillaries were discovered you could until recently find them dealt with in a few lines in most textbooks on physiology, and the references to their structure, given in textbooks of histology, were likewise of the most summary character.

In the last twelve years, however, the capillaries have been, so to speak, "rediscovered" as a subject worthy of study and experimental research. Interest in them must have been "in the air," for the study was taken up independently and almost simultaneously in different countries and has been developed at a rapid rate by quite a number of new workers. It is now, therefore, possible and desirable to review our position, to take stock of the results obtained, to coördinate them into a sort of system, however provisional, and thereby to try and indicate fields in which further work is especially needed and to mark out lines along which progress is to be expected. This is what I shall attempt to do in this series of lectures, and I wish to say at once, in order to avoid misunderstanding, that what I propose to give is not a monograph, aiming at a complete presentation of the literature of the subject, but just lectures, in which my personal views are allowed to dominate, and the statements of the literature are dealt with in so far as they have come to my notice without any exhaustive search and in so far as I think them relevant to the problem discussed.

By way of introduction I propose to describe in some detail the observations which can be made on suitable parts of living animals brought under the microscope, but not experimentally interfered with. This should serve to give you a provisional idea of the problems to be more fully dealt with in succeeding lectures.

Observations of the capillary circulation have been made from very early times. The exquisite beauty and variety of the living pictures, presented by a number of organs when viewed in this way, have fascinated many trained observers even more deeply than they impress the casual onlooker who sees them for the first time. A large number of facts have been recorded and, while the method has its obvious limitations as a means of causal analysis, it must be admitted that a great deal of insight into the processes of circulation can be gained by simple inspection.

The methods for arranging a number of organs for microscopic observation are given in the appendix (p. 369) and it is only necessary here to emphasize the difference in appearance between transparent organs or membranes viewed by transmitted light, and more or less opaque organs, the surface of which can be studied by reflected light. In the first case only, is it possible to study the whole of the circulation from (microscopically) large arteries to the corresponding veins and to correlate observations on capillaries s.str. with changes taking place in larger vessels. In the latter case the fragments of the circulatory system which can be clearly seen are generally too small to admit a definite interpretation.

Examining at a power of, say, 50 diameters transparent organs like the web, tongue, bladder, or thin muscles of frogs, the ears of small white mammals, the wings of bats, mesentery with small glands of various animals, one notices first a meshwork of capillaries in which the blood corpuscles are flowing at very variable rates. The capillaries coalesce into venules and veins which are usually very conspicuous. Provided the tissue has not been stimulated by any interference and is in a resting condition, the corresponding arteries and especially the arterioles are generally very narrow and sometimes difficult to find. The bore of an arteriole may be as narrow as that of a single capillary, but more often it is about double that of a normal capillary. The relatively thick walls and the extremely rapid current are responsible for the fact that they are less conspicuous than the smaller vessels.

On hydrodynamic principles the rate of flow is inversely proportional to the transverse section of the bed, and in accordance with the observations given above the rate of flow in the capillaries is seen to be slow compared with that in the arterioles. The difference in rate between the capillaries and the venules on the other hand is not at all pronounced, though in most systems the current certainly becomes more rapid in the veins than it is in the capillaries. The general picture differs in a very significant way from that presented by an injection preparation. One is often reminded of a relatively broad stream (running at first in a number of separate channels) supplied by a system of pipes—the arterioles—and it is impossible to doubt that the main resistance to be overcome lies in the arterioles where, therefore, the main fall in pressure must take place. That this is generally so will be shown quantitatively in a later lecture (XIII) where pressure measurements will be dealt with. There are exceptions, however, to be observed for instance in the tongue or mesentery of the frog in which the arterioles are wider, the capillary bed narrower and the rate of flow from arteries to veins more uniform.

The pulse in the small vessels.

When a fairly large artery is watched under a low power it is sometimes possible to observe the changes in diameter corresponding to the pulse. On sinuous arteries definite movements of the loops due to the same cause are of frequent occurrence, and such movements are shown in the cinema film photographed in my laboratory to illustrate these lectures (Krogh and Rehberg, 1924). In the smaller arteries and arterioles the pulse causes no visible movement of the walls, but only variations in the velocity of the flow. Although these variations are often considerable the mean rate of flow is normally so high that the corpuscles can be seen only as stream lines during the whole cardiac cycle, and the velocity variations cannot be made out.

In the capillaries the pulse does not as a rule cause any variation in diameter of the vessels, but the velocity variations can often be very distinctly seen and are practically always present when the flow is too rapid to render them visible, as shown by Heimberger (1925)[1] for the human nail fold capillaries. The pulsating flow is generally equalized in the venules, because the capillary paths are of unequal length; the phases of the pulse waves arriving are different and the pulse is extinguished by interference. Occasionally, however, the capillary network is sufficiently uniform to allow the pulse to penetrate to the small veins and this may be the case especially when the pulse amplitude is exceptionally high.[1]

The axial flow of corpuscles.

When, at a fairly high magnification, the walls of the small vessels are distinctly visible it is seen that in all vessels having a diameter of two corpuscles or more the red corpuscles are flowing in a definite axial stream, surrounded by a layer of clear plasma. In somewhat larger vessels the occasional white corpuscles are on the outside of this stream and they generally show a rolling movement.

It is well known that in a fluid moving along a tube or channel, the velocity increases regularly from the resting layer along the wall toward the axis of the tube. Particles suspended in the fluid will, therefore, obtain a greater velocity on the side nearest the axis. Their movement will tend to be rolling and they will be drawn in toward the axis as can be shown in experiments on blood or artificial suspensions flowing along capillary glass tubes (Schklarewsky, 1868; Fülleborn, 1925; Fåhraeus, 1928).

The extent of the zone of clear plasma depends upon the rate of flow and the size of corpuscles and vessel.

It can be stated that as soon as a tube is wider than the diameter of the red corpuscles these travel along without generally touching the wall, provided the rate of flow exceeds a certain minimum.[2] In larger vessels the plasma zone widens and may become nearly as broad as the largest diameter of the corpuscles.

Fülleborn (1925) has made some interesting experiments on the flow of filariform Strongyloides larvae in glass tubes and in pieces of arteries with a number of branches going off in different directions. These

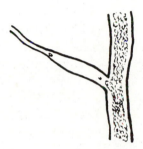

Fig. 1. Plasma skimming by
contraction of a branch
of an artery.

larvae have a length of 530μ with 15μ thickness. When flowing in tubes of 1.5 or 1 mm. diameter they occupied an axial stream of 0.95 and 0.45 mm., respectively, leaving a plasma zone 275μ broad in both cases. When the suspension flowed in an artery very few larvae would enter small branches going off at right angles, and the bulk would be reserved for the final branches in which the artery would split up. Similar though less pronounced variations will take place with regard to the distribution of erythrocytes in the smaller arteries and are not without significance when blood-samples are taken to determine the red cell count.[3]

A special reduction in the number of corpuscles, which may even amount to their complete washing away from a certain capillary field is sometimes brought about by the process which I have termed *plasma skimming* (Krogh, 1921): When a small artery branching from a larger vessel is partly contracted as indicated in the diagram, Fig. 1, the current of blood through it may seem to cease altogether, and at the same time the corpuscles are washed out from the corresponding capillaries which become empty and can easily be supposed to have contracted. In favorable circumstances it can be observed how at each pulse the column of corpuscles bulges into the mouth of the branch artery and retreats again immediately afterward, leaving only a few corpuscles which become detached and are passed swiftly along through the contracted portion of the artery. Plasma skimming is a further development of the unequal distribution of corpuscles between the smaller arterial branches, referred to above, and there is, of course, a complete gradation between a branch artery giving clear plasma and an end artery showing a cell number well above the normal.

The deformation of red corpuscles in capillaries.

The capillaries in a microscopic field often vary considerably in diameter. When examined under a fairly high power, so that the capillary walls can be distinctly seen, some are found which allow the corpuscles to pass in a continuous current, and these generally exhibit a definite axial stream surrounded by a plasma zone through which a white corpuscle will occasionally come rolling along. Others are so narrow that the corpuscles have to pass in single file and come continuously in contact with the wall. Others again are even narrower, and the corpuscles can pass only in a deformed state. The simplest deformation is observed in capillaries down to about 4-5μ diameter (in mammals) where the edges of the flat disklike corpuscles are bent in (Fig. 2, 5) while the length of the corpuscle measured during the passage does not exceed its diameter in the free state. In still narrower capillaries the red

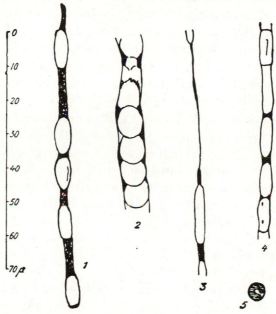

Fig. 2. Muscle capillaries from guinea pig, vitally injected with Indian ink. Walls of capillaries not shown.

corpuscles are greatly deformed and compressed into a shape like sausages the length of which may be double the normal diameter. Fig. 2 shows such corpuscles from muscle capillaries of a guinea pig, vitally injected with Indian ink. When they escape from such narrow vessels their shape immediately becomes normal again and free deformed corpuscles are never observed.

The pressure necessary to bring about the deformation in narrow capillaries must be comparatively low, since the flow does not stop in a single narrow capillary, even when the same arteriole supplies several others through which the corpuscles can pass freely, but a definite estimate cannot be attained.

It is well known that red corpuscles will pass through filter paper, the pores of which will hold back quantitatively precipitates consisting of particles which are much smaller than the corpuscles. There can be no doubt, though the passage has never been directly observed, that the corpuscles are greatly deformed during the passage. The pressure available for such a passage cannot exceed the height of fluid in the funnel.

The most direct evidence of the wonderful plasticity and elasticity of red corpuscles is obtained when they are watched in a current, where they can be caught against a projecting edge and bent by the pressure of the current flowing past them. This happens very often in the lungs where the circulation is of a peculiar character and appearance. The small arteries open through holes or very short branches into a close-meshed network of comparatively wide capillary channels on the surface of the alveoli. These channels occupy a very large percentage of the surface, but in the meshes there are small cellular islands of very varying shape. With each beat of the heart the flow in the capillaries becomes greatly accelerated, while it slows down gradually between beats.

On the cinema film of the flow of blood through the alveolar capillaries in the frog's lung, we find a corpuscle caught on a very sharply projecting edge, as shown in Fig. 3, copied from the film. It remained hanging on the edge during about four seconds (seventy pictures). At first it is riding nearly along the short axis, and both ends are bent down in the direction of the current, but the pressure is not sufficient to press the content of the corpuscle out toward both ends. Somewhat later it slides along toward one of the ends and becomes rather sharply bent into the shape of a large and a small sac. Finally, when the current becomes slack in the interval between two beats of the heart, the corpuscle slides off the edge. The four lower figures show four consecutive stages of this

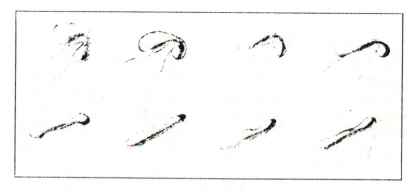

Fig. 3. Red corpuscle riding on projecting edge in frog's pulmonary capillaries and finally sliding off in four lower pictures. From moving picture film.

process with an interval of 0.06 second. In the last figure, about 0.3 second after the release, the shape has practically returned to normal, in consequence of the elastic properties of the corpuscle.

When a riding corpuscle is watched on the cinema film or directly through a high-power microscope, the current appears to be so rapid that it is not very surprising to see such effects, but it must be remembered that the rate of flow is magnified in the same proportion as the objects. On the film the actual rate can be approximately measured by noting the shifting posi-

tion of free swimming corpuscles from one picture to
the next. In the case now described, the rate, during
the period the corpuscle remained hanging, did not
exceed 0.12 mm. per second, corresponding to about
400 mm. per hour, a rate which is too slow to be followed by the naked eye. I am not familiar enough with
hydraulic problems to venture upon a calculation of
the actual pressure to which a current of this rate has
exposed the corpuscle, but it is evident that it must be
of a very low order.

The nonexistence of "vasa serosa."

Capillaries may sometimes be so narrow that they
cannot admit red corpuscles even when these are compressed ad maximum. Such "empty" capillaries were
observed early in the last century and have played a
prominent part in the discussion on the peripheral circulation under the designation *"vasa serosa."* Even as
late as 1888 Cohnstein and Zuntz described vasa serosa
as normal constituents of the frog's web, and in recent
papers (Smith, Arnold, and Whipple, 1921) their possible existence is sometimes used as an argument to explain discrepancies in blood counts, etc. It should be
pointed out, however, that capillaries can only under
exceptional circumstances and for short periods admit
a slow current of plasma without admitting corpuscles.
This is an unavoidable consequence of the extreme
softness of the red corpuscles. When a capillary containing one or more red corpuscles contracts to such
a degree that the corpuscles cannot pass along, they
will be squeezed into a form which fills up entirely the
lumen of the vessel and prevents any passage of
plasma along it. It is only when a capillary happens to
contain no corpuscles at the moment of becoming so
narrow that these elements can no longer be squeezed
through, that it may for a time admit a current of

plasma which must necessarily be very slow. Even in that case it will generally not last long before a corpuscle is carried into the mouth of the vessel and blocks the passage. In my observations of the circulation in specimens vitally injected with Indian ink, I have found that the submicroscopical particles of this substance can pass, as a rule, through only those capillaries which are also open to the passage of corpuscles.

Irregularities of the flow of blood in the smaller vessels.

When a microscopic field in any organ is watched for some time many slight variations in the flow are usually observed. These are due to local contractions and dilatations, very often too slight to be directly observed or measured. In single capillaries the flow may become retarded or accelerated from no visible cause; in capillary anastomoses the direction of flow may change from time to time. Similar changes in the direction of flow are sometimes seen also in arterial anastomoses and more often in veins. The mechanism of all these apparently spontaneous changes is unknown, but their effect certainly is an extremely nice adjustment of the general uniformity of the circulation. When an organ like the tongue of a frog is pinned out the mechanical tension on the different parts varies greatly, and one would expect certain areas to be cut off from the blood supply, but such a thing has never happened within my experience, and whether a membrane is stretched, folded, or bent in sharp angles the blood finds its way to any part where the actual pressure in the tissue does not exceed the pressure available in the arteries supplying that part.

Cases have been described, especially with regard to the nail capillaries in certain patients (Hinzelmann, Otfr. Müller, 1922), in which the flow at frequent, but quite irregular, intervals, often several times per minute, will stop altogether to resume its course after a period of one to many seconds. Sometimes the flow will come to a simultaneous standstill in all the capillaries in one nail, sometimes the flow stops only in a small group of capillaries. This is a further and pathological development of what is seen normally in most tissues as well as along the nails of human subjects, viz., irregular variations in the tone of arteries of different size. The condition obtaining when an artery has contracted completely is called stasis by several authors, but this terminology is very unfortunate, leading as it does to confusion of a simple suspension of flow with the quite different condition of true stasis, characterized by the packing of corpuscles presently to be described.

When the flow in the capillaries and small veins is slowed sufficiently it is often, in observations on mammals and especially on man, described as granular, and when the flow stops the corpuscles are seen to agglutinate into large lumps with spaces of clear plasma between them. These phenomena constitute an in vivo demonstration of the agglutination taking place in shed blood and brought back from oblivion by the beautiful researches of Fåhraeus (1921) on the ''Senkungsgeschwindigkeit'' of red corpuscles. With a rapid flow the turbulence is sufficient to counteract the mutual attraction and adhesiveness of the corpuscles, which bring about agglutination when the blood is quiescent.

Even when agglutination is very complete the apparently massive columns of corpuscles offer very little resistance and are swept away into the veins and broken up as soon as the flow is resumed (Tannenberg, III, 1925). True stasis, which shows a striking similarity to the complete agglutination described in so far

as the red corpuscles are seen to be closely packed,
shows a very different form and degree of resistance
to the resumption of flow.

Concentration of red corpuscles and stasis.[4]

At a fairly high magnification it is sometimes possible to observe how the corpuscles become concentrated during the passage of a long capillary. Where
they enter, the single corpuscles can be seen to be a
certain distance apart, and there is a distinct zone of
clear plasma along the wall. During their progress
they come much closer to each other and to the walls.
This is the first stage leading up to the definitely
pathological condition of stasis.

The development of stasis can be most easily observed in the tongue and mesentery of the frog and
in the mesentery of mammals (Krogh and Harrop,
1921; Florey, 1926, 2; Tannenberg, III, 1925). In the
first stage the corpuscles at the venous end of a capillary
become so closely packed that they obstruct the flow,
and during the further development we see the blood
enter into this capillary in a distinctly pulsating flow;
the fluid part of the blood disappears during its progress, and the corpuscles are deposited on the already
existing column which grows until the whole of the
capillary is filled up. The process is well shown as a
result of urethane application to the tongue of a frog
in the cinema film.

The column of corpuscles is generally transparent,
which shows that the corpuscles are so closely packed
that the rays of light can pass through without suffer-
ing refraction at the surfaces of the single corpuscles.
In hematocrite tubes this transparency is taken as an
indication of complete separation of the corpuscles
from the plasma, and no amount of centrifuging will
reduce the length of a column of corpuscles so packed.

The corpuscle volume determined in this way corresponds closely to that found by indirect methods, and it must be concluded, therefore, that in a transparent column plasma is practically absent, in spite of the doubt expressed by Tannenberg (III, 1925), who believes that agglutination of corpuscles is the main factor responsible for stasis instead of loss of plasma.

Stasis appears often, or perhaps usually, to be an irreversible process, but Florey (1926, 2) has had the opportunity of observing in the rat's mesentery the resolution of stasis in a number of capillaries. A main factor appears to be the capillary pulsation which will cause a gradual loosening of the massed corpuscles at the arterial end of the column, which loses its transparency, while at the same time the corpuscles are broken loose one by one or in small lumps by the pulsating fluid. In other cases the whole length of a column becomes imbibed with fluid, and apparently a series of contractions gradually forces the content over the lip of the stased capillary into the current of blood, when the liberated corpuscles are washed away.

Diapedesis of red corpuscles.

When the circulation is observed in inflamed tissue, where the blood flow is slow and the capillaries generally dilated, the process of diapedesis of single red corpuscles or parts of corpuscles can be observed along with the emigration of leucocytes of which I shall presently have to speak. Both these processes were very carefully studied long ago by Cohnheim, and I refer especially to the descriptions given in his lectures on general pathology (1877, pp. 120-125, 197-200).

The red corpuscles pass out through the capillary wall sometimes quite smoothly as through a hole, and it happens that two or more corpuscles pass through in the same place one after another. Often, however, a corpuscle may stick in the wall for some time, with the result that one part is carried off by the current of blood, while the other is finally deposited outside the vessel. In capillaries which have gone into stasis the wall of the vessel may slowly bulge out in one or (generally) more places, and suddenly it is found that the corpuscles contained in such a varicose dilatation are outside the vessel.[5] The most interesting point is that the integrity of the wall seems in all cases to be restored very rapidly. Even where a few corpuscles pass out one after another they are not followed by a further number, though diapedesis may take place just afterward close to the point, and when the circulation becomes normal again in a capillary which during stasis has lost a number of corpuscles in many places, the vessel appears to be tight not only to corpuscles but to the plasma fluid as well. Drinker, Drinker, and Lund (1922) have described how in the bone marrow the reverse process takes place and the newly formed red blood cells are pushed into the lumen of capillaries, the walls of which are closed behind them.

Circulation and emigration of white corpuscles.

The white corpuscles circulating in the blood are always spherical. Being comparatively few in number they are usually difficult to observe in the rapid stream in the arteries. They are occasionally seen to pass through capillaries, where the resistance offered to their passage through vessels with a diameter less than their own appears to be greater than that experienced by erythrocytes.

The leucocytes are most easily and most often seen in the small veins, where there is a definite axial flow and a not too rapid current. Here they are found chiefly in the marginal layer of plasma, rolling along the wall, sometimes in a more or less straight course, sometimes in spirals, but without entering the axial stream of more rapidly flowing erythrocytes. Schklarewsky has shown by his experiments in glass tubes that the expulsion of the white corpuscles from the axial stream is a consequence of the fact that their specific gravity is intermediate between that of the erythrocytes and that of the plasma. Their movement is a rolling one by reason of the increase in velocity from the periphery to the axis of the vessels. It appears, however, as if some slight adhesion between the endothelium and the surface of the white corpuscles had also something to do with the peculiarity of the movement. At least the corpuscles are often seen to move much more slowly than the plasma and to stop completely for short periods in contact with the wall. When the tissue is in a state of inflammation the white corpuscles become definitely adhesive to the vessel walls especially in the venules, but also, though generally at a somewhat later stage, in the capillaries. They are then flattened out by the current into a pyramidal or wedge-like shape with the top against the current as described by Tannenberg (IV, 1925). At first a slight impulse like the collision with another corpuscle will be sufficient to loosen the hold and cause the adhering corpuscle to roll on, but a little later it adheres more firmly, and emigration may take place. The tip of the corpuscle bends and penetrates the wall, and slowly the whole of the corpuscle moves through the endothelium, while pseudopodia may be stretched out to a considerable distance outside.

In the circumstances which cause emigration the leucocytes are strongly attracted toward and even beyond the vessel walls, and the smaller veins may be covered inside by a layer of corpuscles several cells deep, while many capillaries become more or less completely blocked. It appears that almost all leucocytes carried to an inflamed spot are held back by the attracting forces and eventually find their way into the tissue spaces.[6] As in the case of the passive diapedesis of the red corpuscles the active penetration of the white leaves the endothelium substantially intact, that is, the opening, which must undoubtedly exist during the penetration, closes again immediately afterward by the elasticity or vital contraction of the cell or cells concerned.

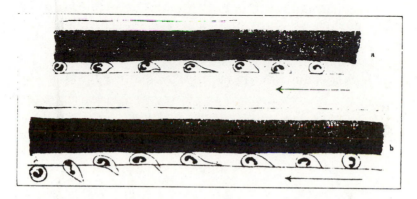

Fig. 4. Stages in the diapedesis of leucocytes. Semidiagrammatic. After Tannenberg.

In the present lecture I have tried to give a simple objective description of some of the outstanding phenomena of the circulation in the small vessels as they are to be observed through the microscope. As many of these phenomena will come up again for study in subsequent lectures I have endeavored here to avoid as far as possible any causal analysis.

A few points on the border line of my subject, but of sufficient interest to be treated a little more closely are referred to in the appended notes.

* * * * * * *

The blood vessels of muscles.

The arrangement of the blood vessels in striated muscles has been studied and depicted very carefully by Spalteholz (1888). The arteries supplying a muscle branch freely, and between the branches there are very numerous anastomoses forming a primary network. Into the meshes of this net small arteries are given off at regular intervals, and these again anastomose freely, forming a secondary cubical net of great regularity. From the threads of this network the arterioles branch off, generally at right angles to the muscle fibers and at very regular intervals (of about 1 mm. in the warm-blooded animal), and these arterioles finally split up into a large number of capillaries running along the

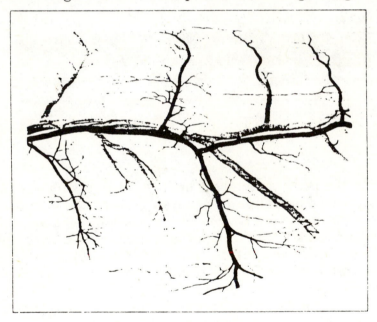

Fig. 5. Small arteries (black), capillaries, and veins from striated muscle. After Spalteholz.

muscle fibers and in the main parallel to them, but with numerous anastomoses, forming long narrow meshes about the fibers. The capillaries unite into venules intercalated regularly between the arterioles, and the whole system of veins reproduces and follows almost exactly that of the arteries. All the veins down to the smallest branches are provided with valves allowing the blood to flow in the direction of the heart only. Short pieces of secondary arteries and veins, with arterioles, venules, and capillaries, are shown in Fig. 5, reproduced from Spalteholz.

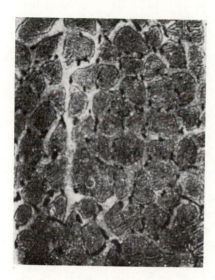

Fig. 6. Transverse section from the injected m. gastrocnemius of a horse. ×156.

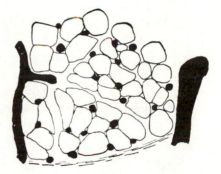

Fig. 7. Transverse section of injected muscle from the tongue of a cat. ×268.

When the muscle contracts its form is greatly altered, the fibers becoming much shorter and proportionally thicker. The whole of the vascular system is beautifully adapted to these changes: the arterial and venous networks insure the supply and drainage of almost every point, even if a number of anastomoses are temporarily blocked. The capillaries, which in the resting muscle are practically straight, become much twisted. The blood is driven out by compression from a number of the venous branches, and, when the muscle relaxes again, these can be filled from their peripheral ends only. Since muscular contractions usually more or less regularly alternate with relaxations, the system of valves makes of the veins of every muscle a very effective pump, capable of maintaining a low pressure in the muscle capillaries. The significance of this arrangement will come up for study later, but at present our attention must be focused on the capillaries. It is apparent from Fig. 5 that sections, cut at right angles to the muscle fibers, must represent the capillaries as dots which can be counted and the distribution of which can be studied. Such transverse sections are given in Figs. 6 and 7; and an inspection of them shows that the capillaries are present in very large numbers and are distributed among the muscle fibers with conspicuous regularity. A quantitative test of the regularity of the arrangement can be obtained by counting the number of capillaries in a large number of small equal areas chosen at random from sections of the same muscle. I give as an example a series of countings, each made on an area of 0.0300 square mm. (mm.²), from five different transverse sections of the m. gastrocnemius of a horse.

	1	2	3	4	5
	45	34	38	38	31
	40	34	42	43	33
	42	40	43	47	43
	41	46	41	49	39
	44	44	46	33	36
	36	41	..	..	..
	49	38	..	..	..
Average,	42	39	42	42	36

An inspection of this table shows the remarkable regularity of distribution, and, when it is treated mathematically, the average number of capillaries in the area measured works out as 40.5 ± 5, a dispersion of not more than 12 per cent. Dividing by 0.03 we get the number of capillaries per square mm. transverse section as not less than 1,350 with a mean error of ± 31. The transverse section of an ordinary pin is about 0.5 mm.² It requires some mental effort to conceive how there can be room within such a pin for about seven hundred parallel tubes carrying blood, in addition to about two hundred muscle fibers.

In other animals the number of capillaries per mm.² may be even larger. It is well known that mammals have a higher metabolism than cold-blooded vertebrates, and small mammals a higher metabolism than large ones, and there appears to be some relation between the metabolic activity and the number of capillaries per mm.² of muscle. In a dog's m. semimembranosus the number worked out from 30 countings as 2,630 ± 51, while the dispersion or "standard deviation" of the single counting was not more than 10.6 per cent.

Even larger figures were found for guinea pigs' muscles, and I have no doubt that in the smallest mammals the number of capillaries per sq. mm. can be above 4,000. In cold-blooded animals, such as the cod and the frog, much smaller figures are found, averaging only about 400.

Stoel has compared (1925) the number of capillaries in white and red muscles in the domesticated rabbit. The figures given by him are remarkably low. He finds for the red m. semitendinosus only 790 capillaries per mm.² and for the white m. add. magnus 1,550, while in the heart he has counted 3,230.[1] The diameters given as averages are very narrow, viz., 5.2, 2.5, and 5.0μ, respectively, but I cannot feel convinced that the diameters measured on injected and fixed specimens are

trustworthy. Quite recently (1927) Duyff and Bouman
have repeated Stoel's countings and extended them to
a number of other muscles in the rabbit. They report
higher figures, from 1,000-2,700 capillaries per mm.²
(not cm.² as they say), but give their numbers as relative only.

To obtain some insight into the meaning of such
figures as those found by my countings let us consider
very briefly the problem concerning the supply of oxygen to the muscular tissue. The oxygen molecules have
to travel outward from the capillaries, and the longest
distance a molecule has to go must be half the distance
between neighboring capillaries, denoted R. This works
out in the case of the frog's muscle (400 capillaries
per mm.²) as $R = 28\mu$ (calculated from the center of
each capillary) and in the case of the dog's muscle
(2,600) as $R = 11\mu$. I shall show later in some detail
how these figures can be utilized for a calculation of
the oxygen pressure head necessary for supplying the
muscles. If we consider the exchange of dissolved substances between the blood and the muscle lymph, this
depends evidently on the available capillary surface,
and, assuming the average diameter of capillaries $2r$
as equal to the diameter of a red blood corpuscle, we
obtain the following figures for the total surface of
capillaries in 1 cubic centimeter of muscle:

Muscle	Weight of animal kilos	Muscle capil- laries per sq. mm.	R μ	$2r$ μ	Capillary surface cm.² per cm.³	Volume per cent	Surface of 1 cc. blood cm.²
Frog,	0.05	400	28	15	190	7.1	2,700
Horse,	500	1,400	15	5.5	240	3.3	7,300
Dog,	5	2,600	11	7.2	590	10.6	5,600

On the same assumptions the volume of blood in the
muscle capillaries works out as between 3.3 per cent
(horse) and 10.6 per cent (dog) of the muscle volume,

and the surface of 1 cc. blood contained in capillaries as 2,700 cm.^{2} (frog) to 7,300 cm.^{2} (horse). It is evident that very large exchanges of substances can take place in a short time through such enormous surfaces. Supposing a man's muscles to weigh 50 kg. and his capillaries to number 2,000 per sq. mm., the total length of all these tubes put together must be something like 100,000 kilometers or 2½ times round the globe and their total surface 6,300 sq. meters.

It is evident that much more work could be done, and ought to be done, on what I should like to term the *quantitative anatomy* of muscle capillaries. A number of different animals ought to be examined and a number of different muscles from each animal. The regularity or otherwise of the capillary arrangement ought to be made out and definite relationships established between the capillary supply and the amount of work required of muscles. I would suggest, for instance, comparisons between the capillaries in the muscles of the hind legs and the hearts in domesticated rabbits and hares.

* * * * * * *

LECTURE III

THE INDEPENDENT CONTRACTILITY OF CAPILLARIES

IN the preceding lecture I described the wonderful arrangement of the capillaries and tried to make clear the enormous extent of the surfaces they present for the exchange of substances between the blood and the tissues. I alluded also very briefly to the problem with which we are now confronted: Supposing these facilities for exchange to be necessary and just sufficient to provide for the needs of an organ when that organ is doing work at its maximum rate, how can they avoid being wastefully in excess of the requirements when the organ is absolutely or comparatively at rest?

The generally accepted view of the capillary circulation, at least until a few years ago, was that the capillaries are passive, that blood flows continuously through all of them at rates which are determined by the state of contraction or dilatation of the corresponding arterioles, and that the dilatation of an arteriole will cause a rise of pressure in the corresponding capillaries, which will become passively expanded, to contract again by their own elasticity when the pressure is reduced.

By the varying resistance in the arteries and arterioles the supply of blood to an organ can undoubtedly be regulated in accordance with its requirements, but an increase in current must always be accompanied by a corresponding increase in capillary pressure, and when the requirements are small the quantity of blood constantly present in a large number of the capillaries would serve no useful purpose. A much more effective distribution would obviously be obtained if the capillaries themselves were contractile, if in a resting organ only a limited number of capillaries, distributed at suitable regular intervals, were kept open so as to admit blood and provide the necessary surface area for the exchange of substances. This hypothetical conception was to me personally the starting point and guide in the experimental study of capillary contractility. Since, however, I was by no means the first to discover or even to demonstrate that capillaries show independent contractility, the most suitable course will be to present the evidence in the order in which it was published.

* * * * * * *

My own first contribution to the problem of capillary contractility was published in Danish in 1918, about a month after Dale and Richards' paper, and somewhat later appeared in the British *Journal of Physiology* (1919). It was undertaken to test the hypothesis of a regulation of the supply of blood to muscles through the opening and closing of individual capillaries. I found it possible to observe at least the superficial capillaries of muscles both in the frog and in mammals through a binocular microscope, using strong reflected light as a source of illumination. Resting muscles observed in this way are usually quite pale, and the microscope reveals only a few capillaries at fairly regular intervals. These capillaries are so narrow that red corpuscles can pass through only at a slow rate and with a change of form from the ordinary flat disks to elongated sausages. When the muscle under observation is stimulated to contractions a large number of capillaries become visible and dilated, and the rate of circulation through them is greatly increased. When the stimulus has lasted only a few seconds the circulation returns in some minutes to the resting state; the capillaries become narrower and most of them are emptied completely, while a small number remain open. Since capillaries, even in a group fed by the same arteriole, do not all behave in the same way, the changes obviously cannot be due to arterial pressure changes.

In resting muscles of the frog the average distance between open capillaries, observed simultaneously through the microscope, was estimated at 200 to 800μ, but after contractions this could be reduced to 70 or 60μ. In the guinea pig average distances of about 200μ could be observed during rest. The exposure to the air and the strong light always increased the circulation, and it was often possible to see the circulation begin in one capillary after another.

It might be argued that the observations here recorded could be explained as the results of dilatation of arterioles alone, on the assumption that the capillary paths offer various degrees of resistance, that a few are opened by a low pressure, while the majority of capillaries belonging to an arteriole require a higher pressure and are opened only when that arteriole is dilated. Such an assumption would involve as a consequence that a reduction of the pressure to 0 by cutting the artery must produce an elastic contraction and emptying of the postulated high-pressure capillaries. Numerous observations have shown that all the capillaries may remain open when a piece of muscle is cut out after stimulation.

The measurement of distances between open capillaries made upon living specimens could not, of course, be very accurate, and the degree of regularity of their distribution could not be satisfactorily made out by simple inspection. I had, therefore, to try and devise a method by which the state of the vessels at any given moment could be studied after fixation. This I succeeded in doing by injecting an Indian ink solution, dialyzed against a Ringer solution to make it isotonic with the blood and deprive it of the toxic substances present in the commercial preparation. When a suitable quantity of Indian ink is introduced into the circulation of a living anesthetized animal it is evenly mixed with the blood, and if the animal is suddenly killed by stopping the circulation a few minutes later, and preparations are made from the muscles and other organs, these show the capillaries which were open at the time.

On frogs I found by this method that there were large differences between different organs in the number of open capillaries. The skin, liver, and brain were always well injected, with all, or nearly all, capillaries open. The tongue was generally white and nearly bloodless, when not stimulated before being removed. The empty stomach and intestines had only a small number of open capillaries. The injection of muscles was variable, but in most of the resting muscles few capillaries only were open, while muscles which had been tetanized before stopping the circulation were almost black from the large number of injected capillaries. Countings of the open capillaries on transverse sections of muscles injected vitally in this way demonstrated the fairly regular distribution of open capillaries. In stimulated muscles I counted in one case of an extensor tarsi muscle 195 capillaries per mm.^{2}, while the corresponding unstimulated muscle from the other leg had so few that an accurate count could not be obtained. There were certainly not more than 5 in a mm.^{2} Other resting muscles showed higher numbers, however, especially the rectus abdominis muscle, which had also been observed in the living state to be always well supplied with blood, and three countings from which gave, respectively, 115, 155, and 180 open capillaries per mm.^{2}, which is from 30 to 40 per cent of the total number. On guinea pigs considerable differences were observed between the degrees of vascularization of different resting muscles, probably connected with the length of time since they had been in activity. Some flat muscles were examined provisionally in the fresh state by counting under a low power the capillaries visible in a single field without using the vertical adjustment. When the positions of capillaries along the eyepiece micrometer are noted, a fairly good idea of the regularity of their distribution can be obtained. I give some instances of such countings on muscles from the abdominal wall and from the diaphragm of the guinea pig.

Capillaries at scale divisions

Muscle from abdominal
wall upper layer:
1 division = 21.8µ.

10 13 16 21 24 28 31 33 35 38 44 50
55 61 65 67 72 75 78

Largest distance 6 divisions, smallest 2, average 3.8 = 83µ.

Diaphragm: 20 22 23 25 27 30 32 35 37 39 41 42 44 46 48 50
1 division = 8.8µ.   51 53 55 57 59 62 64 66 68 70 71 73 75 77 79 81

Largest distance 3, smallest 1, average 1.96 = 17µ.

The first muscle had been at rest, but the diaphragm, being the chief respiratory muscle, had been working vigorously up to the death of the animal. Several

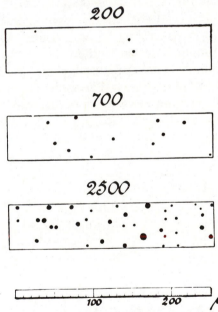

Fig. 20. Preparations from vitally injected
muscles from guinea pig. Optical
transverse sections.

countings of optical transverse sections of the same muscles, which is, of course, a more accurate method, gave for the muscle from the abdominal wall the figures 86, 70, 92 capillaries per mm.^{2}, corresponding to a distance of 125μ between them, and for the diaphragm 2,700, 2,550, 2,450 capillaries per mm.^{2}, corresponding to a distance of 18μ.

Fig. 20 shows equal optical sections from three different muscles with the number of capillaries per sq. mm. as noted. In this figure the approximate diameters of the open capillaries are also indicated, and it should be noted that in the working muscle they vary considerably, while in the resting muscle, with 200 open capillaries, these are extremely narrow. The table gives a number of measurements in micromillimeters. When it is remembered that the red corpuscles of the frog are on an average 22μ long, 15μ broad, and 4μ thick in the middle, while those of the guinea pig are 7.2μ in diameter and about 2μ thick, it seems almost incredible that they can pass through capillaries of the smallest dimensions given and even that they can pass through the average open capillaries of resting muscles. That they do so can be easily observed in the living muscles, as mentioned in the first of these lectures.

I have said enough, I believe, to make it abundantly clear that capillaries are not merely passively distended by arterial blood pressure, but possess a tone of their own and may show contractions and relaxations independently of the corresponding reactions in the arteries. I think it right, however, to record one more experiment which demonstrates in a crucial manner that the whole length of a capillary from an arteriole to a venule can be contractile, that it cannot, when contracted, be forced open by the available arterial pressure, but can be made, by suitable stimulation, to relax and open up to a pressure which is much lower.

Frog, m. sartorius.				Guinea pig.			
Resting		Stimulated		Abdominal wall		Diaphragm	
7.3	5.2	7.2	7.4	2.2	4.0	4.4	4.2
3.5	2.4	7.6	7.3	4.1	1.8	4.8	4.0
2.5	4.1	6.0	8.0	3.0	3.8	7.4	2.8
10.6	3.6	7.0	4.3	4.2	3.0	8.2	5.8
2.9	4.3	7.6	4.2	4.5	3.5	3.3	7.4
4.6	2.1	4.1	6.7	2.7	6.5	6.7	10.4
5.6	2.7	9.6	6.7	3.7	3.1	2.2	3.5
5.5	3.3	5.5	10.7	2.5	2.9	4.2	4.6
4.0	2.9	7.4	5.6	2.9	5.0	4.7	5.5
4.4	4.0	4.9	7.0	2.8	3.3	3.1	5.4

Average,					
4.3μ	6.8μ	3.5μ	5.0μ

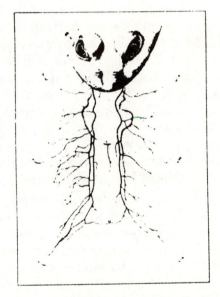

Fig. 21. The frog's tongue pinned out
for microscopic examination.
Natural size.

The lower surface of the frog's tongue is covered
by a smooth mucous membrane and, when suitably

stretched, shows a very wide-meshed network of capillaries, small arteries, and veins. While in the mouth the tongue is usually pale and almost bloodless. When the tongue of narcotized frog is pinned out, as shown in Fig. 21, it becomes stimulated by the process and a large number of vessels appear. When the tongue is left to itself in a moist atmosphere the vessels contract again, the tongue becomes pale and many of the capil-

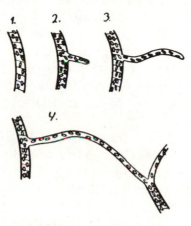

Fig. 22. Opening up of a capillary by
repeated weak stimulation.

laries are completely closed and cannot be seen at all with the magnification practicable with the binocular erecting microscope. If the surface of the tongue is now very lightly scratched with a hair or a fine glass needle along a small vein (Fig. 22, 1) a reaction can be obtained like that shown in Fig. 22, 2. A small branch opens up and is filled with blood, which becomes stagnant. By continuing the stimulus in front of the column of stagnant blood the relaxation is carried further (Fig. 22, 3), the blood flows slowly on in the direction from the vein and at last connection is established

with an arteriole, resulting, of course, in a sudden onset of current in the opposite direction, toward the
vein.

*The effect of internal pressure on the caliber of capil-
laries.*

According to the old conceptions regarding the regulating mechanism of the circulation, the arteries and
arterioles were almost exclusively responsible for the
state of dilatation of capillaries which were opened up
by the pressure transmitted to them when the arterial
vessels dilated. According to our new conception the
caliber of capillaries is mainly determined by their own
tonus, but they must, of course, be affected also to a
certain extent by the pressure of the blood upon their
walls.

It is worthy of note that the direct effect of pressure
upon the walls of capillaries is normally very small or
even negligible. Ordinarily the pressure which can be
brought to bear upon capillaries by dilatation of arterioles is but low, because the integral transverse section of capillary beds and their veins is large compared
with that of normal or even greatly dilated arterioles,
and we find further that most capillaries are able to
withstand a considerable pressure without giving way.

These points will be discussed in some detail in later
lectures and here I shall only give a few examples revealed by the preliminary study of capillary circulation which has been the subject of this lecture.

When the main artery supplying one side of a frog's
tongue is completely blocked before an area is stimulated no visible dilatation takes place until the blood is
admitted. When the arterial pressure is greatly diminished by compression of the artery the dilatation after
mechanical stimulation will take place slowly, and after
the opening of the artery a further slight dilatation

will take place and a few capillaries may be opened up which had up to that time remained closed.

In the frog's web the arteries can be brought to dilatation by the application of a drop of acetyl-choline and to a partial contraction by adrenaline, and when the capillaries are watched during these changes the effect upon their caliber is seen to be very slight and sometimes scarcely noticeable. When the femoral artery is blocked completely there is a general contraction of the capillaries in the web amounting to some 20 per cent (Oinuma, 1924).

When muscles, especially those of mammals and fishes, are artificially injected in the fresh state it is found to be very difficult to obtain a complete injection, and microscopic examination of some of the injected specimens has revealed the fact that of the number of capillaries supplied by the same arteriole a minority only have become injected, in spite of the high pressure employed.

The power to resist an internal pressure is developed to a very different degree in the capillaries of different tissues. It appears to be very high in muscles and comparatively low in the frog's skin and web. The cutaneous capillaries and venules in the arm of man become somewhat dilated when the venous pressure is raised by means of a Recklinghausen cuff to about 30 cm. water pressure. They appear to resist the pressure for some minutes before they give way.

NOTE

[1] The experiments of a single author from this period, Heubner (1907), will be referred to in a following lecture.

LECTURE IV

THE STRUCTURE OF THE CAPILLARY WALL

HAVING established the fact of independent capillary contractility we are again face to face with a problem, this time mainly histological: By what means can the contractions be carried out? If we turn to the histological textbooks for information we get a rather disappointing reply. The walls of the arterioles and small veins consist generally of three histologically different layers, viz., an inner tube made up of flat polygonal endothelial cells, an outer coat of connective tissue fibers, containing cells, and a middle portion consisting of one or more layers of smooth, ring-shaped muscle cells. When we approach the capillaries the outer coat first disappears, the muscle fibers become fewer in number and do not form a continuous layer, and finally we have left only the endothelial tube. This is built up of very thin cells of a polygonal or usually of an elongated rhomboidal shape, compared by Stöhr to steel pens pointed at both ends. The cells are cemented together at their edges to form a completely closed tube. The delimitation of the cells can be made very distinctly visible microscopically by treatment with nitrate of silver and subsequent reduction (Fig. 23). The cement will then show up as black lines. By suitable staining each endothelial cell can be shown to possess a nucleus, generally of an oval form and projecting somewhat above the internal as well as on the external surface of the cell.

A structure like this makes it easier to understand why the majority of physiologists have for a long time declined to accept any evidence for capillary contractility, and leads, when the evidence becomes overwhelming, to the assumption of a mechanism of contractility entirely different from that possessed by the larger vessels. The mechanism assumed, I believe, by

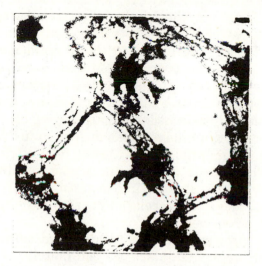

Fig. 23. Capillaries from frog's web. Border lines of endothelial cells silvered. Black pigment cells. ×300.

most of the physiologists who have observed the contractility for themselves (Hooker, 1920), was suggested by Stricker (1876) on the basis of his observation that the outside diameter of capillaries did not become appreciably altered, even when the lumen was greatly diminished. This observation leads almost unavoidably to the conclusion that the decrease in internal diameter must be brought about by a swelling of the protoplasm; that, in other words, osmotic or imbibition processes are responsible for the variations in the internal diameter of capillaries.

The existence of contractile cells in the capillary wall.

There exists, however, another and very different conception regarding the contractile mechanism of capillaries.

A few years after Stricker's first communication, Rouget (1873), who had independently observed the contractility of capillaries in young tadpoles, studied histologically the capillaries in the hyaloid membrane of the frog's eye and found on the outside of the endothelial tubes certain oblong nuclei, arranged in the direction of the tube and surrounded by a zone of protoplasm with ramified elongations which embrace the capillary in a number of places like so many hoops. In a second communication (1879) he states having observed these cells also on the living capillaries of young newt larvae and having seen them contract.

He takes them to be related to the smooth muscle cells of larger vessels.

Rouget's papers were practically completely disregarded and soon, as it seems, completely forgotten. Nearly thirty years later Sigmund Mayer (1902) rediscovered the branched cells on the capillaries of the hyaloid membrane and also on those of the intestine of amphibia and stated that a continuous series of cells of intermediate form could be demonstrated between these and the normal spindle-shaped cells of the arterial muscular coat. It did not inspire confidence, however, that these interesting structures could be made visible only by vital staining with methylene blue, and even then only occasionally, and the further statement, that a system of branched cells, similar to that on capillaries, or even isolated cells of the same kind, could occasionally be found where no capillaries could be detected, could not fail to arouse the suspicion that they had no real physiological connection with capillaries. The suspicious attitude of histologists was probably further strengthened by the fact that, although Mayer concluded his preliminary paper by the announcement that a detailed publication, accompanied by figures, was to appear shortly, this promise was never fulfilled.

Mayer's paper gave, however, the immediate impulse for the physiological investigations undertaken by Steinach and Kahn, and although these authors have not made any positive contribution to the histological problem, they have shown conclusively by measurements of dilated and contracted capillaries that the rival theory of capillary "contractility" by imbibition of the endothelial cells cannot be correct, since they find that the outside diameter of contracting capillaries, far from remaining constant or even increasing, as that theory demands, is very considerably diminished. They give a number of examples, of which I reproduce a few.

Outside diameter of capillaries in frogs' nictitating membrane		Lumen when contracted
Dilated	Contracted	
μ	μ	
26	12	still open
24	7	closed
22	6	very narrow
19	3	closed

These observations have been repeatedly verified in my laboratory, and the situation shortly before the first edition of these lectures appeared was the following: Of the two theories brought forward to explain the capillary contractility, one—the imbibition theory—was untenable for physical reasons, while the existence of the histological elements demanded by the other was, to say the least, extremely doubtful. Evidently a solution of this difficulty was essential for a successful attack on the many physiological problems connected with capillary contractility. If the contractility were due to muscles, the innervation, for instance, or the reactions to stimuli must be supposed to be very different from what one would expect if it were due to imbibition processes in the endothelial cells or to a mechanism as yet undiscovered. I, therefore, asked a young histologist, Dr. Vimtrup, to take up the problem, and he reached very definite conclusions (1922) regarding the existence of muscle cells in the capillary wall.

Utilizing the fact that it is possible to bring about experimentally in certain tissues, and notably in the muscles and mucous membrane of the tongue of the frog, any desired degree of capillary contraction and dilatation, Vimtrup has examined sections from such tongues suitably fixed and stained. On the outside of the capillaries he finds certain nuclei slightly, but distinctly, different from the ordinary endothelial nuclei. The form of these nuclei varies with the state of contraction of the capillary. On a dilated capillary they are broad and very thin; by contraction they become narrower and thicker, their cross-section approaching the form of a circle.

The protoplasm belonging to these nuclei is very difficult to stain by ordinary histological methods though Vimtrup has succeeded in obtaining a fairly good staining with iron trioxyhematein. Even when stained the protoplasmic structure can only be observed by means of high power immersion lenses, and very good illumination, which must often be made excentric, is necessary.

The best results were obtained by supravital staining with methylene blue, the method first employed for

this purpose by Mayer and further elaborated by Vimtrup. The application of this method is limited, however, to thin membranes which can be examined in toto
without being cut into sections, such as the web, bladder, and nictitating membrane of frogs. The general
results obtained by Vimtrup are as follows.

On a dilated capillary the protoplasm surrounds the
nucleus as a continuous layer on the capillary wall,
but it diminishes in thickness toward the periphery,
which is very irregular and sends out a number of very
fine branches along and especially around the capillary wall. The branches show at their base a definitely
triangular cross-section, but soon become flat. Sometimes they become broader and divide, but the ends
are always very thin and pointed. Most of the branches
lie athwart the capillary and are of such length that
they reach those from the other side. Some of the
branches, however, run along the capillary, and both
the protoplasm and the nucleus are, as a rule, stretched
in this direction. From the ends of the continuous protoplasm a broad branch usually runs along the capillary, giving off very fine secondary branches encircling
the vessel. The distance from the last of these branches
to the center of the nucleus can, in large cells, amount
to about 100μ.

On a capillary of normal diameter, which will allow
the red corpuscles to pass without much deformation,
the appearance of the protoplasm is rather different.
The continuous mass around the nucleus is distinctly
thicker, with a more conspicuous structure; the contours of the branches are more distinct; the triangular
form of their cross-section is very pronounced, the
sides being somewhat concave. On very narrow capillaries these changes are further accentuated. The protoplasm is packed about the nucleus and the branches

are short and stout, though still encircling the capillary and ending in sharp points.

When the branched cells are followed along a capillary toward an arteriole or a venule their shape gradually becomes different. They become shorter; the nuclei do not lie exactly in the direction of the capillary, but more or less slantingly around it; the branches are reduced in number and length along the capillary. On the arterioles themselves every stage of transition can be found between normal spindle-shaped muscle cells with an elongated nucleus, encircling the vessel, and others with an oblique nucleus and the protoplasm split up into a few ramifications. These latter become more numerous on approaching the capillaries, and there is no sharp distinction between them and the richly branched cells characteristic of the capillary.

By supravital staining with methylene blue the pericapillary cells take up the stain only at a certain stage, while later it disappears and is probably decomposed. The cells are not stained in their entirety, but the nuclei and certain fibrils in the protoplasmic branches take up the stain and deposit it as fine granules. From the analogous staining of the undoubted smooth muscle cells on arterioles it is concluded that the fibrils represent the contractile elements in the cells.

I reproduce three of Vimtrup's figures showing smooth muscle cells from an arteriole and the complete series of transitional cell forms connecting these with the typical branched cells on a capillary.

Fig. 24 shows the point of branching of an arteriole with circular, smooth muscle cells around the endothelial tube. A few of these cells are simple spindles, while the protoplasm of others is broken up into two or more parallel threads, and others again show a quite irregular ramification. The nuclei (a) of the more or less regular forms are arranged as arcs of a circle at right angles to the direction of the vessel, while the nuclei of the others occupy a slanting position. The nuclei of the endothelial cells (*b*) are visible in the figure, but are not very distinct.

Fig. 25 shows a large capillary with typical branched cells in considerable number, though much fewer than on the arteriole. The threads, which run from the nuclei (*a*) round the circumference of the capillary, probably represent the muscle fibrils and not the entire

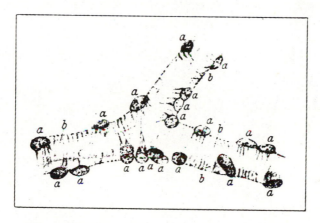

Fig. 24. Transition between arteriole and capillary.

protoplasm of these cells. The granular appearance of the threads has probably nothing to do with the structure of the fibrils, but is a simple deposition of methylene blue. In Fig. 26, which shows a small and slightly contracted capillary of 8μ diameter, the cells are fewer in number. Their nuclei are arranged lengthwise on the vessel, and in one place the elongation of the cell along the capillary wall can be distinctly seen. Red blood corpuscles, *r*, are also shown.

Vimtrup's methylene blue preparations have been examined by several very competent histologists

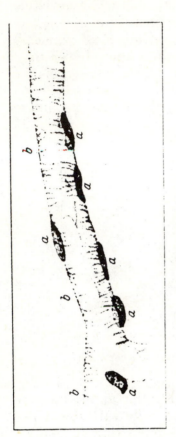

Fig. 25. Large capillary.

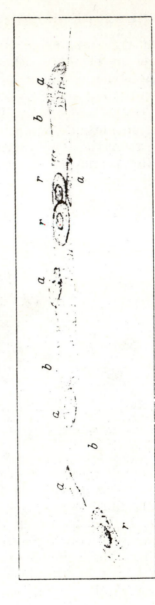

Fig. 26. Small, somewhat contracted capillary. *a* Muscle cells, *b* Nuclei of endothelial cells, *r* Red corpuscles. From nictitating membrane of frog. Supravital staining with methylene blue. ×500. After Vimtrup.

(F. C. C. Hansen, Spalteholz, Bensley, and others) who have declared themselves entirely convinced regarding the muscular nature of the cells stained.

As there can be no doubt that the richly ramified muscle cells on the capillary wall are the same as those originally found by Rouget in the hyaloid membrane,

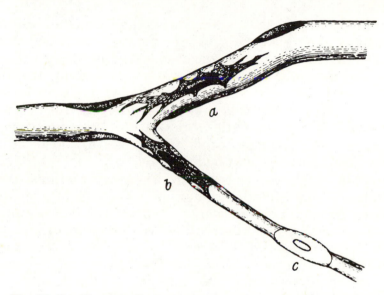

Fig. 27. Two Rouget cells (*a* and *b*) as seen on capillaries in living newt larvae. *b* is contracting, *c* is a red corpuscle.
×500. After Vimtrup.

Vimtrup has named them after the first discoverer, and we shall speak of them, henceforward, as *Rouget cells*.

After having studied these cells in stained preparations so as to be completely familiar with their distribution and appearance, Vimtrup has further succeeded in observing them on living capillaries and has been able to follow in a single cell the changes of form taking place by contraction. The best object for these observations he has found to be the tail of young newt larvae (Triton punctatus), which can be arranged for observation even with oil immersion lenses. By a simple and ingenious arrangement Vimtrup has been able to immobilize these larvae and keep them in excellent condition for hours without having recourse to narcosis.

In these animals spontaneous contractions and dilatations of single capillaries or parts of capillaries are of frequent occurrence, and it is a significant fact that a contraction always begins just where the nucleus of one of the Rouget cells is located. During the process of contraction the cell shows the different forms described as characteristic in the case of stained preparations, but the movements themselves are generally too slow to be followed by the eye.

This can be done, however, when contractions are induced by stimulation of nerves in the web of a small frog. After a latent period of about fifteen seconds the Rouget cell under observation will show an increase in the refraction of light, and a few seconds later the contraction proper will begin. The nucleus of the cell is observed to sink a little into the capillary, and on the opposite wall several small indentations make their appearance. Some of the ramifications, as a rule, become distinctly visible, when the capillary is already somewhat contracted, and it can be observed that their positions correspond to the indentations seen in the endothelial wall. After two to three minutes' stimulation a maximum, though usually incomplete, contraction is generally obtained, but about this time a very curious change takes place in the tissues, which lose their normal transparence and become so opaque that no structural details can be observed. When the stimulation has ceased the tissues regain their normal transparence and the contracted Rouget cells relax in the course of a few minutes.

*   *   *   *   *   *   *

*The direct communications between arteries and veins
and their significance.*

In the anatomical literature of fifty years ago there
are a number of references to the existence of *"derivating channels,"* represented by small arteries opening directly into somewhat larger veins. Such connections have generally been observed on injected
specimens and without verification by a study of the
structure of the vessels in question. As single capillaries can easily become greatly dilated by injection
under pressure and give the appearance of wide
channels, evidence of this kind is obviously untrustworthy.

Hoyer (1877) describes the existence of direct anastomoses between arteries, generally of about 0.02 mm.
diameter, and slightly larger veins as occurring only
in certain places in the body of mammals. He has
found them near the edge of the ears in rabbits, dogs,
and cats, in the tip of the snout in several animals, as
well as in the tip of the tail, and finally in the tips of
fingers and toes in man and other mammals. In many
of his cases he has studied the structure of the vessel
wall in the places of anastomosis after suitable staining, and he describes and pictures vessels of undoubted
arterial structure opening directly into others which
must be accepted as veins. He has made a search for
these "derivating channels" in many other places, but
apart from the well-known case of the arteries opening
directly into the corpora cavernosa, he has found them
only in such projecting parts as might require a considerable supply of blood to keep them warm, when
exposed to low temperatures.[3]

Grosser (1902) confirms Hoyer's results as to the
existence of derivating channels in the skin of the ex-

tremities and gives a careful description of their structure. They are numerous in the skin of human fingers where they are arranged in small groups 1-2 mm. apart. Their musculature is twice to thrice as strong as that of arteries of the same bore (about 0.02 mm.) and they are imbedded in connective tissue with numerous nuclei. They are common also within the digital bones, where they are surrounded by a venous plexus which allows them to open and close freely. They are especially large (0.1-0.2 mm.) in the thumb of bats. Grosser has made a search for them in appropriate places in reptiles, where they appear to be absent.

In the last few years evidence has been brought forward for the existence of arterio-venous anastomoses from intra vitam observations of the circulation in the human skin. Heimberger (1925, 1) has been able to observe such connections directly and in considerable numbers in the fingers of persons having a very delicate skin. He describes them as short connections between peripheral arterioles and venules, short-circuiting the long capillary loops, and gives a number of figures of which I reproduce one (Fig. 37). He finds these channels normally closed, to be opened up for a short period by weak mechanical stimulation.

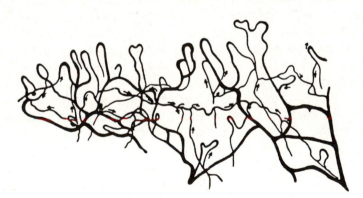

Fig. 37. Arterio-venous anastomoses. After Heimberger.

I should not attach much weight to these observations, which must be exceedingly difficult to verify, but for the two facts that Heimberger is an observer of quite extraordinary ability and patience, and that his direct findings are supported by observations of the blood flow in superficial venules and capillaries which are explicable only if arterio-venous anastomoses exist in close proximity to the vessels under observation. In a few cases Heimberger (1925, 2) has seen pulsation of the blood in venules when the corresponding arterioles were closed and the blood in the capillaries quiescent. This is possible only when the venule in question possesses another connection with the arterial system, through which the pulse is admitted. In other cases the blood is seen for some time to flow back from a venule through the capillaries to an arteriole, which postulates that the venule is connected directly with a somewhat larger artery, transmitting sufficient pressure to carry the blood back into an arteriole which must also be in direct communication with a larger vein.

It follows from the observations of Heimberger that his "derivating channels" which are distal to those of Hoyer and Grosser must be able to contract and expand and to close up entirely.

It must be borne in mind that the arterio-venous anastomoses here dealt with have nothing in common with the pathologic arterio-venous fistulas of the gross anatomy. Though wider than capillaries, when fully dilated, they are much too small to be seen with the naked eyes and cannot in any way imperil the circulation even when present in very large numbers. The blood passing through them will probably fail to give off the normal amount of oxygen and other substances which it is supposed to carry to the tissues, because it is not exposed to the thin walls and large surface of the capillaries, but for the dissipation of heat the surface available in vessels of less than 1/10 mm. diameter is ample.

It seems unnecessary to show this by an elaborate calculation of the rate at which heat can be given off from the surfaces of capillary tubes, when it is remembered that according to the calculation first made by Stewart (1895) 1 cubic millimeter of blood takes over 6 hours to pass a capillary of 10μ diameter when flowing at the high rate of 0.5 mm. per sec. For the equalization of the temperature of 1 mm.³ of blood with the surrounding tissue 1 second is probably more than

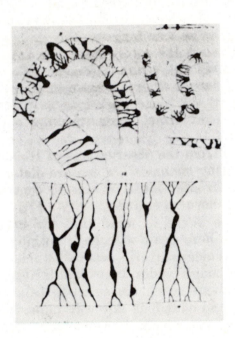

Fig. 38. Blood vessels of Nereis.
After Retzius.

sufficient, and this would be provided in a vessel of 100µ diameter, when the rate was 12 mm. per sec. That is why small arterio-venous anastomoses must be considered extremely efficient for keeping up the temperature of exposed parts, and I cannot doubt, considering the location of derivating channels described by Hoyer, that the main function of these vessels is to supply enough blood to projecting parts of warm-blooded animals to keep them warm when exposed to low temperatures.

It would probably be worth while to make a search for such anastomoses in the ears, feet, and snouts of arctic mammals and in the feet of certain birds. When the penguins brooding on the South Polar Continent at temperatures far below 0° keep their one egg raised upon their own feet, there must certainly be a rush of blood through the web of those feet, and the existence of large and numerous arterio-venous anastomoses would seem extremely likely.

IV
The Renaissance After Krogh

Editor's Comments on Papers 8 Through 14

The papers in Part IV are primarily concerned with new *in vivo* techniques for the microscopic study of minute vessels. In essence, four types of studies have evolved: (1) the tissue chamber technique, exemplified by the rabbit ear chamber designed by Sandison and Clark and Clark, (2) the *in situ* organ study, available because of Knisely's development of the quartz rod technique to visualize the borders of spleen, liver, and lungs, (3) the exteriorized tissue technique, the models being the rat cecal mesentery developed by Zweifach and the hamster cheek pouch developed by Lutz and Fulton, and (4) the transparent membrane technique, seen in the experimental model of Nicoll and Webb, who used the wing of the bat.

Each method has its special usefulness and each group has contributed new and useful information, although they are not always in agreement about what features constitute "typical" structures, nor are they in accord about anatomical design, nomenclature, or control mechanisms. Every current investigator, however, can find some support for his favorite concept or special interest. The accuracy of the descriptive material is never in question, and the anatomical and physiological significance of the material is still open to individual preference.

Eliot R. Clark and his wife wrote many splendid descriptive articles based on what they saw in the transparent chamber in the rabbit ear. This innovative technique, which was developed in their laboratory, proved to be a very efficient method for advancing the knowledge of capillary beds.

One topic of immediate interest in the Clarks' paper is their discussion of the contraction of blood vessels. They mention that:

> there seems to be no general knowledge among physiologists of the spontaneous rhythmic contraction of branch arteries and of the smaller arterioles, which the present method reveals as occurring normally and in most cases practically continuously in the vessels of the rabbit's ear and as playing an immensely important role in the regulation of blood flow.

It is with a sense of dismay that one realizes that this sponteous rhythmic contraction of arterial vessels is not, 40 years later, generally recognized, although autoregulation has become a favorite theme. The Clarks were aware that anesthesia could adversely affect spontaneous contractile activity and that, therefore, it was not prominently visible in every preparation.

This paper also suggests, although no definitive statements are made, that capillaries do not show contractile activity. It is obvious that the intent to disprove the function of the Rouget cell in capillary contractility is forthcoming.

J. C. Sandison, while a graduate student with the Clarks, designed and implemented the rabbit ear chamber.

The paper by Sandison is presented to conclude the controversy of the contractile activity of mammalian blood vessels. He states in the introduction that the major purpose of the study is to determine what elements of the minute vessels are responsible for the regulation of the flow through capillaries: capillary endothelium, Rouget cells, or smooth-muscle cells. The vessels under observation were new ones that had grown into the ear chamber, and he mentions that no nerves were seen.

Sandison makes it explicit that smooth-muscle cells, easily distinguished from the "adventitial" cells that lie along the arteriolar vessels, are alone responsible for diameter changes. Capillary diameter changes and flow, he thinks, are secondary to the arteriolar changes. Vascular contraction is described in great detail. Having observed the development of muscle cells on newly formed vessels, he notes that contraction of blood vessels occurs only in the areas where muscle cells have appeared.

He also discusses plasma skimming, platelet skimming, and the reaction of vessels to changes in temperature, to adrenalin, and to histamine, and uses such induced changes as further proof of the importance of smooth-muscle cells as the regulators of flow.

Melvin Knisely developed a technique that allowed microscopic observation of living tissues *in situ,* having solved the problem of transillumination by the use of a quartz rod that could be positioned beneath the organ to be studied.

The usefulness of the technique is demonstrated in this paper on circulation in the spleen, a controversial topic owing to artifacts that appeared in fixed tissue. There was, at that time, a continuing controversy over the means by which blood moved from the arterial to the venous side in the spleen. One group supported the theory that blood moved through completely endothelium-lined pathways from its entrance into the spleen to its exit in a closed circulation system. A second group proposed the theory of open circulation in which the arterioles or capillaries poured blood into the intercellular spaces of splenic pulp and the blood eventually found its way into the veins. Transillumination and microscopic observation of the living tissue should have settled the argument; instead, they served to initiate a flood of investigations. Knisely states that neither "open" nor "closed" are appropriate terms.

Knisely makes the important observation that there are "physiological sphincters" located along the arterial tree. He also describes contractile activity in venous sinuses and concludes that the distribution of blood in the spleen is controlled through the action of sphincters located at strategic positions on the vasculature.

Benjamin W. Zweifach introduced a new area for microscopic observation of blood vessels in a living mammal that was to become one of the most widely used techniques for a long period of time. It has been said that Zweifach made the rat cecal mesentery more important to physiologists than it ever was to the rat.

The Zweifach article presents the concept of the muscular capillary, or a–v bridge, thought by Zweifach to be the backbone of an anatomical unit characteristic of capillary beds; the a–v bridge concept was the forerunner of the preferential, or thoroughfare, channel concept. A number of new terms and definitions are introduced, and capillary diameter changes are discussed, and another minor controversy is in the making.

The presence of a thoroughfare channel was neither confirmed nor supported by other investigators using tissue other than the mesentery as a site for observation. The terminology appears occasionally in the current literature, but the idea was not accepted by the majority of *in vivo* microscopists. Nonetheless, Zweifach's work dominated the field for several decades and provided many useful and lasting contributions to the understanding of microcirculation.

Paper 12, again by the Clarks, is on observations of the growth of new blood vessels into a rabbit ear chamber. The detailed account of the formation, or regeneration, of a vascular bed with all its variables makes interesting reading. The influence that the rate of blood flow has on the characteristics of a newly formed vessel is surprising, as is the fact that vessels can change from arterial to venous or venous to arterial, depending on the demands placed on them in a specific anatomical location in a vascular network. The advent of spontaneous contractile activity is also described, as is the acquisition of tone in the new vessels.

Although Zweifach's paper dealing with the muscular capillary had already been published, the Clarks did not refer to the presence of any such structure in their developing vascular beds, although they do note their agreement with Zweifach's earlier papers on amphibian beds. The Clarks make quite clear the differences in behavior between the vessels of amphibia and those of mammals.

Two new techniques for *in vivo* microscopic observation of blood vessels appeared in the mid-1940s. Fulton and his coworkers at Boston University found the hamster cheek pouch to be well suited for a variety of studies on small blood vessels. The impressive list of investigations demonstrates both the imagination of the researchers and the adaptability and usefulness of the technique. The article reproduced here (Paper 13) is included because it contains a description of the technique, as well as an overview of the numerous areas of exploration that had been undertaken.

Paper 14, by Nicoll and Webb, contains a precise description of the architecture of the vasculature in the bat wing as well as a detailed description of spontaneous contractile activity in the arterial and venous vessels. The advantage of this preparation for studying normal behavior and responses to external influences is, of course, that the animal is not anesthetized. The information that the researchers gathered regarding control of blood flow into capillary networks is the forerunner of current beliefs.

8

Reprinted from *Am. J. Anat.*, **49**(3), 441–474, 476–477 (1932)

OBSERVATIONS ON LIVING PREFORMED BLOOD VESSELS AS SEEN IN A TRANSPARENT CHAMBER INSERTED INTO THE RABBIT'S EAR [1]

ELIOT R. CLARK AND ELEANOR LINTON CLARK

Department of Anatomy, University of Pennsylvania, Philadelphia, Pennsylvania

SEVENTEEN TEXT FIGURES AND TWO PLATES (EIGHT FIGURES)

INTRODUCTION—METHOD

By the method of inserting transparent chambers into the rabbit's ear, it has been possible to carry out long-continued studies of blood vessels, as well as of other cells and tissues, with high microscopic magnifications, for the first time in the living mammal. The original chamber, worked out by Sandison ('28) in this laboratory, was designed for the purpose of obtaining records in the living mammal of the growth and reactive powers of vessels and other tissues, similar to those made in the transparent tail fin of Amphibia (Clark, '09, '18). Sandison ('28) has published accounts of the growth and reactions of blood vessels in such a transparent chamber. In developing the technique further and adapting it to the many types of morphological and physiological problems which can best be attacked by this method of study in the living animal, the question arose as to whether newly growing blood vessels and those which had recently grown into such transparent chambers were comparable in their morphological character-

---

[1] A preliminary account of living preformed blood vessels as seen in this type of transparent chamber in the rabbit's ear, including observations on the contractions of arteries and of arteriovenous anastomoses, was presented at the meeting of the American Association of Anatomists, held at the University of Virginia in April, 1930, and the living vessels present in such 'preformed-tissue' chambers were demonstrated at the same meeting as well as at the International Anatomical Congress at Amsterdam in August, 1930 (Clark and Clark, '30).

441

istics and in their reactions to normal preformed vessels. In order to determine this point as to the resemblance of newly formed and growing vessels to those already present in the ear, and, in addition, to obtain a transparent region for physiological studies in which normal vessels with their original nerve supply were known to be present, the 'preformed-tissue' chamber was designed.

The details of the construction and the operation for the insertion of the standard chamber of this type have been described recently (Clark, Kirby-Smith, Rex, and Williams, '30). In brief, the method consists in the retention of the skin on the outer side of the ear with the vessels and tissues adherent to it, the removal of cartilage and skin on the inner side of the ear over an area about 1.5 cm. in diameter, and the substitution for it of a depressed ring with a thin mica cover, in immediate contact with the surface of the tissue, through which the observations are made. The remaining tissue is retained between two parts of the chamber which are constructed in such a way as to maintain a uniform pressure just sufficient to keep the area as thin as possible without impeding the circulation. The use of small bolts and nuts to hold the two sides of the chamber together and of small rubber washers to prevent excessive pressure makes possible accurate adjustment of the chamber to secure normal circulatory conditions. Albino rabbits are best for this type of chamber in which the skin of one side is retained.

In making observations in this type of chamber the most brilliant pictures are obtained with the use of a binocular dissecting microscope and transmitted light from a lamp such as the 'Point of light' or Delineascope, passed through a water filter containing copper sulphate or through blue-green heat-resisting glass. This method allows a precise study of a large area of the original arteries, veins, and capillaries of the ear, and of the circulatory phenomena involved, which can be carried on continuously for weeks or months under normal and experimental conditions in the living animal. The vessels, including the outline of their walls, stand out in beautiful detail, and the direction, volume, and speed of the blood flow may be seen with striking clearness. In cases where it is desirable to concentrate upon a single vessel or a few vessels the compound microscope is used. For studying the finest cytological details of vessel walls, a second operation has been performed, in which the outer skin is dissected away carefully under the binocular microscope and the chamber replaced.

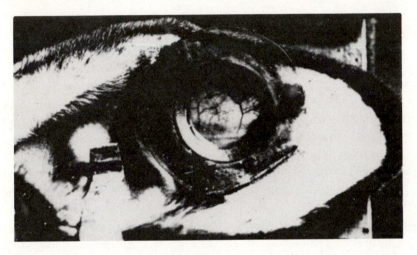

Fig. 1 Photograph of the ear of a rabbit in position for observation on the stage of the microscope, with a chamber of the 'preformed-tissue' type inserted in the ear. Natural size. (Reproduced from The Anatomical Record, November, 1930.)

During the past year over fifty of the 'preformed-tissue' chambers have been inserted. In all of them, the vessels were available for study immediately after the operation. In over twenty of the chambers long-continued observations of one month to six months were carried out.

From an intensive study of these chambers with the aid of frequent photographic records it has been found that the blood vessels of the operated area undergo a regular series of changes and reactions in their recovery from the operation and adaptation to the chamber, after which they become physiologically stable. These changes in the blood vessels of such an area have now been studied and recorded in a sufficient number of cases to make it possible to determine the time at which a given chamber is available for physiological experiment with a reasonable assurance that the vessels and tissues are normal.

GENERAL REACTIONS—RECOVERY FROM OPERATION

Immediately after the operation, the rabbit is removed from the operating room and the chamber examined under the binocular microscope. The field is then pale—except for small patches of extravasated blood which are frequently present. The main artery of the ear and its branches are narrowed down—the circulation through them is slow and frequently stops altogether. The veins are pale and there is little or no blood flowing through the capillaries. After several minutes to an hour, the arteries relax somewhat, the movement of blood through them becomes faster, but very little blood enters the capillary plexus of the skin.

Twenty-four hours after the operation, the circulation becomes more rapid, although the arteries still remain relatively narrow, the veins become distended, and a large amount of blood rushes through direct communications from artery to vein, while the arterioles supplying the capillaries of the skin remain tightly contracted so that no blood passes through the capillaries. These arteriovenous anastomoses are invariably present in the preformed tissue of the chamber area, and some of them are always visible and show an active flow of blood immediately after the operation. Although the presence of such direct connections had been described by anatomists, notably Hoyer ('77) and Grosser ('02) from the study of sectioned and of injected specimens, the large numbers regularly present in a region such as the rabbit's ear (forty to fifty in the area of the 1.5-cm.-in-diameter chamber) and their undoubted physiological importance have not been generally recognized.[2] A number of studies have been made

[2] Since the completion of these studies a recent article of Grant ('30) on arteriovenous anastomoses in the rabbit's ear has come to our attention. Grant

upon living arteriovenous anastomoses in preformed chambers, studying the same ones by daily observation over a period of weeks under normal and experimental conditions, and upon their formation (which has been observed in the other types of chamber containing new growing vessels), and these will be reported separately.

After the stage of enlarged veins and relatively narrow arteries, a period of one to several days follows in which the arteries and arterioles of the chamber dilate and remain distinctly wider than the veins and in which there is a gradually increasing flow of blood through the smaller vessels, which are now conspicuous even with low magnifications (fig. 20). Coincident with this widening of the arteries and increased flow through the capillary plexus the arteriovenous anastomoses become relatively smaller, i.e., they show frequent active contractions and often remain narrow for long periods. During this time the extravasated blood is gradually absorbed and the whole chamber becomes clearer (fig. 21).

During the next few days the arteries and arterioles again become relatively narrow and show frequent active spontaneous rhythmic contractions, and at the end of seven to twelve days the chamber reaches what may be termed a stable condition. From this time on, photographs taken at weekly intervals show relatively little change in the pattern and caliber of the larger vessels (figs. 22 to 24).

The time at which any given chamber attains the stable condition varies considerably and appears to be dependent largely upon the amount of trauma sustained at the time of operation. In a chamber inserted recently in which the entire operation was performed under the binocular loupe,

confirmed the observations of the earlier investigators on the richness of muscle and nerve supply of these direct connections between artery and vein and of the large number of them present in the rabbit's ear. By using thin ears of albino rabbits and bright transillumination, he was able to identify a few of the arteriovenous anastomoses in the living animal by means of the regions of pulsation in the vein with which they communicated. Grant has carried out some interesting experiments on the reactions of arteriovenous anastomoses with and without their sympathetic nerve supply which we will discuss later in connection with our studies.

with practically no haemorrhage or other objective sign of injury to the tissues which were left, recovery of the chamber area took place much more rapidly than usual. Fairly rapid circulation through the larger vessels was observed in the first half-hour following the operation, circulation through the smaller vessels returned fully twenty-four hours earlier than was the case in any other chamber of the series, frequent active periodic contractions of many of the arteries were seen on the fourth day, and the chamber area attained stability on the sixth day after the operation.

These studies established definitely the possibility of making microscopic studies on preformed vessels in the living mammal under comparatively normal physiological conditions and showed that a week to ten days after the operation the region contained in the typical observation chamber has reached a stable condition in which the same vessels are available for study and experimentation over a period of months.

Although the vessels of the chamber always became stable in their appearance and reactions in the manner just described, a general slow shifting of the tissue in relation to the chamber was observed in specimens kept over a period of months. The chamber tends to move gradually toward the tip of the ear, so that vessels located on the proximal side of the chamber may be lost to view, while other vessels may appear at the opposite side of the observation area. This shows in figures 21 to 25, where the arterial arch present in the center of the chamber at the time of operation is seen to be located well toward the left after the passage of a month's time. A method has been devised recently for preventing this shifting in cases in which it is necessary to preserve all the vessels of a large area over a long period.

CONTRACTION OF BLOOD VESSELS

The most striking phenomenon noticed in the study of the preformed chambers is the contraction of the arteries and arterioles. Two varieties of contraction were observed: first, spontaneous rhythmic contractions, which occur normally about one to three times a minute when the rabbit is quiet but not sleeping, and the tempo of which varies for each vessel and even for parts of the same vessel; and, secondly, contraction in response to artificial stimulation which occurs simultaneously in all the arteries and arterioles of the region.

The rhythmic contraction of the main artery of the ear is of course a well-known phenomenon, since it is so marked as to be visible (at least as evidenced by blanching followed by reddening) through the unoperated skin, and there are references to it in the literature (Feldberg, '26; Kuntz, '30). However, there seems to be no general knowledge among physiologists of the spontaneous rhythmic contraction of branch arteries and of the smaller arterioles, which the present method reveals as occurring normally and in most cases practically continuously in the vessels of the rabbit's ear and as playing an immensely important rôle in the regulation of blood flow. This is, of course, not surprising, in view of the fact that a sufficiently transparent region has not been hitherto available in the mammal in which long-continued microscopic observation of the same vessels in the living animal could be made under normal conditions.[3]

With the recovery of equilibrium, a week to ten days after the operation, typical spontaneous contraction may be studied. The contractions were found to be conspicuous and surprisingly varied. As the main artery of the ear contracts the amount of blood flowing through the whole area is diminished, while, when it relaxes, the area becomes noticeably redder. However, the distribution of the blood to all parts of the chamber is not equal, for the different arterial branches and even parts of the same branch may be undergoing con-

---

[3] Grant ('30) has recently published the results of his interesting experiments on the reaction of the arteries of the rabbit's ear to local mechanical stimuli and to drugs such as adrenalin and histamine. The contraction and dilatation of arteries which he could see through the skin all appear to belong to the second category, i.e., response to stimulation, as he makes no mention of the spontaneous rhythmic contractions. Very probably the anaesthetic which Grant used may have interfered with the normal periodic contractions. See footnote 4, p. 450.

tractions each at a different tempo and quite independently
of the contraction of the main artery as well as of each other.
An artery or arteriole may constrict tightly and shut off all
blood to the capillaries which it supplies, while at the same
time a neighboring vessel—often another branch from the
same artery—remains distended and permits the passage of
a rapid and full amount of blood. Again, the artery or
arteriole may contract partially and allow a rapid flow with
diminished volume to reach the capillaries which it feeds. At
times contraction waves proceed peripherally from the main
artery, but in general the initiation of contraction is irregular
as regards individual vessels and portions of them. We have
frequently made simultaneous records of two arteries of the
same size and also of the main artery and one of its branches,
and again of a large branch artery and one of its smaller
branches, and found that although the number of contractions
per minute might or might not average the same, the initiation of contraction rarely occurred simultaneously in the two
vessels under observation. Our records show in many cases
a tendency toward more frequent contraction of the smaller
arteries than of the larger branches or of the main artery.
For example, in one animal we made observations on the
main artery, a large branch, and a smaller secondary branch
on three different days and found the contraction rate to
average 3 per minute for the main artery, $3\frac{1}{2}$ for the large
branch, and 5 for the smaller branch on one day, 2, 2, and
$2\frac{1}{2}$ and 2, 2, and 3 on the two later days.

At the same time that the arteries, their branches, and the
arterioles supplying the capillaries are undergoing spontaneous contractions at different rhythms, the arteriovenous
anastomoses are contracting actively. In fact, these direct
communications from artery to vein are the most actively
contractile of all the portions of the vascular system in this
region. Following the preliminary period after the operation, when the arterioles remain constricted for hours and the
arteriovenous anastomoses wide open, the latter often contract very vigorously and at frequent intervals. When the

arteriovenous anastomoses relax, they permit the passage of a relatively great volume of blood into the vein.

The rhythmic contractions of individual arteries and parts of arteries, together with the very active contraction of the arteriovenous anastomoses, not only cause great changes in the distribution of blood to different capillary areas, but also cause continuous alteration in the direction of flow in many of the large veins as well as in all the smaller vessels. Frequently the blood in a vein may be seen to flow steadily for a minute or more in a given direction; then, following the contraction or relaxation of one of the arteries or with the contraction or relaxation of an arteriovenous anastomosis, the flow oscillates and then reverses for another period, after which this is repeated. The irregular contractions of individual arteries and parts of arteries can be seen in these chambers to cause a temporary shutting off of the blood from different networks of small vessels. This results in the intermittent paling of localized areas, which observers of the intact ear have interpreted as being due to contraction of capillaries (p. 452).

Although almost all of the rabbits tended to lie quietly on the especially constructed animal board in use in this laboratory, with no real struggling unless disturbed or startled, they often showed intervals of slight restlessness, as evidenced by small jerks and chewing movements, while at other times they actually seemed to go to sleep, judging from the closed eyes and slower respiration. We found that the periodicity of arterial contraction was altered by changes in relative drowsiness and wakefulness. For example, we have observed a periodicity of two to two and one-half contractions per minute in a given vessel change to three or four when the rabbit became more wakeful, while later, on the same day, it dropped to one contraction per minute when the rabbit became sleepy. In the sleepy animals, with an average of one contraction or less per minute, the duration of the dilatation period was increased, while in the more wakeful animals the contraction time was lengthened. But although relatively

wide arteries are characteristic of the drowsy state, the rate
of blood flow is very slow, so that the total amount of blood
passing through the whole chamber is obviously less than in
the wakeful state, for in the latter, although contractions are
more active, the blood flow during the periods of dilatation
is extremely rapid—the differences in the two conditions
being probably due to differences in the strength of the heart
beat. We have made several observations on rabbits which
apparently fell into deep sleep and in such cases the main
arteries and all of their branches remained wide and several
minutes passed with no perceptible contraction. During this
time the speed and volume of blood flow diminished. On the
other hand, we have observed in rabbits which passed from
a stage of quiet wakefulness to a state of definite irritability
that the periodicity again disappeared and the vessels remained narrow for periods of several minutes. In this latter
case the character of the contraction corresponds more nearly
to the second type—the response to stimulation.

We have observed that these spontaneous rhythmic contractions, so characteristic of arteries which have reached a
state of equilibrium (a week to ten or twelve days after the
operation), are seriously interfered with and even temporarily abolished by the local anaesthetic (cocaine) and the
shock and injury attendant upon the operation.[4] As stated
(p. 444), every chamber in the arteries all became very narrow for several minutes to an hour after the insertion of the
chamber and showed a tendency to remain narrow for a number of hours thereafter. When the vessels of a newly inserted
preformed-tissue chamber were watched continuously for several hours after the operation, and records kept, it was found
that at about the end of one hour the main artery and the
larger branches relaxed rather suddenly, allowing active circulation to start, and that, following this, periods of narrow-

[4] We have as yet made no systematic observations on the effect of anaesthetics
on the rhythmic contractions. Mrs. Wilson and Dr. R. G. Williams, who have used
sodium amytal as a general anaesthetic in several rabbits with chambers in the
ear, have noted that these spontaneous contractions ceased during the anaesthesia,
as was the case in natural sleep.

ing alternated with periods of widening. During the first twenty-four hours such spontaneous contractions were infrequent, averaging less than one in five minutes, in contrast to one to three per minute seen in the same vessels a week later. At this period the duration of the contraction phase was greater than that of the relaxation, averaging four minutes for contraction in contrast to one and one-half minutes for dilatation. On the first few days following the operation, in one chamber watched continuously, it was found that the periodic contraction of the main artery and large branch arteries averaged about one contraction or less per minute. In contrast to the longer duration of the contraction in the period immediately after the operation, the duration of each contraction in the main artery now, i.e., on the fourth day, averaged only 4.5 seconds and the period of dilatation, 50 seconds. In the same chamber records of the same portion of the main artery showed rhythms of $3\frac{1}{2}$, 3, 2, $2\frac{1}{2}$, 2, and 2 contractions per minute on the tenth, twelfth, thirteenth, seventeenth, eighteenth, and nineteenth days, respectively, after operation, while the duration of contraction in this stable phase then averaged 10 seconds and that of dilatation, 15 to 20 seconds.

Frequently some of the vessels of the chamber recover their typical periodic contraction before others. For example, in one chamber studied on the fourth day after the operation, there were periods in which the main artery remained wide for five to eight minutes with no contraction, while during the same period a branch artery continued to contract at the rate of two to three times per minute.

The contraction in response to stimulation, in contrast to the spontaneous rhythmic contraction, involves *all* the arteries from the main artery down to the smallest arteriole either simultaneously or in a peristaltic wave starting at the main artery and spreading out to its branches, and is so marked as to cause a distinct paling of the whole ear. After the contraction a period of maximum distention intervenes in which all the arteries relax and blood reaches the whole capil-

THE AMERICAN JOURNAL OF ANATOMY, VOL. 49, NO. 3

lary plexus. The paling and flushing are so marked as to be evident to the naked eye and to be visible in intact ears (Krogh, '22). Feldberg ('26) has used this phenomenon in a physiological study of the nerves of the ear. Observers (such as Krogh and Rehberg) have interpreted the paling and flushing as evidence of capillary as well as arterial contractility. However, it is quite impossible to see the walls of even the larger vessels through the intact skin and all conclusions must be based on the distribution of the blood alone. In the transparent chambers the constriction and relaxation are obviously much more striking and the detailed reaction of all the different vessels can be studied (p. 470).

Such generalized contraction of the arteries may be caused by a number of different stimuli—mechanical, tactile, auditory, etc. It was found that rabbits differ greatly in temperament—some of them reacting violently with a jump, invariably accompanied by marked contraction of the arteries, at the slightest touch or at any sudden noise, while in other more phlegmatic animals a much stronger stimulus is necessary to elicit the same response.

The time interval before the constriction of arteries in response to stimuli and the subsequent relaxation is quite definite for any one animal. This fact has been used in the taking of photographs, where it is desirable to show the effect of constriction and relaxation, as in figures 2 and 3, and also where it was desirable to obtain comparable daily records of the maximum number of vessels present in a given field. In some of our earlier records we failed to secure complete photographs of all the vessels of the region, owing to the occurrence at the time of taking the picture of spontaneous contraction of different portions of the branch arteries, thereby shutting off the blood from many of the small vessels, which then failed to register. In all of our more recent records the camera is placed in position and the animal then stimulated by a touch, whereupon the arteries all contract and remain constricted for periods of ten to twenty seconds, after which they all dilate, allowing an increased flow of

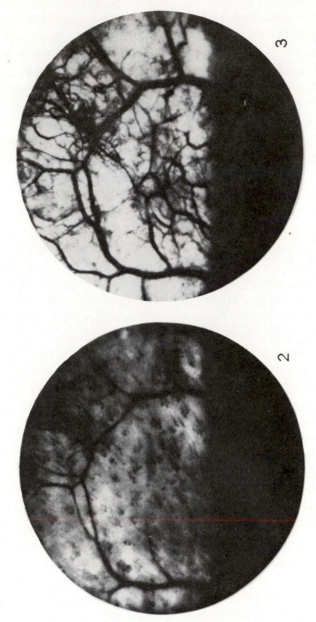

Figs. 2 and 3   Two photographs of the same chamber shown in figures 18 to 25, taken on the same day (twenty-three days after operation).   Shows reaction of vessels to stimulation.   × 6.5.

Fig. 2   (Contraction; picture taken a few seconds after pinching rabbit.

Fig. 3   Dilatation; picture of same chamber taken two minutes after contraction shown in figure 2.

blood through all the vessels of the region, including the capillaries, for a period of ten to twenty seconds or longer. During this period of maximum distention in which all the vessels are conspicuously filled with blood, the photograph is taken. The time interval is so constant for individual rabbits that in making daily photographic records the seconds following the stimulation until the time when the picture is snapped are counted with a stop-watch, after making preliminary counts to determine the reaction time of the arteries of the individual rabbit. Figures 2 and 3, which are two photographs taken two minutes apart on the same day, illustrate the contrast in the vessels of a chamber in the two phases, i.e., marked contraction followed by maximum dilatation after artificial stimulation. Higher-power studies show that even this extreme fading out does not necessarily mean contraction of the smallest vessels (p. 470).

Dr. R. G. Williams is making a comprehensive study of the nerves of the rabbit's ear, including the nerves on the blood vessels of preformed-tissue chambers as well as the regenerating nerves of the new-growth chambers, with correlated observations on contraction of vessels. Dr. Helene C. Wilson also is engaged in a study of the contraction of vessels in response to drugs, such as adrenalin and vasopressin, in such preformed-tissue chambers. Both of these lines of investigation will undoubtedly throw more light on the nature of vessel contraction.

INJURED VESSELS

The operation for inserting the chambers, in spite of the extreme care with which it is carried out, necessarily involves some degree of injury. The haemorrhages at the time of operation are usually caused by the necessary severing of small vessels, two or three of which normally pierce the cartilage. Aside from this unavoidable injury and the reactions already described (pp. 444–446) to the shock of the operation and the adjustment to the new environment of the chamber, more severe injuries may occur in which only one or two vessels are involved. These injuries are of three main varieties: first, squeezing, in which the vessel is temporarily occluded, either in an empty or thrombosed condition; secondly, severing of the vessel; and thirdly, a form of injury in which the lumen and wall of the vessel show no visible change, but in which there is a localized interference with its tonicity and contractile power.

In the first type of injury in which circulation is interfered with by squeezing, the cause may be excess pressure of the walls of the chamber itself. In these cases the vessel concerned is usually empty. If the interference with flow has not lasted for too many days, recovery of the vessel may be instantaneous after release of pressure by loosening one or more nuts slightly. Where the squeezing of a vessel occurred at the time of operation, the vessel usually contains stagnant blood and frequently some extravasated blood is present in the tissue in its vicinity. In several cases of this kind, complete recovery of the vessel with normal circulation was observed to occur in a week's time.

We have records of two instances in which a complete break of an artery occurred and in which the process of healing was watched from day to day. In the first case, the two ends of the artery were joined by several small connections on the second and third days after the operation. On the fifth day there was only one connection and it showed a distinct bend. The bend grew straighter each day, until, on the tenth day following the operation, the artery was straight and smooth and showed no noticeable evidence of any former injury (figs. 4 to 7). In the other case of a severed artery, the joining of the two ends took place in the same manner and just as promptly as in the first instance, and at ten days after the operation this artery also was smooth and straight. However, there was a difference in contractility in this case which persisted for over a month. When this artery contracted, the part of the vessel at the location of the former break failed to contract. At times of partial and complete dilatation and of slight contraction, the artery showed no sign of injury after the first two days, but at times of a marked contraction the area mentioned stood out as a small sausage-shaped widening. After a month this portion of the artery gradually recovered normal contractility.

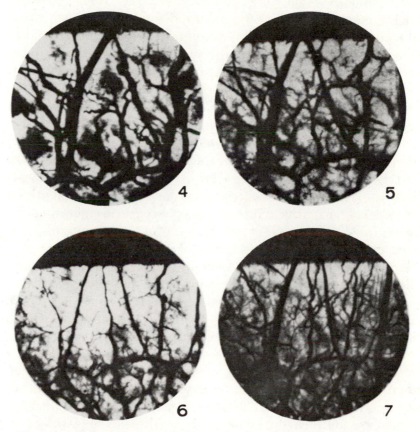

Figs. 4 to 7 Series of photographs of an area of the same chamber, in which one fork (right) of one of the arterioles was severed at time of operation. Showing healing and complete recovery. × 6.5.

Fig. 4 Six days after operation. Severed ends of artery joined (see text, p. 455). Right-angled bend in artery at point of healing.

Fig. 5 Eleven days after operation. Artery completely healed and smooth. Chamber stable.

Fig. 6 Eighteen days after operation. Both branches of the artery strongly contracted at time picture was taken. The right fork shows no sign of former injury.

Fig. 7 Thirty-one days after operation. Right fork (one formerly injured) contracted. Left fork dilated. (Spontaneous contraction.)

The third type of injury noticed in the study of the preformed-tissue chambers is the same as that noticed in the second instance of the healing of a severed artery in which the contractile power was temporarily lost. In about half of the chambers which were studied intensively for a month or longer, one or more arteries showed one or two such areas in which the contractile power was temporarily impaired. In these cases the vessels in question showed no objective signs of injury and their walls were smooth and intact. However, during the periods of arterial contraction, portions of certain arteries retained their wider caliber and thus gave to such vessels a beaded appearance (fig. 12).

In most of these cases, complete recovery was very slow, in spite of the lack of objective signs of injury to the vessel. In four chambers in which such injuries occurred the localized interference with contractility persisted for a month to six weeks. Figures 8 to 11 are photographs showing an artery at different intervals after the operation, in which a restricted area of the vessel was affected in the manner just described and illustrate the mode in which this type of injury still shows up during contraction of the vessel even twenty-seven days after the operation. Figures 12 and 13 show a similar area of injury present after the operation which in this case had disappeared at seventeen days.

In the case of a 'preformed-tissue' chamber inserted recently and still under observation, some interesting facts in regard to the recovery of an artery from injury of this third type were observed. At the time of operation a small portion of a nerve and near-by artery were slightly dislodged by the blunt dissector, although neither of them was severed. After the operation this portion of the artery formed an elongated sausage-like widening. At nine days most of the arteries of the chamber had become narrow and displayed the rhythmic contractions characteristic of the stable chamber, but the injured portion remained conspicuously wide and non-contractile. At eleven days after the operation, although the localized widening was still present, a narrowed portion had appeared in the middle of it. A day later, this narrow mid-portion covered a more extensive area, although none of this region of former injury showed any tendency to contract. At thirteen days after operation the whole region of the former

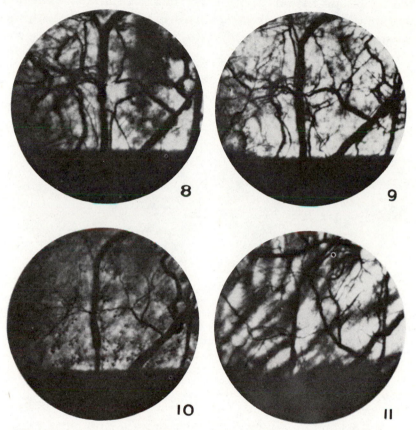

Figs. 8 to 11   Series of photographs of the same chamber, showing an artery injured at the time of operation. Impairment of contractile power which persisted for over a month. × 6.5.

Fig. 8   Six days after operation. Artery at center injured, but not severed.

Fig. 9   Eight days after operation. Chamber stable. Artery, dilated at time photograph was taken, shows greatest widening at site of injury.

Fig. 10   Eleven days after operation. Artery partially contracted. Sausage-like swelling at point of former injury.

Fig. 11   Twenty-seven days after operation. Artery strongly contracted. Swelling at point of former injury still shows, when remainder of artery is contracted, but is less than at eleven days.

widening had narrowed. For many days this portion maintained a fairly uniform, narrowed caliber—wider than the uninjured parts of the artery when they were contracted, and much narrower than the uninjured parts when they were dilated. Now, fifty days after the time of injury, the affected portion of the artery shows changes in caliber along with the periodic contractions and dilatations of the uninjured parts, but it still lags behind, both in time and in extent of narrow-

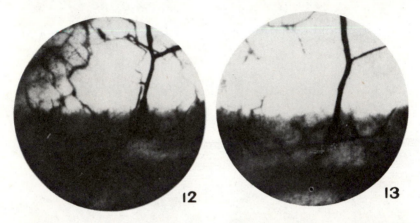

Figs. 12 and 13 Two photographs of the same artery, taken four days apart, showing sausage-like aneurysm at time of contraction in the first record—recovery in the second. In this case there were no signs of injury to this vessel, following the operation, except the localized impairment in the contractile power. × 6.5.

Fig. 12 Thirteen days after the operation. Chamber stable. Contracting artery shows two swellings.

Fig. 13 Seventeen days after operation. Same artery partially contracted—no sign of injury. Injured portions have developed tonicity.

ing and widening, giving the impression that its changes are secondary to the changes in pressure and blood flow regulated by the actively contracting arteries.

This observation has, we believe, given the probable key to some of the arterial phenomena which follow the operation. The great widening of arteries and of arteriovenous anastomoses is probably due to injury or exposure of nerves. The duration of the widening evidently depends upon the extent of such injury, and may be from two to twelve days. During this time there is apparently a loss of tonicity in all vessels near the exposed surface, which becomes excessive in those severely injured. Tonicity returns and the ability to perform definite active contractions and dilatations reappears from three days to two weeks in the case of mild injury or exposure. In more severe injuries tonicity returns between the eleventh and fourteenth days after the injury, and this tonicity may persist for weeks in the absence of a resumption of active contraction and dilatation.

It is quite remarkable that, when the recovered portions of the artery dilate, their caliber exceeds appreciably that of the injured portion which has developed tonicity. Is this apparently complete and rather sudden relaxation of the muscle due to special nerve stimulus, or to inhibition of constrictor nerve stimulus? We believe this type of preparation offers an opportunity to test this point.

REACTION TO INFECTION

In these preliminary observations on vessels in the preformed-tissue chambers, no studies have yet been carried out which involve the experimental production of inflammations or infections of various types, although such experiments have been planned. Up to the present our efforts have been directed toward obtaining the most normal conditions possible in the chambers, and obviously one of the most necessary elements contributing to such a result is the exclusion of all sources of inflammation. With the technique now employed infections of the area included in the chamber are so rare as to be negligible. However, among the fifty chambers of this type we have had a number of cases, particularly at a time when the technique was in a more experimental state, in which infections developed a week or longer after the operation, usually starting outside the chamber around one of the screw holes or under the edge of the protective collar, which, if neglected, gradually invaded the chamber from the periphery. Such abscesses in some instances spread over the surface and eventually destroyed the whole tissue of the chamber; in others they became walled off, while in some cases, chiefly in those in which drainage to the exterior was established, there was complete recovery. Cultures made from this type of infection showed them to be due to staphylococcus albus.

In general the reaction of the blood vessels to localized infection of this sort consists in the dilatation of the near-by arteries and arterioles accompanied by an increased flow of blood through all the vessels of the region and later in the persistent distention of the near-by arteries (figs. 15 and 16). If the abscess is of such a size as to cause pressure at the side of the chamber, the near-by arteries become tortuous. In many cases where the infection is outside the chamber distention without tortuosity results.

If the infection persists, new capillaries usually grow out and form a border of loops around the edge of the abscess.

The widening of the arteries near such an infection has many points of similarity to the reaction of such vessels toward heat. For example, we observed that the periodic contractions do not disappear as a rule, although the duration of the individual contractions is shorter and the interval of dilatation greater, and the arteries expand to a much wider caliber between the periodic constrictions than in normal chambers. The chief differences in the case of such infections are: 1) the localized character of the reaction (only those vessels of a comparatively restricted area near the small abscesses remaining dilated), and, 2) the persistence of the reaction (one group of vessels remaining dilated for days or weeks with little or no response to lowered temperature or stimulation of the whole animal, which cause the rest of the vessels in the chambers to constrict). In one chamber, however, in which a small abscess was present near the edge, a lessening of the periodic contractions of the neighboring artery was noted in addition to a lessening in their duration and extent. Records showed that the vessel situated near the abscess averaged one contraction per minute at the same time that the main artery and a corresponding branch artery

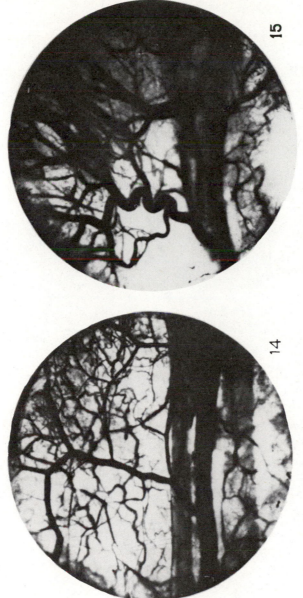

Figs. 14 to 17 Selected photographs from a series of records of the same chamber, showing reaction of vessels to an infection (a small abscess outside area of chamber) with recovery. × 6.5.

Fig. 14 Sixteen days after operation. Chamber stable.

Fig. 15 Forty-eight days after operation. Infection had been present for a few days in region outside the upper part of the chamber as shown in photograph. Enlarged arteries, especially those in 'upper' part of chamber nearest region of infection.

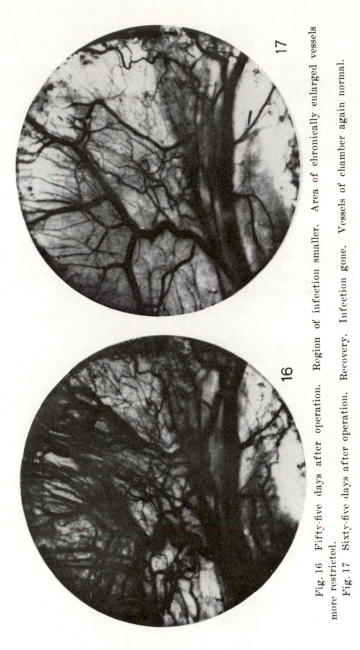

Fig. 16 Fifty-five days after operation. Region of infection smaller. Area of chronically enlarged vessels more restricted.
Fig. 17 Sixty-five days after operation. Recovery. Infection gone. Vessels of chamber again normal.

at the opposite side of the chamber were contracting two to three times per minute. This same vessel the day previously had shown no such difference in contraction rhythm. Two days later—at a time when the infection had diminished—the same artery, although still remaining wider than the other arteries of the chamber, averaged two contractions per minute, which was then the rhythm of contraction for the main artery.

In one instance it was possible to observe the first reactions of blood vessels to a beginning infection. This particular chamber had been under observation for three weeks and the pattern and reactions of the main blood vessels followed by daily observation, with frequent photographic records. The vessels had shown the usual series of responses to the insertion of the chamber described (p. 444) and had reached a stable condition at seven days after the operation. On the day of this observation the chamber became slightly loosened at one side, allowing the entrance of leucocytes and débris from a small unhealed abscess under the outside collar. An immediate response of the previously normal vessels in the chamber was noticed following the floating in of the material from outside. The main artery and its branches dilated at once, became tense, and pulsated violently, and a half-hour later the main arterial branches became very tortuous. An increased volume of blood entered the small arterioles and capillaries. The periodic contractions of the arteries continued and their frequency was not diminished, although the duration of individual contractions was shorter and the distention period longer than before the beginning of the inflammation. In general, this acute phase of the reaction to infection resembled very closely the reaction of vessels to increased heat. (Observations on the reaction of vessels to temperature changes will be reported separately.)

In the cases in which infections diminished and disappeared, recovery showed strikingly in the return of the blood vessels to their normal contour and caliber. Figures 14 to 17 illustrate such a typical reaction of blood vessels to infection.

They show the vessels of the chamber in the stable condition before the development of the abscess, which in this case was located near the chamber area but outside of it, and the subsequent changes in the vessels, in this case becoming chronic, coincident with the formation and persistence of the abscess, over a period of twenty days, and, finally, the return of the vessels to normal associated with the final clearing up of the abscess following treatment.

SMALLER VESSELS

As stated (p. 442), the type of chamber used in these experiments is best adapted for low-power study of a large circulation area, while cytological details of vessel walls can be seen to much better advantage in the new-growth chambers, the 'combination chamber,' or in the present type after a reoperation to remove the outer skin. Although the present observations have been concerned chiefly with the larger vessels and with the more general circulatory phenomena involved in a relatively extensive area, we have made a sufficient number of preliminary observations on the small vessels of the preformed tissue to be sure of two characteristics which it seems to us have not been sufficiently emphasized in physiological studies.

The first of these is the extreme *lability* of the vascular system, which is shown most strikingly in the great capacity for formation of new capillaries, in the tendency toward retraction and disappearance of others, and in the continuous alteration in caliber, form, length, and thickness of wall of individual small vessels.

The growth of vessels, accompanied by the processes of formation of new capillary sprouts, frequent anastomoses, and subsequent retraction of many of the capillaries, and by the alteration in form and size of vessels, was described by one of the authors (E. R. Clark, '18) for the transparent tail fins of living amphibian larvae, and Sandison ('28) has given an account of the new growth of blood vessels studied in the transparent chambers in the rabbit's ear in which similar phenomena were observed. A number of workers in this laboratory have been engaged in a study of the newly growing blood vessels in standardized chambers in which the size of the observation tables is uniform and the space into which new vessels grow can be regulated and retained or altered to any desired thickness and the details studied with highest magnifications over a large area. Here we find the process of new growth of mammalian blood vessels, as seen in the transparent chamber in the rabbit's ear, by formation of new capillary sprouts and loops, retraction of others, and the enlarging of certain vessels more favorably placed in relation to blood flow, the whole resulting in constant remodeling of the vessel pattern to be similar in all essential particulars to that observed in amphibian larvae (Clark et al., '31).

In the study of the vessels in 'preformed-tissue' chambers it has been possible to see clearly that similar changes to those described for Amphibia and for the rabbit in the other type of new-growth chambers are a matter of common occurrence in the case of the small vessels of the preformed tissue. Our observations show that although the same large arteries and veins, seen at the time of operation, continue to occupy the same relative position and retain approximately the same form for months, the smaller vessels are much more labile. Not only does the appearance of the capillary plexus change constantly, due to the alterations in the amount of blood entering it from the arteries, but, when a small region is watched with higher magnification, it can be seen that formation of new vessels and retraction of others are a matter of common occurrence. The slightest loosening of the nuts, resulting in a small increase in the space enclosed in the chamber, is the signal for the formation of numerous new capillaries. A whole new plexus may be formed in the space of two or three days. In fact, the new growth of vessels is so constant a mode of response to such relatively minute stimuli that it would seem quite impossible in most physiological studies of capillaries of adult mammals to be certain whether the individual vessels studied had been in existence for years, months, or only days, unless the same vessels had been watched in daily studies such as those made possible by the present method. Normal stimuli, such as those afforded by slight changes in diet or exercise or in external temperature or sunlight, not to mention small scratches, contusions, burns, and other minor insults to which the superficial tissues are constantly subjected, undoubtedly call forth growth responses on the part of mammalian capillaries with great frequency.

The other noticeable characteristic of the small vessels, in this instance one in which they appear to differ from those of Amphibia, is in the specialization of their contractile power. It has been well known since the time of Stricker ('79) that spontaneous contractions of the capillaries of Amphibia occur which are important in regulating the flow of blood. Krogh ('22) attributed the contraction of capillaries to the activity of the so-called 'Rouget' cells—longitudinally placed adventitial cells first described by Rouget ('73), and more recently studied by Vimtrup ('22), working in Krogh's laboratory. The present writers watched the formation of these cells on the outside of vessels from stellate connective-tissue cells, by continuous observation of individual cells in the transparent tails of living tadpoles, and showed that in capillaries of the tail fin of frog, salamander, and Hyla larvae they are not necessary for contraction, since the vascular endothelium itself, of early vessels on which these cells have not yet developed, contracts in the same manner as that of older capillaries, and that, following the development of adventitial (Rouget) cells on the wall, vessel contractions tend to be initiated more frequently *away* from these cells than in their neighborhood (Clark and Clark, '25). In the tadpole's tail there is no formation of smooth muscle cells on the capillaries or arterioles in the transparent fin expansions. In his studies of newly formed blood vessels in the transparent chambers in the rabbit's ear Sandison ('28, '29) found that, although active contractions of small vessels could be seen, they were confined to the arterioles—vessels with smooth muscle cells on their walls—while there was little if any

THE AMERICAN JOURNAL OF ANATOMY, VOL. 49, NO. 3

active contraction of true capillaries. His observations have been repeated during the past year by a number of workers in this laboratory in over sixty of the standardized new-growth 'round-table' chambers, which had been in the ear for varying periods of a few weeks up to fourteen months and longer.

In the case of the capillaries of 'preformed tissue' our studies are still incomplete. Careful, high-power observation is necessary in order to distinguish with absolute certainty the terminal arterioles from capillaries, since many of the small vessels with muscular walls are consistently narrower than true capillaries. Such cytological details are best seen in reoperated specimens either of the 'combination' type (devised for comparison of preformed and newly growing vessels in the same ear) or in specimens in which the outer skin has been removed, and an additional period of a week or more must then elapse before the vessels again become stable, while, as pointed out (p. 466), very slight disturbances are the signal for the formation of new capillaries. Hence, it is evident that the problem of determining the presence or absence of contractility of 'preformed' capillaries—by which is implied capillaries of the normal ear tissue in contrast to newly formed or regenerating capillaries of so-called 'scar tissue'—is by no means a simple one.

However, in addition to numerous observations on the small vessels of typical preformed chambers, we have studied the small vessels of several reoperated chambers in which the outer skin had been dissected away so that the endothelial wall of the minutest vessels could be seen with the greatest clearness. In two such specimens the vessels were observed every day for several weeks, and for two or more weeks of this time it was clear that the larger vessels had attained a stable physiological condition as evidenced by the typical spontaneous rhythmic contraction of the arteries and arterio-venous anastomoses in the field of observation. In none of these cases were we able to see a sign of active contractility on the part of the true capillaries. Moreover, in some of the preformed chambers we were able to identify the same vessels—in this case a line of capillaries accompanying a large nerve trunk—and to be sure that the vessels watched were the same ones which had been present before the operation. In these cases also no evidence of independent capillary contractility was found. However, many more observations are necessary before this point can be considered as definitely settled.

At present, therefore, although it is impossible to state positively—as is the case in the new-growth chambers of different ages—that there is *no* active contraction of true capillaries of the preformed tissue, in the rabbit's ear, it is evident from repeated observations that if present, such capillary contraction (in contrast to the condition in amphibian larvae) is rare and quite negligible in its influence on the circulation. It appears from our studies and from those of Sandison that vascular contraction is more highly specialized in mammalian blood vessels than in those of Amphibia (where undoubted contractions of naked endothelium can be observed directly in the transparent tail fin), since it appears to be confined in the mammal, for the most part at least, to arteries and arterioles, while capillaries and venules possess tonicity and elasticity, but little if any active contractility. This conclusion is not necessarily in disagreement with the conclusions of Thomas Lewis ('27) from his interesting studies on the reaction of the human skin nor of those of Dale and Richards ('18), since in both cases the authors refer for the most part to active contraction of 'minute vessels,' and since according to our observations the terminal arterioles, which certainly display active independent contractility, are as small as true capillaries and frequently even narrower.

The methods of study with the aid of the transparent chambers afford the first satisfactory opportunity to differentiate *cytologically* between the smallest arterioles and true capillaries under normal conditions, in the living mammal. Previous observations on the so-called contraction of mammalian capillaries have been made largely on the shaved ears of rabbits and cats (Krogh) and upon the vessels at the base of the human nail (Hooker, Carrier, etc.). In such regions conclusions were necessarily based merely upon paling or flushing—although the recent improved method of Vonwiller ('27) permits the observation of the blood in the living vessels with higher magnifications than had been possible previously. Our observations made with high microscopic magnification, in which the *walls* of the vessels can be clearly seen, have shown us that paling and flushing, which indicate merely the absence or presence of erythrocytes inside the vessels of a region, give no indication as to the condition of the vessel lumen (whether open or closed) or as to the occurrence of active contraction or passive narrowing or flattening of a vessel which is temporarily deprived of its erythrocytic content.

In our studies on the preformed-tissue chambers, it can be seen clearly that the spontaneous paling of the whole observation area (such as illustrated in fig. 10) follows active contraction of all the arteries, while localized palings follow irregular localized contractions of individual arteries or parts of arteries (pp. 449, 452). High-power microscopic observations of thin areas in chambers of both varieties ('new growth' and 'preformed tissue') in which the endothelial walls can be seen, show clearly that, following the contraction of an artery, the small vessels supplied by it either continue to remain open with circulation of serum and blood platelets through them (the phenomena of 'plasma skimming,' described by Krogh) or, in cases in which the artery closes completely, they flatten out and the blood is squeezed through into the larger veins, in the manner described by Sandison. That such 'flattening out' is a pressure phenomenon due to sinking of the elastic cover-slip or skin, which is lifted at the time of active circulation, has been demonstrated conclusively by Sandison and by other workers in this department in the case of specially constructed chambers in which a small rigid 'box' has been made for the vessels to grow into and in which no lifting of the cover-slip was possible. In such cases, at the times of shutting off of blood flow, caused by contraction of the supplying artery, the small vessels did not flatten out, but remained round and unchanged in caliber, while the blood cells inside them remained stagnant or merely oscillated slightly and did not squeeze on into the veins.

These observations appear to account for the fading out of blood from a region of small vessels in most cases. As already stated, we have not yet observed a real instance of active contraction of a true capillary in any of the chambers studied so far. More extended observations on contractility of blood vessels are being carried on at the present time with correlated studies of the development of adventitial cells on their walls. Dr. R. G. Williams is engaged in a parallel study of the regeneration of nerves correlated with differences in the contractility of newly formed arteries and veins. It is expected that these studies will throw more light on the problem of vascular contractility in the mammal.

SUMMARY

In the 'preformed-tissue' chamber inserted in the rabbit's ear a thin transparent area is obtained in which is included a portion of the main artery of the ear and an area of the original tissue 1.5 cm. in diameter, including the preformed arteries, veins, and capillaries. The construction of the chamber and the operation for its insertion have been so standardized that uniform results are now obtained. This type of chamber is available for observation immediately following the operation, and the form and distribution of blood vessels and all of their circulatory changes in the observation area can be seen in beautiful detail and followed with frequent continuous records in the same living animal over a period of months. The 'preformed-tissue' chamber is especially valuable for observation and experiment in which it is important to be sure that vessels with intact nerve supply and normal surrounding tissue are present. Over fifty such preformed-tissue chambers have been inserted to date and a number of them studied in daily observations over a period of one to six months.

The larger blood vessels show a regular series of reactions to the operation and to the new environment presented by the presence of the chamber. After a week to ten days, they become stable, and from that time on they are available for daily observation in the living and for physiological experiment with the assurance that the vessels and surrounding tissue are normal.

Changes in the amount, rate, and direction of the blood flow through the vessels of chambers which have reached a state of equilibrium and changes in the caliber of such vessels can be seen in the living with marvelous distinctness and observed *directly* without resort to interpretation from indirect physiological methods or to the uncertainties involved in observations in which blanching and flushing are taken as criteria of contraction or distention.

Preliminary observations on the pattern and circulatory conditions in vessels of a stable area have been carried out and also upon the reaction of such vessels to different physiological states of the animal, such as sleep and excitation, as well as to localized injuries and to small local infections.

Three striking points have been observed in this study. The first of these is the normal occurrence of spontaneous rhythmic contractions of arteries, involving the main artery down to smaller and smaller branches. The different arteries and even parts of the same artery each contract at a different tempo. These periodic contractions of arteries and parts of arteries have a profound influence on the distribution of blood to different areas, and on the direction of flow in different vessels.

The second point is the normal presence of numerous arteriovenous anastomoses, which are very contractile, each with an individual rhythm, and which also have a great influence on the circulation.

The last point is the extreme lability of blood vessels, particularly of the smaller ones, as evidenced by the tendency to the formation of new capillaries and the retraction of others upon very slight alteration in the environment. This last point is best studied in the other type of chambers, designed for the study of growing vessels and tissues in a specially constructed thin space, but the present observations show that the same remodeling of the capillary network by the processes of formation of new capillary sprouts and anastomoses accompanied by retraction of some of the vessels already formed, together with the change from capillaries to arterioles or venules and the continuous alteration in size and form of individual vessels, are phenomena characteristic of the normal vascular system of adult mammals.

Our studies have added further confirmation to the observations of Sandison upon new-growing capillaries, that, contrary to the condition in the vascular system of amphibian larvae, active contractility of true capillaries (i.e., vessels composed of simple endothelium in contrast to small vessels with a layer of muscle cells on their walls), if present at all, is so slight as to be negligible as a factor in the control of circulation in the rabbit's ear.

BIBLIOGRAPHY

CARRIER, E. B. 1922 The reaction of the human skin capillaries to drugs and other stimuli. Am. Jour. Phys., vol. 61, no. 3, p. 528.

CLARK, E. R. 1909 Observations on living growing lymphatics in the tail of the frog larva. Anat. Rec., vol. 3, p. 183.

————— 1918 Studies on the growth of blood vessels in the tail of the frog larva by observation and experiment in the living animal. Am. Jour. Anat., vol. 23, p. 37.

CLARK, E. R. AND E. L. 1925 A. The development of adventitial (Rouget) cells on the blood capillaries of amphibian larvae. Am. Jour. Anat., vol. 35, no. 2, p. 239. B. The relation of Rouget cells to capillary contractility. Am. Jour. Anat., vol. 35, no. 2, p. 265.

————— 1930 a. Observations on living preformed blood vessels. b. Arteriovenous anastomoses. Proc. Amer. Assoc. Anat., Anat. Rec., vol. 45, p. 211.

CLARK, E. R., KIRBY-SMITH, H. T., REX, R. O., AND WILLIAMS, R. G. 1930 Recent modifications in the method of studying living cells and tissues in transparent chambers inserted in the rabbit's ear. Anat. Rec., vol. 47, no. 2, p. 187.

CLARK, E. R., HITSCHLER, W. J., KIRBY-SMITH, H. T., REX, R. O., AND SMITH, J. H. 1931 General observations on the ingrowth of new blood vessels into standardized chambers in the rabbit's ear, etc. Anat. Rec., vol. 50, no. 2, p. 129.

DALE, H. H., AND RICHARDS, A. N. 1918 The vasodilator action of histamine and of some other substances. Jour. Phys., vol. 52, p. 110.

FELDBERG, W. 1926 The peripheral innervation of the vessels of the external ear of the rabbit. Jour. Phys., vol. 61, p. 518.

GRANT, R. T. 1930 Observations on local arterial reactions in the rabbit's ear. Heart, vol. 15, no. 3, p. 257.

————— 1930 Observations on direct communications between arteries and veins in the rabbit's ear. Heart, vol. 15, no. 3, p. 281.

HOOKER, D. R. 1921 Functional activity of capillaries and venules. Phys. Rev., vol. 1, p. 112.

HOYER, H. 1877 Ueber unmittelhare Einmündung Kleinster Arterien in Gefassäste venösen Charakters. Arch. f. mikr. Anat., Bd. 13, S. 603.

KROGH, A. 1922 The anatomy and physiology of capillaries. Yale University Press.

KUNTZ, A. 1929 The autonomic nervous system. Lea & Febiger, Philadelphia.

LEWIS, THOMAS 1927 The blood vessels of the human skin and their responses. London.

ROUGET, C. 1873 Mémoire sur le développement, la structure et les propietés physiologiques des capillaires sanguins et lymphatiques. Arch. de Phys. norm. et path., T. 5, p. 603.

SANDISON, J. C. 1928 The transparent chamber of the rabbit's ear, etc. Am. Jour. Anat., vol. 41, no. 3, p. 447.

————— 1928 Observations on the growth of blood vessels as seen in the transparent chamber introduced into the rabbit's ear. Am. Jour. Anat., vol. 41, no. 3, p. 475.

————— 1928 Contractility of blood capillaries of the rabbit as seen in the transparent chamber of the ear. Proc. Phys. Soc. of Phila., Am. Jour. Med. Sci., vol. 3, 1927–1928, p. 21.

————— 1929 Observations on the contraction of blood vessels as seen in the transparent chamber introduced in the rabbit's ear. Proc. Amer. Assoc. Anat., Anat. Rec., vol. 42, p. 62.

STRICKER, S. 1879 Untersuchungen über die Contractilität der Capillaren. Sitz. d. Wienerakad. d. Wiss., Bd. 74, Abt. 3, S. 313.

VIMTRUP, B. 1922 Beiträge zur Anatomie der Blutcapillaren; über contractile Elemente in der Gefässwand der Blutcapillaren. Zeits. f. Anat. u. Entw., Bd. 65, S. 150.

VONWILLER, P. 1927 Beiträge zur Anatomie der lebender Blutkapillaren und des lebenden Blutes des Menschen. Sond. a. d. Schweiz. Med. Wochschr., Bd. 57, H. 46, S. 1093.

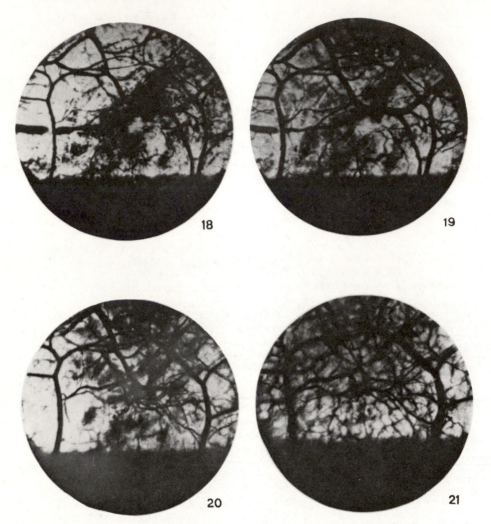

18 to 25 Selected photographs of the blood vessels of the same chamber from a series of records made at frequent intervals over a period of two months. × 5

18 Two days after operation. Extravasated blood still present. Arteries narrow.

19 Four days after operation. Arteries still narrow. Veins wide.

20 Six days after operation. Extravasated blood nearly gone. Arteries wide, veins narrow.

21 Ten days. Chamber almost stable. Arteries distended at time photograph was taken.

476

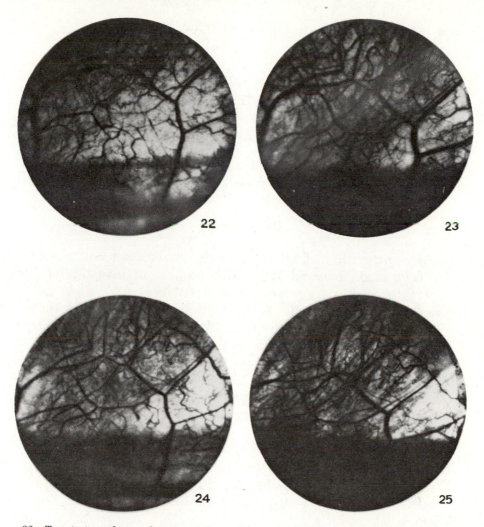

22   Twenty-two days after operation.   Right branch of arterial loop contracting spontaneously, left one moderately dilated at time of photograph.

23   Thirty-four days after operation.   Arteries moderately dilated at time photograph was taken.

24   Forty-four days after operation.   Main artery dilated (at bottom of chamber). Others moderately contracted.

25   Fifty-five days after operation.   Chamber area has shifted.   Right branch artery still shows.

477

Reprinted from *Anat. Rec.*, **54**(1), 105–127 (1932)

CONTRACTION OF BLOOD VESSELS AND OBSERVATIONS ON THE CIRCULATION IN THE TRANSPARENT CHAMBER IN THE RABBIT'S EAR

J. C. SANDISON

Laboratory of Anatomy, Medical School, University of Pennsylvania, Philadelphia, Pennsylvania

SEVEN FIGURES

The contractility of small blood vessels is a subject which has been studied in the living by a number of investigators during the past sixty years. Before Stricker ('65) saw the phenomenon of independent contraction of capillaries in the nictitating membrane of the frog, these vessels were thought to respond to circulatory changes in a passive manner only, the flow of blood through them being regulated entirely by the contraction and dilatation of vessels surrounded by muscle cells. Lister ('58) had noticed a dilatation of capillaries in inflammation. The further studies of Golubew ('69), Rouget ('73), Tarchanoff ('74), Roy and Brown ('79), Steinach and Kahn ('03), and many others, established the fact that capillaries are contractile as well as elastic. Most of these observers studied the capillaries of amphibians and obtained contractions by using mechanical, electrical, or chemical stimuli.

Renewed interest in capillary contractility has recently been aroused by the studies of Vimtrup ('23), working under Krogh ('22). Vimtrup made a careful study of the adventitial cells of capillaries which were first described by Rouget, and which he termed 'Rouget' cells. Using the transparent tails of living amblystoma larvae, he observed definite contraction of capillaries without any special stimulus, and

105

described it as being inaugurated by the contraction of Rouget cells. Parker ('23) and Federighi ('28) described, in certain invertebrates, the active contraction of endothelium of capillaries on which no adventitial cells could be seen. E. R. and E. L. Clark ('25), repeating Vimtrup's studies on larvae of Amblystoma and of Anurans, found active contraction of capillary endothelium, but failed to corroborate Vimtrup as regards the part played by the 'Rouget' cells, since they observed contraction of capillaries on which there were no 'Rouget' cells, and since, in capillaries on which sparsely distributed 'Rouget' cells were present, the inauguration of the contraction occurred much more often away from the 'Rouget' cells than in their immediate neighborhood. Moreover, they noted that the endothelium contracted away from the 'Rouget' cell, leaving a clear space between.

It is, then, clearly established that in Amphibia capillary endothelium possesses the property of active contractility, and that capillary contraction plays an important rôle in regulating blood flow.

For the mammal, until recently, nothing has been definitely known, in spite of a large number of studies by Hooker, Krogh, Rich, Hill, Florey and Carleton, and others. The reason for this uncertainty has been the unavailability of any region in a mammal in which the smallest blood vessels could be seen with sufficient clearness in the living under normal conditions. This need has been supplied by the artificial production of a tissue so thin and transparent that the individual cells of the walls of arteries, veins, and capillaries may be seen clearly with the highest microscopic lenses, and in which prolonged studies may be made of the same vessel similar to those carried out in the tail fins of amphibian larvae. The method developed in this laboratory, under the direction of Dr. Eliot R. Clark, consists of the introduction into a hole made in the ear of the rabbit of a thin, transparent, double-walled chamber with its sides open to the deeper tissues of the ear, and into which new blood vessels and connective tissue grow, forming a tissue which is permanent and which is essentially similar to the subcutaneous tissue of the ear (Sandison, '24, '28; Clark, Kirby-Smith, Rex, and Williams, '30). As described in a previous paper (Sandison, '28), the newly formed blood vessels undergo a complete differentiation into arteries, arterioles, capillaries, and veins. Recently (Clark et al., '31), a description has been given of the ingrowth and differentiation of blood vessels in sixty standard chambers under controlled and approximately uniform conditions, with a correlated study of the circulation, and the subsequent changes in the vascular pattern over a period of months (over a year in several cases).

The studies to be described here were made on chambers constructed entirely of kodaloid (Sandison, '28). The vessels were all new ones which had formed by ingrowth into the chamber from the subcutaneous vessels of the ear, and the observations were carried out largely on a chamber in which the vessels were from two to four and one-half months old. The major purpose of the study was to find out, if possible, just what elements of the minute vessels are responsible for the regulation of flow through the capillaries, whether the capillary endothelium is contractile, what part the adventitial or 'Rouget' cells may play, to what extent the flow is regulated by the smooth-muscle cells, and what other factors may be concerned with the capillary circulation. It should be mentioned that nerves were not seen in the present observations on the new vessels, and it was uncertain whether they were present or not. However, important as this question may be from many standpoints, it does not seriously affect the primary object of this study. A preliminary account of these observations was presented before the Physiological Society of Philadelphia, May, 1928.

OBSERVATIONS ON CONTRACTION

It was early noted that, in a well-developed plexus, there were frequent changes in the circulation; periods of active flow alternating with periods of marked slowing or even of actual stasis. Careful study showed that the circulation in any given plexus of vessels changes in an almost rhythmical manner.[1] On the average, about twice in each minute, the free, active flow of blood is interrupted by a slowing or stasis of a few seconds duration. Examination of the various parts of the system to discover the factors responsible for this periodic slowing brought out certain interesting facts. It became clear that it is the contraction and relaxation of the smooth-muscle cells of the arteries and arterioles which cause the changes in the circulation. The adventitial or 'Rouget' cells, which are present in abundance on the precapillaries, play no part whatsoever in the contraction, and the endothelium of the capillaries displays a power of contractility so slight that it is not a factor in the regulation of the blood flow.

The contraction sometimes appears first in the main artery of the ear, which narrows markedly, and may extend as a wave along the arteries and their branches and the arterioles until the last smooth-muscle cell is reached, three or four seconds being taken up in the passage of the wave from large artery to small arteriole. The narrowing in the different parts of the arteries may be partial or it may be sufficient to block completely the flow of blood. Contractions of the smooth-muscle cells around the arterioles do not occur simultaneously in all arterioles, and as a result of this alternating contraction, the blood may flow first in one and then in the opposite direction in the same vessel (fig. 1). The smooth-muscle cells on the larger arteries may remain contracted for long periods of time under certain conditions, while the mus-

---

[1] Clark and Clark ('32) have made observations on the living preformed blood vessels, using the 'preformed tissue' chamber (Clark et al., '30), in which the main artery of the ear is retained and a thin, transparent area about 1.5 cm. in diameter, including the preformed arteries, veins, and capillaries. They describe the normal occurrence of spontaneous rhythmic contractions of arteries, involving the main artery of the ear, down to smaller and smaller branches, and find that the different arteries and parts of the same artery each contract at a different tempo and that the periodic contractions have a profound influence on the distribution of blood to different areas and on the direction of flow in different vessels.

cle cells on the arterioles rarely remain contracted for more than a few seconds.

That it is the smooth-muscle cell which is almost exclusively responsible for the contraction of vessels comes out most strikingly from a study of the smaller arterioles and capillaries. In the arterioles the continuous sheet of smooth-muscle cells is succeeded by muscle cells in groups, and these in turn by pairs, and finally by isolated single cells. They can be readily seen, especially with the oil-immersion lens, as small round structures outside of and encircling the endothelium. They can be distinguished easily from the adventitial cells which lie longitudinally along the vessel, and which

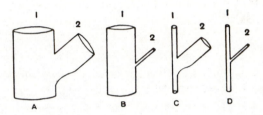

Fig. 1 Camera-lucida tracings, showing the size of the lumen of an artery (1) and its branch (2), in different phases of dilatation and contraction. A, both 1 and 2 dilated; B, 1 partially, 2 completely contracted; C, 1 completely, 2 partially contracted; D, both 1 and 2 completely contracted. × 310.

are larger in cross section. If such an area is watched it will be seen that the arterioles contract at the places where the smooth-muscle cells are present, and that the vessels beyond the last cell narrow only to a very slight extent, if at all.

It is most fascinating to watch the contraction of a single isolated smooth-muscle cell on an arteriole (fig. 2). When undergoing a contraction, it causes a rapid narrowing so that, in the course of two or three seconds, the lumen may be so constricted that no blood cell can pass. It remains contracted for three or four seconds and rather suddenly relaxes, the relaxation being immediately followed by a rush of blood through the vessel. It remains relaxed for periods of time varying from ten seconds to a minute, and then contracts again. The smooth-muscle cell does not always constrict the lumen completely, for it may contract only partially and narrow the lumen without obliterating it. The periods of relaxation are definitely longer after the partial contraction.

While these definite contractions are occurring in the smooth-muscle cells, which regulate the flow of blood, there are only such general changes in the capillaries as can clearly be explained on the basis of elasticity and of outside or inside pressure. Following the shutting off of the blood flow, there may be a slight general narrowing of the capillary, to be followed by a slight widening when active circulation is re-

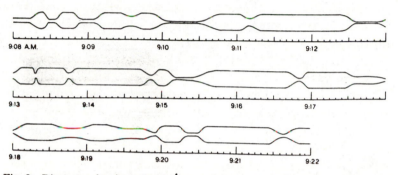

Fig. 2 Diagram showing the degree and rate of changes in caliber of an arteriole following contraction of a single muscle cell which almost completely surrounded the arteriole. The contraction periods of this cell occurred at the same time as did the rhythmical ones of the arteries within the whole chamber.

sumed. But these changes are obviously secondary to the contraction and relaxation of the smooth-muscle cell on the arteriole. At times there has been observed a complete emptying of an extensive capillary plexus, coincident with a reduction in blood flow, and occurring simultaneously with the contraction of the large supplying artery. This simulated capillary contraction, but was found to be due to the pressure exerted on the tissue by the thin, elastic celluloid cover of the chamber, for pressure over the area with a fine glass rod produced an identical picture. Evidently the widening of the arteries raises the cover slightly, permitting easy circulation through the capillaries, while the contraction of arteries allows the cover to spring back and compress the capillaries, particularly over the tables. This was further proved by constructing chambers in which the covering celluloid was cemented in places to the tables to make it rigid. In such chambers the capillaries did not show this peculiar type of emptying.

The circulation is markedly influenced by the development of muscle cells on the newly formed capillaries as they become transformed into arterioles. Changes in caliber were observed in the same vessels both before and after the appearance of muscle cells on their walls. It was found that before the development of these cells the narrowing of such vessels was always very slight, involved the whole vessel uniformly, and followed the rhythmic contraction of the main artery just described. After the appearance of muscle cells, however, the same vessels were seen to display localized narrowings, and such constrictions always occurred in the region of the newly developed smooth-muscle cells.

OBSERVATIONS ON THE CIRCULATION

The manner in which blood flows through vessels and the behavior of the blood cells in the normal blood stream were observed and described many years ago by numerous investigators and only a few new observations have been made on the circulation as studied in the rabbit's ear. However, since most of the previous work on this subject has been carried out on the mesentery of mammals where one is limited to short observation periods, it is of interest to restudy the problem in the transparent chamber, where the same blood vessels may be seen from day to day for months, and the circulatory changes in them observed during both their early formation and their subsequent adult growth.

The different rates of flow in various kinds of vessels at different stages of growth, together with the causes for these variations, have already been discussed and partly analyzed (Sandison, '28). One sees in the blood current in the rabbit's ear the well-known axial stream of cells, and the compara-

tively narrow, clear, plasma layer, or 'randzone,' which surrounds this rapidly moving central core. The throwing off
of the leukocytes into the peripheral layer and their slow
rolling motion along the vessel wall is also a phenomenon
which is readily seen.

In this study it has been observed that the presence of the
clear peripheral stream is dependent upon the rate of flow:
it is widest when the blood is flowing rapidly, and occurs
chiefly in the arteries and arterioles, except when these vessels are so constricted that the single blood cells are squeezed
in passing through. When the circulation slows down or
stops, during a period of contraction of the arteries, this
peripheral layer is absent in all vessels. At such times the
erythrocytes and leukocytes are no longer limited to the axial
stream, but wander at random; or they may settle to the
dependent part of the lumen, leaving only a clear layer of
plasma above. During a period of stasis, which may last for
several seconds or minutes, this sedimentation of blood cells
may be quite noticeable, particularly in the larger vessels.

Then, too, an uneven mixture of cells with plasma has been
observed during a period of sluggish or irregular flow of
blood through the capillaries—a condition which results in
part from an irregular contraction of first one arteriole and
then another. This independent contraction of arterioles
(i.e., one vessel closed at the same time another is open)
causes blood to be fed to the veins through the capillaries
and venules in the form of a broken stream. An uneven
mixture may also occur within an arteriole or an artery itself
as a result of contractions occurring at intervals along their
walls, leaving dilated portions of the vessel in which clumps
of cells collect (*Art. G,* fig. 5). When such contracted regions
again dilate and the circulation is resumed, the clumps of
cells pass on without mixing evenly again until they reach
the larger lumen of the venules. In this connection the work
of Landis ('26) is of interest. He has been able to measure
capillary pressures during capillary stasis in the frog's
mesentery and to watch the flow of plasma through the endo-

thelium as indicated by the passage of injected dye. He finds that wherever such a flow is present there is a considerable change in the proportion of blood cells and plasma within the lumen.

The phenomenon of 'plasma skimming,' a term introduced by Krogh ('22), and that of leukocyte skimming may be exhibited in various ways. The former is seen mainly in partially contracted vessels or in capillaries which are cross connections between the main path of the circulation and which, even though dilated, have no circulation on account of equal pressures at their two ends; it may be seen also in blind-ending, new-growing tips. Not infrequently vessels containing skimmed plasma, i.e., plasma without erythrocytes, are loaded with leukocytes which, along with the plasma, have been skimmed off from the main circulation. In fact, leukocyte skimming may be seen in practically any uncontracted vessel in which the circulation has temporarily ceased, but which remains connected with other circulating vessels.

The following observation on platelet skimming was also made: in a single, very narrow capillary loop, whose two ends were connected to a large circulating vessel, plasma flowed at all times, as was indicated by the passing of the smallest blood platelets. For many minutes only platelets would pass. It was interesting to note that with an increase of blood supply through the large vessel, erythrocytes would be forced through the narrow loop. With a very rapid rate in the larger vessel, accompanied supposedly by an increase in blood pressure, even the largest leukocytes were forced through the capillary, although its entrance was so constricted that the cells, in passing, were forced out into very long and narrow forms.

Plasma skimming is not confined to capillaries, since it has been seen in arterioles which are constricted almost completely at their proximal end and dilated along the remainder of their course, the dilated portion containing only a single blood cell here and there. Such plasma skimming in an arteriole is a rather complicated condition, and certain factors must be present for its occurrence. In the first place, the flow of blood through any arteriole is dependent upon: the degree of dilatation and the rate of blood flow in the artery which supplies it, the pressures in the capillary bed which the arteriole itself supplies, the size of its entrance, and the caliber of its entire lumen. Plasma alone will enter the arteriole when its entire lumen or merely the lumen at its entrance, is constricted to a size much smaller than the blood cells, and when the pressure of its arterial supply is not sufficient to force cells through the constricted opening. When, as indicated by the passage of platelets, plasma flows through a vessel under these conditions, an occasional cell may enter it, but if both the pressure in the capillary plexus beyond it and that at its entrance become equalized (a condition which may result from the passage of blood through another arteriole into the same plexus of capillaries) blood flow will cease in this vessel, the cells will be drawn off, and true plasma skimming will usually follow. Krogh ('22), in studying the frog's web and tongue, saw a washing away of the erythrocytes, when he stimulated a portion of a small artery branching from a larger vessel almost to the point of complete contraction. He stated that the current of blood through the small artery seemed to cease altogether, and that at the same time the erythrocytes were washed out from the corresponding capillaries. In the rabbit's ear one also sees that the cells are washed away from a capillary bed, following contraction of the arterioles or arteries, but there still may be a continuation of the flow of the plasma containing platelets only.

In regard to the capillaries, however, this same plasma skimming may occur as the result of another factor, i.e., the reversal of flow in an arteriole—a phenomenon which occasionally takes place during a short period of stasis in the artery. In this case, the blood cells are drained out of the capillary plexus in the absence of circulation. It will be noted, therefore, that two types of plasma skimming have been observed in the vessels of the rabbit's ear, one in which the vessels contain a circulating plasma and the other in which there is no circulation.

Venous and capillary pulsation have been seen in one plexus or another at all times during the new growth of vessels, particularly in vessels which are either short circuits between those which carry the main flow of blood, or blind-ending tubes. A very slight pulse is usually present in all young capillaries, but it is barely perceptible to the eye except when the rate of flow diminishes. In the older tissue, however, a well-defined capillary pulsation is extremely rare, except when the rate of flow is very rapid or very slow, and even then it is present in only a few vessels. One small plexus of blood vessels, containing a single pulsating capillary, was studied carefully in order to determine the cause of this pulsation. The plexus contained two capillaries which emptied close together into a very large vein, in which the flow was even and constant. When the circulation throughout the plexus became slow, one of these capillaries pulsated while the other did not. It was seen that these two capillaries were each supplied by a different arteriole, one of which supplied several other capillaries with blood, while the second arteriole had no other capillary branchings. In the latter arteriole the rate of flow was diminished, and it was in the capillary connected with it that the pulsation was observed. Blood cells were seen to enter the large vein from this capillary in an interrupted stream, a few cells with each beat of the heart. The flow through the entire vein was perfectly steady and it seemed probable that the pulsation in this particular case was present in the one capillary on account of the short connection between the arteriole and vein, and absent in the other on account of the greater number of capillaries which its arteriole supplied.

As for the venous pulse, it may be due to a transmission of the arterial pulse to the veins, or possibly to the contractions of the right auricle. It is difficult to explain the general pulsation which may occur in veins and capillaries when the circulation is extremely fast, as, for example, when the ear is heated to 38°C. or above. At such a time the arterial wall is distended slightly at each beat of the heart, the arterioles are distinctly narrowed, the capillaries and venules are slightly narrow, and the rate of blood flow in the large veins is almost equal to that in the artery.

While the circulation in a capillary bed is almost entirely regulated by the action of muscle cells on arterial vessels supplying it, it has been found that the flow may be diminished or even stopped by a single leukocyte plugging a narrow vessel. This occurs frequently, but is of minor importance, since it is always temporary. One of the most favorable places for such plugging is at the origin of the small arterioles

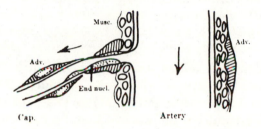

Fig. 3　Camera lucida drawing of a precapillary branch of an artery. The artery has a double layer of muscle cells (*Musc.*); the entrance to the precapillary is almost obliterated by the bulging endothelial nucleus (*End.Nucl.*). Adventitial cell (*Adv.*); capillary (*Cap.*).　× 412.

from their arteries. Normally, this region is constricted partly on account of the bulging of endothelial cells into the lumen. Such a bulging in a capillary is shown in figure 3. At times the constriction is too great to permit the passage of the leukocytes, though the more elastic erythrocytes may pass quite readily. Unless the force of the blood stream (always variable) is sufficient to push the obstructing cell onward, the latter may stop the circulation in the capillaries fed by the arteriole for varying lengths of time—sometimes for several minutes. One such arteriole was watched and the following was observed: With a rapid rate of flow, a condition which was always caused by a dilatation of the artery, both the erythrocytes and the leukocytes were forced through the narrow lumen in the form of an unbroken stream, even though they were enormously distorted in passing. With a moderate rate of flow the erythrocytes passed through easily, though again distorted, but the leukocytes went through the constriction in a jerking manner, apparently due to the effect of the systolic waves upon them, and each one plugged the vessel for a certain length of time. Occasionally the leukocytes' own ameboid activity would assist their passage. The time required for the passage of a leukocyte through such a constriction depended upon the activity (blood pressure) of the general circulation, being greater with a feeble blood stream. At periods of a steady, rapid rate of flow, the number of leukocytes which passed through this arteriole was an average of forty per minute.

REACTION OF BLOOD VESSELS TO TEMPERATURE CHANGES

In addition to the factors just described, which change the rate of flow and the amount of blood distributed through the vascular system, one other phenomenon has been studied in this connection, namely, the reaction of vessels to temperature changes (figs. 4 and 5). The higher temperatures were produced by an ordinary 60-watt electric-light bulb, the degree of heat being regulated by the distance of the bulb from the ear. The temperature was measured by placing a thermometer a few millimeters above that part of the ear which received the greatest amount of heat. The vessels were studied at three different temperatures: 37°C., 26° to 32°C., and 20°C. (produced by placing sponges dipped in ice water directly on the surface of the chamber).

While the heat was being applied, the circulation gradually became more regular and faster, until, by the time the maximum of 37° was reached, it was quite regular in rate of flow and the speed was exceedingly rapid, being almost as fast in the veins as in the arteries. In addition to the rapidity of flow, a general pulsation of the vessels could be seen. The rhythmical contractions previously described now occurred only at very long intervals and lasted for a very brief period of time. After the light bulb was removed and as soon as the ear became accustomed once more to room temperature, the circulation continued as it did previous to the experiment. The sticking of leukocytes to the walls of capillaries and their emigration through the vessel walls, following heating of the ear to 37°C., has already been described (Sandison, '31).

When the ice packs were applied, the branches of the larger arteries contracted completely, and all circulation in the chamber stopped. Very occasionally the arteries would open slightly and permit a sluggish flow of blood, but this partial dilatation had very little effect upon the capillary circulation. The exact point on the arteries where this marked contraction ended varied in all of them, but it rarely extended to the arterioles, most of which were slightly dilated. When the ear was brought back to room temperature, the circulation again returned to its normal condition.

The specific reaction of the different types of vessels during these experiments may be followed in figures 4 and 5. Here it is seen that the main vessels concerned in the regulation of the blood flow are the artery and arteriole. At 20°C., the artery, by its contraction, is alone responsible for the stasis which develops, the arterioles are incompletely dilated in the region of their muscle cells, while all other vessels are wider than at any other temperature. The rhythmic contraction of the arteriole disappears. The small vessels at 32°C. are on the whole narrower than at 20°C., and the rhythmic contraction of the arterial vessels is more regular at this temperature. At 37°C., the capillaries, the arterioles, and the arteries are smaller than at any other temperature; the veins, though larger than at 32°C., are smaller than at 20°C.

Fig. 4 Camera-lucida drawings, showing changes in the caliber of all types of vessels with three different degrees of temperature. The insert at the upper right corner shows the parts of the plexus from which the segments of different vessels shown in figures 4 and 5 were taken. *A*, arteriole; (*H*, origin of arteriole *A*); *B*, a precapillary; *C*, a loop of the prepostcapillary; *D*, a venule; *Dil.*, greatest degree of dilatation; *Con.*, greatest degree of contraction; *No Con.*, no contraction; *a* and *a1*, same group of muscle cells; *b* and *b1*, the same adventitial cell. × 310.

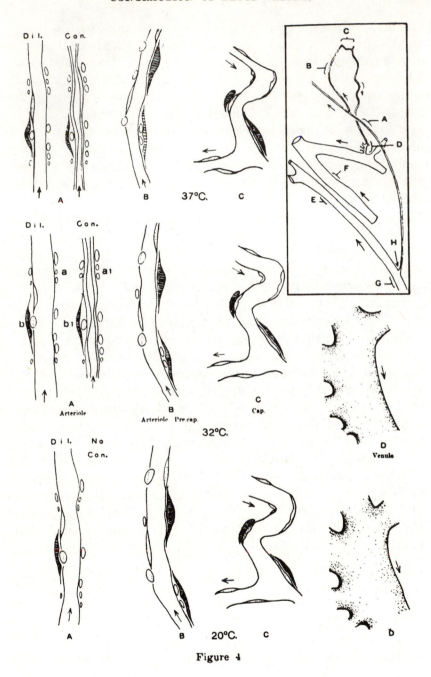

Figure 4

158

REACTION OF THE BLOOD VESSELS TO ADRENALINE AND HISTAMINE

For these experiments a preparation was used containing adrenaline, 9/20 grain; chloretone, 2¼ grains, and physiological salt solution, 1 fluid ounce. For intravenous injection a dilution of 1:100,000 was employed. Observations of the blood vessels in the transparent chamber were made during the injection of the drug into a vein of the opposite ear, and a region among these vessels was selected where an artery of a caliber of over 125 µ, with its arterioles, capillaries, venules, and veins could be watched. This artery had at least three layers of muscle cells around it. Before the injec-

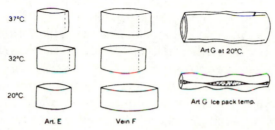

Fig. 5 Camera-lucida sketch, showing changes in caliber at different temperatures of three other vessels of the same plexus shown in the inset figure 4. *E*, an artery having two layers of muscle; *F*, a vein; *G*, the more proximal portion of the artery; *E*, point beyond which contraction did not occur at 20°. × 206.

tion was begun, the normal changes in caliber of this vessel and of its arteriole branchings were noted, and they conformed to the changes which have been previously described. At no time did this artery constrict more than one-half of its fully dilated caliber and the rhythm of its contraction was similar to that which has also been previously described for arteries in this chamber. Surrounding the wall of the proximal half of the visible portion of this large artery were numerous macrophages which contained a dark yellow-brown pigment. The vessel had slight local contractions here and there along its wall.

The injection needle was quickly thrust into the vein with one movement. Almost immediately the arterial vessels constricted slightly more than normal, and in a few seconds they dilated fully. This is the usual response to any disturbance to the animal. Then, after one minute, at the end of which time these vessels were still dilated, a slow injection of the adrenaline was begun. The large artery began constricting one and one-half minutes after 0.3 cc. of the 1:100,000 solution had entered the vein. Injection was then stopped. A few seconds later the large artery constricted to about 25 μ in caliber (one-sixth its dilated caliber) along its proximal half. The degree of constriction was less along the remainder of its course, being less marked the more peripherally one followed it. The normal, locally contracted regions were the points of greatest constriction in any one segment of the vessel. The lumen, even though greatly constricted by contraction of the muscle cells which were much thicker than normal, widened slightly with each beat of the heart.

The arterioles were greatly constricted along most of their course, but they showed only a partial contraction near their capillary terminations, even though they were surrounded in that region by a single layer of muscle cells (fig. 6). They were most constricted at the point where they took origin from the large artery—a point where they are normally narrower (fig. 3). The venules also narrowed, but to a slight extent only. The capillaries were apparently unaffected, except for the usual very slight changes which normally accompany changes in blood pressure, i.e., a slight dilatation with decreased rate of blood flow. The flow of blood in the capillary bed varied in different capillaries from a complete stop to a moderate rate, depending upon their proximity to an arteriole. In most of the main pathways which lie between the arteriole and the venule a slow circulation prevailed.

One interesting observation during the contraction of the large artery was the effect upon the pigmented macrophages which surrounded a part of this vessel. They were apparently unchanged in regard to their position—a wide clear space between them and the muscle cells of the vessel wall being quite evident, whereas previous to the time of injection they had lain directly upon these muscle cells.

THE ANATOMICAL RECORD, VOL. 54, NO. 1

The constriction period in all vessels was not over two minutes, and one and two-thirds minutes after the injection was stopped the arterial vessels began to dilate; twenty seconds later, the dilatation was almost complete. At this moment a second injection was begun, the needle having been kept in place, and 1.2 cc. of the adrenaline solution was steadily emptied into the vein over a period of four minutes.

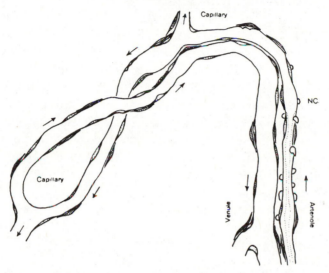

Fig. 6 Camera-lucida drawing, showing effect of an intravenous injection of adrenaline chloride (1:100,000). The arteriole contracts, while the capillaries and venules are unaffected. Dotted line indicates degree and limit of contraction. Endothelial nuclei dotted, adventitial cells cross-hatched, smooth-muscle clear ovals. N.C., no contraction beyond this point. × 316.

One and one-half minutes from the beginning of this second injection, after 0.3 cc. had again entered the circulation, there was a repetition of the change in caliber of the vessels similar to that noted after the first injection. At the end of two minutes, dilatation was not complete, but there was a considerable widening of the arterial vessels. The injection was continued, and one-half minute following this incomplete dilatation a constriction of the vessels again occurred, but to a much less degree than the one which just preceded it. The vessels remained in this state of partial constriction for one and one-half minutes after the injection, at which time they dilated and this dilatation, which was general, lasted at least one-half hour. The effect of this arterial dilatation on the capillary circulation was marked and brought about a great increase in the rate and amount of flow through all vessels with the establishment of circulation in capillaries which were previously open but non-circulating.

Under the action of a more dilute solution of adrenaline (0.3 cc. of 1 : 500,000) the capillaries gave the same response, but there was less of the primary slowing of the capillary circulation, partly on account of a lesser contraction of the arterial vessels. When 2 minims of 1 : 1000 solution were injected subcutaneously, the vessels responded as they did with the intravenous injection, except that the contraction of arteries and arterioles was prolonged for seven minutes or more, and the return of the normal rhythm of these vessels appeared much later. Local application gives such a picture as shown in figure 7.

The effect of histamine upon the blood vessels was also observed. The same method of study as that used with adrenaline was employed, except that only one dilution (1 : 100,000) was used, and only the intravenous route of injection was chosen. The action of 0.004 mg. of this drug resulted in dilatation of arterioles and arteries with almost complete stasis throughout the vessels of the chamber for over two hours. The greatest degree of dilatation occurred in the arterioles, since they widened to twice their usual diameter. The capillaries were unchanged in caliber, except for the usual slight dilatation following lack of flow through them, and all of the previously non-circulating, wide-open capillaries were filled almost to capacity with blood in stasis. The very narrow capillaries, which are the retracting or the new-growing vessels, were observed particularly for dilatation, but they also were unchanged. Frequent reversals of flow in all vessels were noticed. The next day, eighteen hours later, ½ cc. of adrenaline was administered subcutaneously in

the abdominal region, and all of the arterial vessels, which
had dilated with the injection of histamine, then contracted.

The results, therefore, of the action of these two drugs on
the vessels of the rabbit's ear show that the various responses
are chiefly confined to the vessels which are surrounded with
muscle cells. With dilute intraveous injections, adrenaline
causes a fleeting constriction of all arterial vessels in the

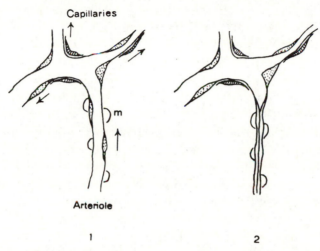

Fig. 7 Camera-lucida drawing, showing degree and limit of action of a local
injection of 1 : 1000 adrenaline chloride. *M*, muscle cell. *1*, preceding, and
2, following injection. × 310.

chamber with diminished capillary circulation, which action
is quickly followed by an arterial dilatation, accompanied by
a much more rapid capillary flow than that usually present in
the normal circulation. Histamine causes a still greater diminution of the capillary circulation, and dilatation of all the
peripheral arteries and arterioles with the strength of solution used. Neither drug acts, apparently, on naked
endothelium.

SUMMARY

Microscopic observations have been made on new blood vessels which have grown into a transparent chamber introduced into the rabbit's ear, and which have persisted for from two to four and one-half months, with the following results:

The local control of blood flow in this newly formed tissue appears to reside in the smooth-muscle cell on the arteriole. Adventitial ('Rouget') cells are present in large numbers, but do not appear to contract.

Capillaries proper, with or without perithelial ('Rouget') cells, have such a limited power of contractility that they seem to play no significant part in the control of circulation. While their caliber manifests changes, the changes seem to be passive rather than active, and brought about chiefly by changes in pressure both within and without, coupled with a certain degree of elasticity of endothelium. However, in the persistent absence of blood flow through a capillary it may gradually narrow until its lumen may permanently disappear —rather a retrogression in growth than contraction.

Nothing was seen which could be interpreted as active contraction of any of the veins or venules under observation.

Application of heat to the ear caused an extremely rapid flow of blood, the arteries, veins, and capillaries maintaining a uniform caliber. Cold applications caused persistent contraction of larger arteries with sluggish flow and slight widening of small arterioles, capillaries, and veins. With both heat and cold there was a marked degree of sticking of leukocytes to the walls of veins and venous capillaries, and, in the case of heat, extensive emigration of leukocytes through the endothelial wall.

Injection of adrenaline was followed by marked contraction of the arteries and arterioles at places where they were obviously provided with smooth-muscle cells, while capillaries and venules showed only slight, and apparently passive, changes in caliber. Contraction of arterioles was followed, after a few minutes, by a half-hour's dilatation.

Intravenous injection of histamine produced relaxation and widening of the small arteries and arterioles, coupled with diminution in blood flow. Capillaries and small veins showed no appreciable change in caliber.

Many of the interesting pictures to be seen in watching the circulation are described, most interesting of which are perhaps 'plasma skimming' (Krogh), platelet 'skimming,' and leukocyte 'skimming.'

Whether the new vessels under observation were supplied with nerves was not determined.

LITERATURE CITED

CLARK, ELIOT R. 1932 A new method for the microscopic study of cells and tissues in the living mammal. Int. Clinics, vol. 1, series 42, p. 301.

CLARK, ELIOT R., AND ELEANOR LINTON CLARK 1925 A. The development of adventitial (Rouget) cells on the blood capillaries of amphibian larvae. Am. J. Anat., vol. 35, no. 2. B. The relation of Rouget cells to capillary contractility. Am. J. Anat., vol. 35, no. 2, p. 239.

———— 1932 Observations on living preformed blood vessels as seen in a transparent chamber inserted into the rabbit's ear. Am. J. Anat., vol. 49, no. 3, p. 441.

CLARK, ELIOT R., H. T. KIRBY-SMITH, R. O. REX, AND R. G. WILLIAMS 1930. Recent modifications in the method of studying living cells and tissues in transparent chambers inserted in the rabbit's ear. Anat. Rec., vol. 47, p. 187.

CLARK, ELIOT ROUND, W. J. HITSCHLER, HENRY TOMKINS KIRBY-SMITH, RICHARD ORLANDO REX, AND J. H. SMITH 1931 General observations on the ingrowth of new blood vessels into standardized chambers in the rabbit's ear, and the subsequent changes in the newly grown vessels over a period of months. Anat. Rec., vol. 50, no. 2, p. 129.

FEDERIGHI, H. 1928 The blood vessels of annelids. J. Exp. Zoöl., vol. 50, p. 257.

FLOREY, H. W., AND CARLETON, H. M. 1927 Rouget cells and their function. Proc. Royal Soc., vol. 100, p. 23.

GOLUBEW, A. 1869 Beiträge zur Kenntniss des Baues und der Entwicklungsgeschichte der Capillargefässe des Frosches. Arch. f. mikr. Anatom., Bd. 5, S. 49.

HILL, LEONARD 1921 The pressure in the small arteries, veins and capillaries of the bat's wing. Proc. Physiol. Soc., J. Physiol., vol. 54.

HOOKER, D. R. 1920 The functional activity of the capillaries and venules. Am. J. Physiol., vol. 54, p. 30.

KROGH, A. 1922 The anatomy and physiology of capillaries. Yale University Press.

LANDIS, E. M. 1926 The capillary pressure in frog mesentery as determined by micro-injection methods. Am. J. Physiol., vol. 75, p. 548.

PARKER, G. H. 1923 Are there Rouget cells on the blood vessels of invertebrates? Anat. Rec., vol. 26, p. 303.

RICH, A. R. 1921 Condition of the capillaries in histamine shock. J. Exp. Med., vol. 33, p. 287.

ROUGET, CH. 1873 Mémoire sur le developpement, la structure et les propriétés physiologiques des capillaries sanguins et lymphatiques. Arch. de Physiol. norm. et path., T. 5, p. 603.

ROY, CH., AND GRAHAM BROWN 1879 The blood pressure and its variations in the arterioles, capillaries, and veins. J. Physiol., vol. 2, p. 323.

SANDISON, J. C. 1924 A new method for study of tissues in mammal. Anat. Rec., vol. 28, p. 281.

———— 1928 The transparent chamber of the rabbit's ear, giving a complete description of improved technic of construction and introduction and general account of growth and behavior of living cells and tissues as seen with the microscope. Am. J. Anat., vol. 41, no. 3.

———— 1928 Observations on the growth of blood vessels as seen in the transparent chamber introduced into the rabbit's ear. Am. J. Anat., vol. 41, no. 3.

———— 1928 Contractility of blood capillaries of the rabbit as seen in the transparent chamber of the ear. Proc. Physiol. Soc. of Phila., Am. J. Med. Sc., vol. 3.

———— 1931 Observations on the circulating blood cells, adventitial (Rouget) and muscle cells, endothelium, and macrophages in the transparent chamber of the rabbit's ear. Anat. Rec., vol. 50, p. 355.

STEINACH, E., AND KAHN, R. H. 1903 Echte Contractilität und motorische Innervation der Blutcapillaren. Pflüger's Arch., Bd. 97, S. 105.

STRICKER, S. 1868 Untersuchungen über die capillaren Blutgefässe der Nickhaut des Frosches. Sitzungsber. d. Wiener Akad. d. Wissensch., Bd. 51, Abth. 2, S. 16.

TARCHANOFF, J. F. 1874 Beobachtungen über contractile Elemente in den Blut und Lymph Capillaren. Pflüger's Arch., Bd. 9, S. 407.

VIMTRUP, B. 1922 Beiträge zur Anatomie der Capillaren: über contractile Elemente in der Gefässwand der Blutcapillaren. Zeitschr. f. Anat. u. Entw., Bd. 65, S. 150.

Reprinted from *Anat. Rec.*, **65**(1), 23–50 (1936)

SPLEEN STUDIES [1]

I. MICROSCOPIC OBSERVATIONS OF THE CIRCULATORY SYSTEM OF LIVING UNSTIMULATED MAMMALIAN SPLEENS

MELVIN H. KNISELY

Hull Laboratory of Anatomy, The University of Chicago

EIGHT FIGURES

INTRODUCTION

Repeated study of the problem of splenic circulation by the classical histologic procedures of injection, fixation, and sectioning has failed to elucidate either the structure of the splenic vascular system or the course of the blood through it. So I have studied living transilluminated mammalian spleens microscopically in an attempt to learn how blood circulates through this organ.

Study of some fixed spleens has led to the development of the concept of a 'closed' circulation. This conception is, that blood is always inside of preformed, interconnected, lined channels. Study of other fixed spleens has yielded the concept of the 'open' circulation, which postulates that the arterioles, or capillaries, pour blood freely into the intercellular spaces of the splenic pulp tissue, and from these spaces the blood finds its way into the veins again. There are a variety of modifications of these two antagonistic concepts. The modifications of the concept of the 'open' circulation are especially numerous. The modifications of each of the two views are based

[1] This work was aided by a grant from the Rockefeller Foundation to the Biological Sciences Division of The University of Chicago.

The studies of living transilluminated organs are being made under the direction of Dr. R. R. Bensley. Dr. William Bloom suggested that the spleen be studied by this method. The assistance and counsel of Doctor Bensley, Doctor Bloom and the other members of the staff of Hull Anatomical Laboratory have been invaluable in this work.

23

largely upon different results which have been obtained in attempting to deduce the course of the blood through the spleen by observing the post mortem position of various injected foreign materials.

One point of controversy relates to the length and ultimate connections of the splenic arterioles, arterial capillaries and capillaries. Some investigators can trace lined arterioles only as far as the ellipsoids of Schweigger-Seidel, while others find that after passing through the ellipsoids, the arterial vessels divide, some branches connecting directly with venous sinuses others penetrating the pulp 'cords' for various distances. MacNeal ('29) traced these 'long, curved' capillaries a long way into the pulp 'cords.' Why is it that these arterial capillaries can be traced a long way by some, only a short distance by others, and cannot be traced past the ellipsoids by other investigators? Why cannot everyone find the connections of arterial capillaries with venous sinuses?

Another difficult point is the presence of a variable number of erythrocytes in the intercellular spaces of the pulp 'cords' in fixed spleens. If the vascular system is 'closed,' then how do erythrocytes get into these intercellular spaces? On the other hand, if the system is 'open,' why is it that there is not as great a concentration of red cells in the pulp 'cords' as there is in hemorrhagic tissue?

A number of investigators have injected colloidal sols into the splenic arteries and studied the position of the injected colloid in the splenic pulp. Sections of spleens so prepared almost always show the colloidal material in the intercellular spaces of the pulp 'cords.' How can this kind of result be explained in terms of the 'closed' splenic vascular system?

It has been postulated by some investigators that a 'closed' circulation in a contracted spleen may become an 'open' circulation when the organ is dilated. And it has been suggested that physiological variations—other than the degree of dilatation of the organ—might account for the structural variations reported.

This is the first of a series of papers dealing with the structure and activities of the splenic vascular system. In this first paper the unstimulated spleen will be described; that is, the structure and activities which are observed while the spleen and its attachments are as carefully protected from external manipulative stimulation as possible.

Another paper will describe, 1) the reactions of the splenic circulatory system to the stimulation of experimental manipulation and trauma, and 2) the changes which rapidly take place in the spleen during the brief period while the animal is dying.

Subsequent papers will probably take up the reaction of the spleen to injected foreign materials and a review of the literature which relates to some of the problems of the splenic vascular system.

MATERIALS AND METHOD

The spleens of seventy-five white mice, thirty white rats and fifteen cats were studied. The cats were all between 3 and 12 weeks old. Mice and rats of all ages, from nurslings to adults were used, in order to see if there were age variations in the splenic vascular system. Because it had been postulated that dilated spleens have an 'open' circulation and contracted spleens a 'closed' circulation, spleens have been studied in many different degrees of dilatation. The spleen is very large during and immediately after the ingestion of food, and progressively decreases in size thereafter. So, to study dilated spleens, animals were taken from the feeding trays and observations of the spleen begun immediately. Other spleens were studied, beginning after various intervals had elapsed since the animal's last meal; the elapsed time intervals varied from a few minutes up to and including overnight, 14-hour fasts.

Because the spleen contracts when an animal is exercised or in some emotional states (Barcroft and Stephens, '27), it was necessary to be sure that the animals used were not in an exercised or frightened condition. For that reason most of the animals were accustomed to being freely handled and to living in the laboratory before they were used in this study.

The spleens of frightened and exercised animals were also observed. To frighten and exercise an animal it was placed in a pail and frightened into running by noisily rapping the pail with a stick.

Sodium amytal, injected subcutaneously at the back of the neck or over the buttocks was the anesthetic. If a fine sharp needle is used, sodium amytal solution can be quickly injected without frightening a tame animal enough so that its spleen contracts. In the longer observations the animals have been given small extra doses of sodium amytal from time to time to maintain that concentration in the animal necessary for light anesthesia.

The position of the spleen is determined by very gentle palpation, and an incision then made in the abdominal wall, just posterior to the ribs in such a position that the incision just crosses the area under which the spleen lies. The incision is made between small hemostats to prevent blood loss. (The hair has been clipped off this area a day or two earlier.) The slit in the body wall is now pulled posteriorward to the posterior-inferior end of the spleen and the posterior lip of the incision depressed until it passes under the end of the spleen. As the tissue of the body wall shortens again the spleen remains in its usual position except that its posterior-inferior end is now outside the body. During this manipulation the spleen itself is not touched with fingers or instruments. (The only instrument ever used to touch the spleen is a smooth, paraffin-coated, wooden probe.) All tension and torsion of the spleen and its mesentery (gastrolienal ligament) are carefully avoided. The best results are obtained in cases in which only a small portion of the ventral end of the spleen is exposed through a hole which is almost filled by the protruding spleen. Precautions are taken in each case to insure that the incision is large enough so that the blood vessels to the spleen are not compressed and that the incision is no larger than is necessary (fig. 1). The spleens were transilluminated by means of the fused quartz rod previously described (Knisely, '36). The vascular system of the spleen is more sensitive to temperature variations than is the vascular system of most other organs, so it is necessary to take strict precautions to maintain the temperature of the exposed portion of the spleen at the temperature of the abdominal cavity of the animal. One cannot use metallic instruments to touch the spleen because of the rapidity with which metal at room temperature conducts heat from tissue

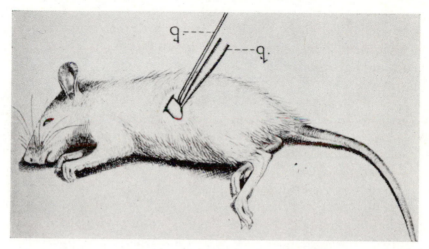

Fig. 1 Young rat with posterior-ventral end of spleen exposed for study. Quartz rod (q) and glass tube (g) in position to illuminate a small area of the spleen.

which is at mammalian body temperature. Also metallic instruments in the Ringer's solution act as electrodes, so developing electrical potentials which sometimes bring about vasomotor reactions.

The structures of the circulatory system were studied by focusing into the thinner portions (medial and lateral surfaces of the sides and ends) of the organ. One can be certain of studying structures well below the surface of the organ by focusing first on the surface, noting the fine adjustment reading, then focusing deep and noting the fine adjustment reading again. A low power binocular dissecting

THE ANATOMICAL RECORD, VOL. 65, NO. 1

microscope and monocular and binocular microscopes were used in the work. The magnifications secured with the latter varied from × 60 to × 600. The higher magnifications were secured by using a long focus × 40 water immersion objective lens in combination with × 10 or × 15 oculars. Most of the observations were made or checked with the × 40 water immersion objective and × 10 oculars.

The majority of the observations were made using the whole visible spectrum. However, a green filter aided in differentiation in many cases.

The preliminary observations showed that the tissue of the spleen is more sensitive and more reactive than had previously been suspected. So, in attempting to observe the routine activities of the splenic vascular system (rather than its reactions to the stimuli produced by the manipulations of experimental procedure) it was necessary to arrange the experiment so that the animal could be undisturbed for as long a time as possible. When an area was found that was especially favorable for study, the illuminating apparatus was adjusted, and from that time on the spleen and the whole animal were carefully left undisturbed while the particularly favorable area was watched continuously until some change (usually in the position of the spleen) took place, which necessitated a readjustment of the apparatus. The microscope could be freely moved from field to field, and the temperature of the wash solutions could be read and adjusted without disturbing the spleen or the animal.

OBSERVATIONS ON UNSTIMULATED SPLEENS

I. The general appearance of living splenic tissue

The capsule and trabeculae are practically transparent when brightly illuminated. The positions of larger trabeculae can be determined by noting the position of the larger veins and the position of the small pits where trabeculae exert tension on the capsule. The pulp tissue is transparent or translucent, depending upon the intensity of illumination used.

The malphighian bodies are irregularly ovoid. Near their surfaces they are translucent but they are more opaque toward their centers. I have not yet been able to observe an exact limiting surface between them and the surrounding tissue. The structures of the living splenic vascular system stand out like the injected vascular systems of 'whole mount' preparations of other organs. So, as in studying a whole mount, one has to focus up and down, and move along the vessels to trace out their connections.

The sheaths of Schweigger-Seidel are also transparent but their position can be determined because they are at or immediately beyond the penicilli tips, and the penicilli are easily recognized.

The venous sinuses are seen to be definite anatomical units, shaped roughly like sweet potatoes, or like cucumbers. They penetrate the tissue in all directions, each like a short, narrow-ended tunnel drilled in a cheese. Their connections to arterial and venous systems, interconnections, and activities are described below. The shape and size of a sinus varies, depending upon which phase of its physiological activity it is in. Venous sinuses are specific anatomical units and are not to be confused, either structurally or functionally, with capillaries, venules or arterio-venous anastomoses.

The tissue between the sinuses consist of thick or thin partitions; the thickness of a given partition at a given time depends upon how much it is squeezed between, and stretched by, the adjacent venous sinuses. The increase in size of the sinuses during some phases of their activity concomitantly decreases the thickness of the partitions, and vice versa. In cutting sections of the spleen this set of irregular partitions is cut in various directions thus creating, by the act of cutting, the appearance of irregular rods and bars known as 'Billroth cords.' The splenic pulp of mice, rats and cats does not consist of a three-dimensional network of cords suspended in blood.

There are relatively few red cells in the pulp partitions (that is, 'Billroth cords')[2] of the living unstimulated spleen.

[2] The term 'pulp partitions' will be used from here on, rather than the terms 'Billroth cords' or 'pulp cords.'

In the experiments in which the greatest care has been taken in preparing the spleen for observation the number of red cells in the pulp partition tissue is very small. Each of the few red cells seen in the pulp partitions of an unstimulated spleen travels slowly across the partition. Each travels by itself. No two follow each other as if they were in a common channel. An erythrocyte does not travel by 'fits and starts' as though it were being washed along, and catching and breaking away from the corners of an irregular patent labyrinth made up of interconnected patent intercellular spaces. The rate of red cell movement across the pulp partitions is nearly uniform and quite slow, as though they were traversing very narrow or potential spaces. As a red cell moves along it may change shape somewhat, but usually its shape does not alter greatly.

When a red cell passes through the lining of the vascular system its shape is distorted in a characteristic manner as it begins to penetrate the lining, and the red cell 'snaps' forward suddenly, as soon as the major part of its protoplasm has passed through the lining membrane. (This snapping forward is like the snapping forward of a moist apple seed when pinched between one's thumb and forefinger.) The initial distortion of the red cell I take to be evidence that the lining membrane offers resistance to the penetration of the erythrocytes and the snapping forward to be evidence that the lining membrane is elastic and exerts pressure on the erythrocyte which is traversing it.

This characteristic 'distortion and snap' has been used as one of the criteria in determining whether the membrane lining a blood vessel was continuous or had gaps in it. Each time that an erythrocyte has been seen to pass through a visible blood vessel lining it has been seen to 'distort and snap.' A red cells does not behave in this way when traversing pulp partition tissue, nor when passing through a visible gap in a visible blood vessel lining.

The lining of arterioles, arterial-capillaries, capillaries, venous sinuses and venules appears in the living spleen as a narrow, clear, sharply refractile line. This line is visibly distinct from, and cannot be confused with, the peripheral plasma layer of the flowing blood stream, for one can see the peripheral plasma layer and the lining of the vessel, a line marking their mutual surface, and one can sometimes see leucocytes rolling along the internal surface of the vessel lining. Pairs of these refractile lines mark the position of the vessel both during the flow of blood and during periods in which there is no blood in the vessel. The refractile linings of the vascular system of the living unstimulated spleen are as continuous as, but thinner than, the refractile linings of arterioles, capillaries and venules in most other tissues, such as smooth muscle, for instance. Each vessel traced was attached to other vessels at each of its ends.

II. Observations on the anatomical relationships of the vascular system of the living spleen

The artery of the malpighian body divides into three or four (occasionally as many as seven) branches, each of which subdivides into from two to four very straight secondary branches, which are penicilli. From each of the penicilli from two to four short branches are given off, the subdivisions of which divide into arterial capillaries.[3]

The branches of the penicilli are connected with each other by a few lateral anastomoses of capillary diameter. These anastomoses are not limited to interconnecting the branches of a single penicillus, but interconnect branches of adjacent penicilli as well.

The sides of the malpighian bodies are sufficiently transparent so that the outer capillaries of the body can be traced a considerable distance inward. The capillaries of the malpighian body form an anastomosing three-dimensional network. (The term 'loops' which was applied to this network by Nisimaru and Steggerda ('32) is misleading, for the term implies that this capillary network has no efferent connections.) The pattern of this network is not essentially different

[3] This is the general pattern of the branching of the splenic arterial system. In the spleen, as in other parts of the mammalian vascular system, there are variations from the general pattern of branching.

from that of the capillary system of several other tissues. The capillaries of the malpighian body (which are frequently said to end by opening out into and connecting with intercellular pulp spaces) peripherally join the capillary network which interconnects the branches of the penicilli (fig. 2).

The branches of the penicilli divide into two or three or four arterial capillaries.

There are two anatomically different types of preformed, lined, vessel systems in the red pulp which connect arterioles or arterial-capillaries to venules. One type consists of venous sinuses and venous sinus systems. The other consists of long, straight or somewhat curved, capillaries. No anastomoses between these two types have yet been found.

Many of the arterial capillaries after a short course connect directly with the afferent ends of venous sinuses. A smaller number enter laterally. There are sinuses which have no other type of afferent, and connect directly with a venule (as at sinus *a* in fig. 2). This type of connection constitutes a single sinus route. There are also multiple sinus routes. Thus the efferent end of a venous sinus may be connected to the end or side of a second sinus as at *b* and *c* in figure 2. The multiple sinus routes have two or three or more consecutive venous sinuses interposed between arterial capillary and venule. (Compare sinuses I, II, III and III a of fig. 2, which constitute a multiple sinus route.) There is a functional as well as a structural difference which distinguishes single from multiple sinus routes.

Each single and each multiple sinus route is a definite anatomical unit. The anatomical connections of a given route have remained constant throughout all observed physiological cycles of that route.

For consideration of fluid flow, it is important to note that, though some sinuses have side afferents and some do not, each sinus has an end afferent.

Many arterial capillaries derived from the subdivisions of the penicilli pursue a long, somewhat curved, unbranched

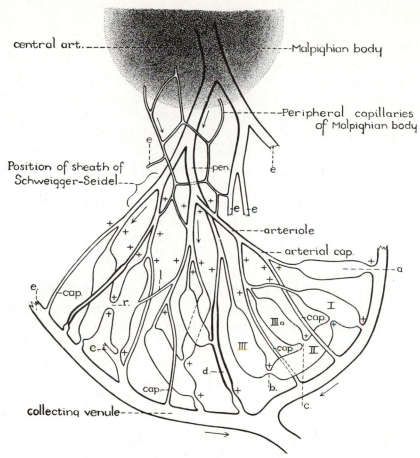

Fig. 2 Diagram of the types of vascular connections which have thus far been seen in the spleen.

I, II, III and *III a* are the individual venous sinuses making up a multiple sinus system. All four are shown in storage phase. *a,* marks the open efferent end of a single sinus route in early emptying phase. *b,* shows where efferent end of sinus III connects to afferent end of sinus II. *c,* shows where efferent end of sinus III a connects to side of sinus II. *d,* shows a venous sinus in conducting phase to distinguish it from pulp partition capillary. *e,* in different positions marks the end of the diagram. At each of these positions the blood vessels would connect to other blood vessels if the diagram were extended. *l,* shows an arterial-capillary entering the side of a venous sinus. *r,* indicates a rare type of connection between sinuses. *cap.,* indicates the long relatively straight capillaries which extend lengthwise through the pulp partitions and end by connecting to venules. Plus signs indicate the positions of the sensitive reactive physiological sphincters whose coordinated actions play so large a part in the control of the circulatory processes of the spleen. The arrows show the direction of blood flow.

In this diagram no effort has been made to show the relative frequency of occurrence of each kind of connection.

33

177

course.   They pass lengthwise through the pulp partition tissue between the sinuses and connect directly with venules. Many authors have described the first portion of these capillaries, but as far as I know, their ultimate termination has not been previously described.   For consideration of function it is to be noted that these long capillaries are connected in shunt with the sinus systems.

The afferent connections of the smallest venules are of three kinds: 1) Efferent ends of single sinus routes, 2) efferent ends of multiple sinus routes, 3) efferent ends of the long, relatively straight capillaries.   The smallest venules join together to make larger venules, the structure and connections of which are well known.

Each vessel traced in the living spleen was connected to the arterial system and to the venous system.   No vessels have been seen to open out into, or pour blood into intercellular pulp spaces in living unstimulated spleens.   No vessels have been seen to end in culs de sac.   In the living unstimulated spleen the vascular system consists of a series of completely interconnected, preformed, lined channels.

From the visible structure alone, one might easily conclude that the splenic vascular system is 'closed.'   But, that the usual concept of the 'closed' circulation is not adequate to include the functioning of the system becomes quite apparent from a consideration of the cyclic and continuous types of activity of single venous sinuses and multiple sinus routes.

III. Observations of the routine activities of the circulatory systems of spleens that were protected from external stimulation as carefully as possible

A. Control of the distribution of incoming blood.   In the spleen there are a number of active, physiological sphincters located at strategic positions on the arterial tree.   The sheaths of Schweigger-Seidel (ellipsoids) act as particularly sensitive and powerful sphincters.   Müller (1865) traced branches of the post-ganglionic splenic nerves as far as the ellipsoids.   It is frequently stated that the diameter of the vessel lumen is always smaller as it passes through the ellipsoid than at the ellipsoids' ends. This is true only in fixed sections. In the living the diameter varies greatly, depending upon the physiological state of the contractile ellipsoid.

There is also a sphincter on each arterial-capillary which supplies a venous sinus, located a little above the point at which the capillary enters the sinus. And there is one at the efferent end of each sinus.[4] The sphincters above the afferent end and at the efferent end of the sinuses are as sensitive but not as powerful as those located in the arterial tree. The position of these physiological sphincters is indicated by a plus sign ($+$) in figure 2. When one of these physiological sphincters is not constricted, the wall at that point shows no indication that it differs from adjacent segments of the vascular system.

In some organs, other than the spleen, the diameters of the terminal arterioles vary from time to time, thus regulating the volume of blood supplied to capillary beds. However, instead of exhibiting only tonus (namely, being partly open or partly constricted) the physiological sphincters exhibit also a valve-like action, changing from fully open to a completely closed condition in a very short time. Not only that, but the timing of the opening and closing of these sphincters seems to indicate that groups of them are controlled, and their activities integrated, by one or more control mechanisms.

The central artery of the malpighian body can contract strongly enough to obliterate its lumen. The sphincters located on each branch of the arterial tree are also capable of

[4] In connection with the sphincters at the efferent end of the venous sinuses, the question has been raised. "How can there be contraction at this point when no cells have been found here which show the structural characteristics of contractile cells?"

I doubt that we are yet in a position safely to conclude that the only cells which can contract are those showing the same cytological appearance as the units of smooth and striated muscle. Further, the nature of the cells at this point has not been the subject of a specific cytological investigation.

These efferent sphincters have been watched while they contracted sharply, while they opened quickly, and while they remained in a partly closed, namely, in a tonic state. For the description of this, see the sections on the activities of the venous sinuses.

complete contraction. By quickly contracting the sphincters of all but one or two branches of any given stem, all the blood coming in through the stem artery (or arteriole) is directed to one or two open branches. At any given time, blood is directed to small individual areas by being prevented from going anywhere else.

Observations made at the branching of a penicillus in the spleen of mouse series A, no. 1, illustrates the control of the distribution of blood by the integrated action of a set of sphincters. A penicillus having three branches was watched while the animal was completely undisturbed for an hour. A sketch was made and the three branches labeled a, b and d. At any one time, one branch was open and the other two closed. There was a rotation of access to the blood supply. Thus a conducted blood, then d and then b. This order was maintained for 50 minutes in perfect rotation. Each branch was closed twice as long as it was open. One branch opened simultaneously with the closing of another, so that the flow in the stem (that is, in the penicillus) was almost steady and constant. The closed and open phases together in any one branch lasted about 5 minutes.

The control mechanism at this location in this specimen was characterized by integrated mechanical regularity, for 50 minutes, while completely undisturbed. Frequently, however, these sphincter mechanisms exhibit flexibility in responding to minute external applied stimuli, or to unknown stimuli.

Further descriptions of the integrated activity of sets of sphincters will be given later.

The distribution of the blood from the central artery of a malpighian corpuscle to any penicillus, to any branch of a penicillus, to any group of venous sinuses, to any venous sinus and to the red pulp capillaries, is completely and precisely controlled at all times by the coordinated action of these physiological sphincters.

B. The activities of venous sinuses and multiple sinus route systems. Venous sinuses exhibit two types of activity; 'cyclic' and 'continuous.' Both types separate the cells of the blood from the fluid[5] of the blood. Sinuses in 'continuous' activity retain the blood cells for a relatively short time. They are retained during long 'storage phases' of the cyclic activity for various periods, from a few minutes up to several hours.

1. The cyclic activity of the venous sinus. The venous sinus has a cycle of activity consisting of, a) a phase of filtration-filling, during which it swells to several times its previous volume, b) a 'storage' phase, c) a phase of sudden emptying, and d) a conducting phase during which whole blood flows into, through, and out of the sinus. Each phase passes smoothly into the next. The cycle is here separated into phases to facilitate description.

a. The filtration-filling phase. At the beginning of the phase of filtration-filling, the sinus appears as a comparatively thick-walled, slightly widened continuation of its own afferent arterial capillary. Its lumen may be three times as wide as that of its afferent vessel, but is usually not more than twice as wide (fig. 3). The flow through the capillary and sinus into the venule at this time is frequently pulsating, similar to that in an arteriole. Suddenly the blood at the efferent end of the sinus backs up a little, as though the sphincter at the efferent end had constricted and obliterated its lumen; and when one focuses on the efferent sphincter it is seen that this has happened (fig. 4). While the efferent sphincter is tightly closed, whole blood continues to come into the sinus from its afferent vessel; blood fluid passes rapidly through the walls of the sinus, blood cells pack into the sinus as the sinus swells and swells, until it becomes a greatly distended cucumber-shaped structure solidly packed with blood cells (fig. 5). At the moment that a sinus is nearly full of packed blood cells, while whole blood is still flowing in, that is, before there is stasis in the afferent vessel, the sphincter located a little above the afferent end of the sinus quickly constricts, suddenly shutting off the blood supply of the sinus before it is quite

[5] The term 'fluid' is used in this discussion rather than the term 'plasma' because the latter indicates a fluid of known qualitative and quantitative composition. Some of the constituents of plasma may be partly or wholly retained within the sinus, so the term 'blood fluid' is used in order that this question may obviously be left open.

full. I take this as evidence that there is a quantitative control
of the volume of blood supplied to a sinus. By this contraction of the sphincter the venous sinus is relieved of the blood
pressure of the arterial system while it is packed with blood
cells.

In unstimulated spleens red cells have not yet been seen to
pass through the lining of the sinus during the filtering-filling
phase.

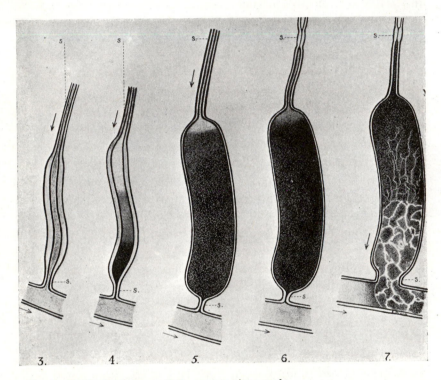

Fig. 3   Conduction phase of the venous sinus cycle.
Fig. 4   Early filtration-filling phase of the venous sinus cycle.
Fig. 5   Late filtration-filling phase of the venous sinus cycle.
Fig. 6   The transition from late filtration-filling to storage phase at the moment
the afferent sphincter closes.
Fig. 7   The beginning of the emptying phase when masses of red cells (a part
of a soft blood cell 'cast' of the sinus) are being emptied into the venule. *S*,
marks the position of sphincters. The arrows show the direction of blood flow.

The separation of cells from fluid is quantitative, for the cells in the sinus are packed so closely together that their individual edges are no longer visible, and, as, the observations of the emptying of the sinus show, there is little fluid in the sinus among the packed blood cells.

While a sinus is in the filtering-filling phase, the finer collecting venules of areas contiguous to that sinus are filled with fluid containing a few red cells which have come from other branches of the venule. It has not yet been possible to discover the exact anatomical position at which blood fluid enters the vascular system again. Because it is transparent, it cannot be seen passing in through the walls of vessels and no holes have been found in the linings of vessels in living unstimulated spleens.

b. The storage phase. The phase of filtering-filling is immediately followed by the 'storage' phase. (This term is used because the retention of blood cells is the visibly prominent feature. However, it is probable that the storage is accompanied by other, much more important processes.) During the storage phase the venous sinus maintains its highly distended condition (fig. 6). This phase usually lasts from a few minutes to 4 hours. However, much longer storage phases have been under continuous observation. In one case (in a young cat) a storage phase lasting for 10 hours was under constant observation. It was followed by several short, apparently normal, complete cycles of activity. This seems to indicate that the tissue was not damaged during the 10-hour storage phase.

During the storage phase while the sinus is highly distended and has a thin wall, some red cells may be seen very slowly passing, individually, from the sinus into the splenic tissue. These red cells are distorted and 'snap' forward as they pass out through the visible membrane-like wall of the sinus.

Specific observation of these red cells in the partitions between the sinuses has thus far failed to show that any of them are phagocytized. In unstimulated spleens the cells of the pulp partitions are so transparent as to be invisible, but, in watching individual red blood cells in the unstimulated spleen I have not yet seen an erythrocyte lose its outline, change its color, and have its pigment diffuse out around it, in the manner in which these visible evidences of the cytolysis of phagocytized red cells are frequently seen while watching the ingestion and cytolysis of red cells during the agonal changes which occur in this organ.

The number of red cells seen in the pulp partitions adjacent to engorged sinuses in living unstimulated spleens is seldom as large as the number of red cells seen in sections of fixed spleens.

c. The emptying phase. At the end of the storage phase the sphincter at the efferent end of the sinus suddenly opens wide. This opening is almost always startlingly abrupt so that continuous close observation of the sphincter is necessary to see it open (fig. 7). At the moment of its opening irregular masses of blood cells (which are fragments of a soft blood cell 'cast' of the sinus) begin to pass down through the sphincter into the efferent venule. After moving a short distance each mass separates into its individual cells. The blood in the efferent venule of a sinus so discharging is thick and pasty, consisting mostly of cells with very little fluid (fig. 8, V_2 and C). Suddenly the afferent sphincter of the sinus opens, letting whole blood into the afferent end of the sinus. After the entering whole blood washes the packed blood cells out of the sinus, the sinus decreases in diameter until it is but little larger than its afferent capillary. Red cells may be seen at this time slowly passing from adjacent splenic tissue back into the sinus. They 'distort and snap forward' characteristically as they pass through the resistant lining of the sinus.

d. The conduction phase. During the conduction phase, which follows immediately, the flow through the afferent capillary, sinus and even the efferent venule is frequently pulsating as in an arteriole. This is evidence that at this time there is very little resistance to the blood flow through the capillary, sinus and venule. In this phase whole blood flows into the sinus and whole blood flows out of the sinus. The sinus does not separate blood cells from blood fluid; it conducts whole blood like most other segments of tubing in the vascular system. During the conduction phase there sometimes are periods during which whole blood stands still in the sinus.

At the end of a conducting phase the sinus enters a filtering-filling phase again, and so the cycle repeats. These cycles

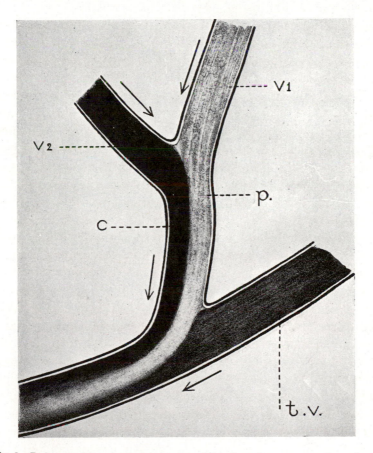

Fig. 8 Redrawn from a sketch made while observing an area in spleen of mouse B3. V_1, venule containing almost cell-free blood fluid coming from an area in which the sinuses are retaining the blood cells. V_2, venule containing thick, pasty blood (many cells, little fluid) from an area where sinuses are pouring out blood cell masses. p, fluid, and c cells, which have not yet mixed in the flowing blood. t.v., small trabecular vein. The arrows show the direction of blood flow.

repeat time after time while the spleen is left entirely undisturbed.

2. Structure of venous sinus walls. In fixed sections the individual littoral cells of the sinus wall appear as rods with slits between them (compare Mollier). Careful focusing on living refractile sinus walls shows that in the living organ the entire wall is continuous and is uniform in thickness at any given degree of distension. No slits have yet been seen in the living sinus walls of the three species studied, even under 400 or 600 diameters magnification. Krogh ('29, p. 9) demonstrated the plasticity and elasticity of the frog's red corpuscles. If we can assume that the mammalian red corpuscle is equally plastic and elastic, we would expect that these corpuscles would easily pass through quite small preformed holes in the sinus wall if preformed holes were present. That red cells do not pass consecutively through preformed holes in the walls but pass through the wall by individual penetration, even when the sinus wall is stretched thin in storage phase, indicates that if holes are present they are very small.

During the filtering-filling phase the sinus wall is freely permeable to the colloids of the blood. Blood coming toward a sinus such as the one marked a in figure 2 would either pass into the sinus, or into the capillary shunt. If the sinus greatly increased the resistance to flow, the blood would take the alternate route through the capillary. When sinuses are in the filtering-filling phase (and the efferent sphincter closed), one sometimes sees blood flowing freely both into the sinus and through a parallel connected capillary. This is the evidence that at this time the sinus wall is freely permeable to the colloids of the blood. For if the sinus wall were impermeable to colloids (like the membrane of an osmometer) the resistance to the passage of colloids through the sinus wall would very soon create sufficient back pressure so that most of the blood would go via the alternate channel.

When a sinus is in conducting phase, its walls do not permit blood fluid to escape for the cells passing through do not become more and more closely packed as they pass along.

From these facts it is obvious that the sinus wall is capable of considerable variability, the entire range of which probably has not yet been observed.

Sinus walls are probably the only place at which fluid leaves the vascular channels. At least there have been no observations so far to indicate that it leaves the lined system at any place other than the venous sinus walls. In the living spleen no slits have been seen in the lining of the vessels which pass through the ellipsoids, such as are described in sections of fixed spleens by Robinson ('26) and MacNeal ('29). At no point have blood cells been seen coming progressively closer together as they passed along a vessel, as they do in the capillaries of frogs' kidney glomeruli.

3. The integrated cyclic activity of a multiple sinus system. Consider the sinus system consisting of the four sinuses marked I, II, III and III a in figure 2. Sinus I has independent afferent and efferent connections. It can have independent cyclic activity. Sinuses II, III and III a can discharge into the vein only while the efferent sphincter of I is open, that is, when it is in an 'emptying' or 'conducting' phase. Number II does not have an independent arterial-capillary afferent, but III and III a do. Beginning with all four sinuses of the system in conducting phases, the efferents of I, II and III a close. I, II and III a go into filtering-filling phase, followed by storage phase. Whole blood flows through III which remains in conducting phase while II fills. When the afferent sphincter of II closes, III enters its filtering-filling phase and then goes into storage phase. By this time no. I may be emptying, or may already be in conducting phase. Sinus I may go through several independent cycles before II, III and III a discharge. But at some time while no. I is in conducting phase, the efferent of no. II opens wide and it discharges into I, and so out into the venule. Nos. III and III a then discharge through II. All the sinuses of the system are then washed out with arterial blood and the system stays in a common conduction phase for a period. This complex cycle of the multiple sinus system then repeats. The dependent sinuses of a multiple sinus route (as nos. II, III and

THE ANATOMICAL RECORD, VOL. 65, NO. 1

III a) differ functionally from independent sinuses (no. I) and single sinus routes, in that they have proportionately longer storage periods. Some multiple sinus systems consist of other numbers of sinuses. Their complex cycles follow the same general principles as that of the four-sinus system described.

As has been said, a sinus system is a definite anatomical unit; its structure and anatomical connections remain constant through all its observed physiological cycles.

4. Continuous separation of cells from fluid, or acyclic function of the venous sinus. Greatly distended single sinuses are seen which have their efferent sphincters partly closed. In these sinuses whole blood flows rapidly and steadily into the afferent end, blood fluid passes rapidly through the sinus wall and thick pasty masses of blood cells continuously squeeze slowly out the efferent end. Meanwhile, clear fluid, with an occasional red cell, is flowing in small adjacent collecting venules.

This type of filtration has not been seen as often as the cyclic functioning of the sinuses. Continuous filtration, when seen, has usually been at a spot, particularly favorable for observation, in the greatly distended spleen of an animal having food in its stomach. It is more difficult to observe the action of sinuses in a spleen in such a distended state than in thinner ones. So it is probable that the rarity of the observation of continuous filtration is not an indication that this activity rarely occurs.

During the continuous filtering process I have not yet seen red cells pass out through the lining of the sinus.

A few times, while a single sinus was being watched, it was observed to change from cyclic activity to continuous filtration and after a time back to cyclic activity again.

5. The time relationships of the phases of venous sinus cycles. The total time occupied by a venous sinus cycle is variable, short under some conditions, long under others. The proportion of the total time of the cycle occupied by a given phase also varies with different conditions. Of the phases,

the emptying phase is usually shortest and least variable. The filtration-filling phase is a little longer and is also more variable. The conduction and storage phases are longest and most variable. The duration of one or both of these two phases occupies most of the time of each cycle.

a. Short cycles. In short (5- or 10-minute) cycles the conduction and storage phases are about equal and together occupy as much as three- or four-fifths of the time of the cycle.

b. During digestion. In early digestion, when an animal has recently ingested food in its stomach and upper small intestine, the sinuses in storage phase are highly distended, and the storage phases are relatively prolonged. On account of the latter, many sinuses are in storage phase simultaneously. At this time some sinuses are distended in continuous filtration periods. The conduction phases are relatively brief. Because so many sinuses are engorged simultaneously, the whole spleen is dilated during the early digestion period.

At this time much of that part of the whole blood which is conducted through the organ without having its cells separated from its fluid goes by way of the long straight capillaries of the pulp partitions, rather than by way of sinuses in conduction phase.

As the time elapses since a meal was ingested, the long storage phases become progressively shorter and the conduction phases longer, so that fewer and fewer sinuses at a given instant are seen distended in storage phase and more and more are seen in conduction phase; each cycle is shorter; and therefore, the spleen becomes progressively smaller and smaller as more time has passed. (However, in the spleen of an animal that has fasted all night, there are still many sinuses in storage phase at a given time.)

c. In fright and exercise. If an animal has been actively exercised and frightened before the spleen is studied, some of the sinuses and sinus systems have relatively brief storage phases, while in other sinus routes arterial blood flows with little resistance in a pulsating stream through arterioles, capillaries and venous sinuses into venules. That is, in an exercised or frightened animal many of the previously stored blood cells are gone, and a great many of the sinuses are in their conducting phases.

d. Reaction to the *local* application of epinephrin. If on the surface of a partly dilated spleen one drops a little epinephrin (a 1/10,000 solution was used, but this was immediately diluted further by the mammalian Ringer's wash solution flowing over the exposed surface of the organ), many sinuses go into emptying phase followed by a period in which arterial blood flows through capillaries, sinuses and sinus systems into venules, in a pulsating stream. A spleen so treated decreases slightly in size; its circulation has somewhat the appearance of that of the spleen of a frightened and exercised animal.

The control mechanisms (namely, sets of sphincters) at the subdivision of the arterioles into arterial-capillaries, regulate the distribution of blood in the venous sinuses and sinus systems, so that the physiological cycles of neighboring sinuses are usually, but not always, out of step with one another. One is filling while another is in storage phase and still a third is emptying, etc. When many adjacent sinuses are seen in conduction, or storage phase at the same time, continuous observation of that area usually shows that one is in the late part of its phase, another in the mid- or early part of its phase, etc.

This control mechanism so operates that the total volume of stored blood cells can be increased or decreased, or, the total can be maintained at a nearly constant level while incoming cells are stored and stored cells are released.

C. The circulation in capillaries. Thus far the connections of and circulation through venous sinuses and multiple sinus systems has been emphasized. It is well to note that the primary function of the venous sinus circulation is not that of nourishing the tissue. It is rather a system which acts upon blood.

The capillary circulation which nourishes the tissue is also important. The capillaries of the malpighian body connect with the fine capillaries that interconnect the branches of the penicilli. The branches of the penicilli have connections with the long straight capillaries which longitudinally traverse the pulp partitions. This capillary network exhibits the irregularly intermittent circulation common to the capillary beds which nourish various tissues. The intermittency of the circulation in the capillaries of the malpighian bodies is roughly similar to the intermittency of the circulation in some of the smaller inguinal lymph nodes of mice. The long straight capillaries of the pulp partitions intermittently conduct blood through the tissue during the storage phases of the venous sinuses. The capillary system is sufficiently independent of the venous sinus system so that regardless of the conditions in the latter the irregularly intermittent nourishing circulation in the former continues.

D. Observations on the circulatory conditions in venules. At a given time some of the collecting venules, draining a small area containing sinuses, are filled very largely with fluid coming from sinuses in their filtering-filling phase. Other venules are filled with a blood cell paste, containing very little fluid, which is coming from sinuses in their emptying phase. The union of two venules in those two conditions is shown in figure 8. Such a situation has been seen to reverse, that is, a venule having cells later had fluid, and vice versa.

By the time that the cells and fluid reach the larger venules they have been uniformly intermingled. They travel for some distance in this condition and later assume the usual distribution of blood cells and plasma in veins, that is, an axial stream of blood cells in plasma, plus a peripheral layer of plasma.

DISCUSSION

The observations described above show some at least of the routine, physiological activities of the splenic vascular system. Because the animals whose spleens were observed were under an anesthetic—even very lightly under an anesthetic—one cannot be certain that the processes observed constitute the entire range of the splenic vascular system's capabilities. The rate of the activities described is probably more rapid in the absence of an anesthetic.

No significant differences have yet been observed between the structure and activities of living mouse, rat and cat spleens. No differences have been observed in the circulatory systems of spleens of animals of different ages.

The observations of the spleens of these three species negate the hypothesis that a dilated spleen has an 'open' circulation and a contracted spleen a 'closed' circulation.

Each of the terms 'closed' circulation and 'open' circulation represents the crystallization of ideas around a theory. There was a single primary, unconsciously made, assumption behind each of these two theories. This assumption was: The cells and fluid of blood passing through the spleen travel together, uniformly mixed, just as blood travels through the vascular system of most other organs.

The present observations show that this single primary assumption was erroneous.

Because the sinuses and sinus systems quantitatively separate blood cells from blood fluid, the circulatory systems of the unstimulated spleens of these three species cannot be included under the usual concept of the 'closed' splenic circulatory system. Because whole blood is not freely poured into the intercellular spaces of the pulp partitions the system cannot be included in the usual concepts of the 'open' circulatory system.

On account of their historical associations, neither of the terms 'open' or 'closed' can safely be used to describe the splenic circulation.

Observations, to be reported in the next paper of this series, on the reactions of the splenic vascular system to traumatic stimulation and on the changes which rapidly take place in the spleen while an animal dies, show the probable sources of the great variety of 'open' circulatory system patterns described in fixed spleens.

SUMMARY OF OBSERVATIONS ON UNSTIMULATED SPLEENS

The unstimulated splenic vascular system of mice, rats and cats consists of a system of preformed, interconnected, lined channels. The tissue between the sinuses and sinus systems consists of partitions which appear as 'cords' after cutting the spleen into sections. In the unstimulated spleen few red cells are in these partitions. The few red cells that leave the lined vascular system pass through the lining of the sinus by individual penetration. The sinus lining is resistant enough, even when it is stretched thin in storage phase, to distort the erythrocytes and make them snap forward as they penetrate it. Red cells traveling in the pulp partitions have not yet been seen to be phagocytized or cytolyzed in living spleens.

The venous sinuses quantitatively separate the cells of the blood from the fluid of the blood. There are two ways in which sinuses do this: 1) By the filtering-filling process, and 2) by the continuous filtration process. The sinus wall is the only membrane which has yet been seen to separate blood cells from blood fluid. During the filtration-filling phase venous sinus linings are freely permeable to the colloids of the blood. During the conducting phase blood fluid does not pass out through the sinus wall.

The venous sinuses store blood cells for various periods of time. Under some circumstances incoming blood cells are stored and previously stored cells are released synchronously, so that the total volume of stored cells in a given area of the spleen remains nearly constant. Under other conditions the total volume of stored cells may be increased or decreased. Whole blood can pass through the spleen without having its cells separated from its fluid, by two different routes: 1) By the sinuses and sinus systems when they are in conducting phases, and 2) by way of the long, relatively straight capillaries which pass lengthwise through the partitions between the sinuses. The capillaries conduct blood which nourishes the tissues during the long storage phases of the sinuses.

Precise, integrated control of the distribution of blood is one of the dominant features of the activity of the splenic vascular system. The proportion of blood which passes through the spleen without having its cells separated from its fluid, the proportion having its cells separated from its fluid, and the length of time the cells are stored are continuously controlled. This control is secured by the coordinated action of sets of sensitive, powerful, reactive sphincters located at strategic positions. The sheaths of Schweigger-Seidel act as especially powerful sphincters.

The venous sinuses and venous sinus systems are not primarily a system of vessels which conduct blood to nourish the splenic tissue. The sinus systems and pulp partitions constitute, rather, a mechanism which acts upon blood.

On account of their historical associations, and the limited concepts they indicate, neither of the terms 'closed' or 'open' can safely be used to designate the splenic circulation.

LITERATURE CITED

BARCROFT, J. AND J. G. STEPHENS 1927 Observations on the size of the spleen. J. Physiol., vol. 64, pp. 1–22.

KNISELY, M. H. 1936 A method of illuminating living structures for microscopic study. Anat. Rec., vol. 64, pp. 499–524.

KROGH, A. 1929 The Anatomy and Physiology of Capillaries, Yale University Press, p. 9.

MACNEAL, W. J. 1929 The circulation of blood through the spleen pulp. Arch. of Path., vol. 7, pp. 215–227.

MOLLIER, S. 1911 Ueber den Bau der Capillaren Milzvene (Milzsinus). Archiv. f. mikr.-Anat., Bd. 76, S. 608–657.

MÜLLER, W. 1865 Ueber den Fineren Bau der Milz. Leipzig u., Heidelberg.
———— The Spleen, in Stricker's Histology, English translation, New Sydenham Society.

NISIMARU, Y., AND F. R. STEGGERDA 1932 Observations on the structure and function of certain blood vessels in the spleen. J. Physiol., vol. 74, pp. 327–337.

ROBINSON, W. L. 1926 The vascular mechanism of the spleen. Am. J. Path., vol. 2, pp. 341–356.

11

Reprinted from *Anat. Rec.*, **73**(4), 475–495 (1939)

THE CHARACTER AND DISTRIBUTION OF THE BLOOD CAPILLARIES

BENJAMIN WILLIAM ZWEIFACH

Laboratory of Cell Physiology, Washington Square College, New York University, New York City

SEVEN FIGURES

In previous communications (Zweifach, '37 a, '37 b), it was pointed out that two types of blood capillaries can be distinguished according to whether the vessels, along their entire length from arteriole to venule, are either partially or completely denuded of muscular elements. The architecture of the capillary system is such that the two types map out characteristic anatomical units, the arrangement of which is an important factor for the regulation of the local distribution of blood. The present paper represents a further contribution to the existence and functional significance of these two types of vessels and of their mode of branching.

MATERIAL AND METHODS

The living vessels were observed in the mesentery, tongue, skin and intestinal wall of the frog; also in the mesentery and ear of the white mouse. In addition, micromanipulative operations were performed on vessels of the mesentery in the mouse and frog. Fixed and stained preparations of the above tissues and of the omentum of the cat were also studied.

Details of the micromanipulative technique, as modified for the study of living blood capillaries in the frog and mouse, have been described (Zweifach, '37 a, '37 b). In brief, an intestinal loop was withdrawn and placed around a glass ring cemented over an opening in the roof of a horseshoe-shaped moist chamber. The tissue was covered with a glass

475

slip to whose undersurface it adhered and was kept irrigated with Ringer's solution. Mechanically controlled microneedles were brought up from below and inserted through the naked mesothelial layer into direct contact with the blood vessels of the mesentery (fig. 1).

The degree and rapidity of coloration of perivascular tissue by Congo red was used as an index of capillary permeability.

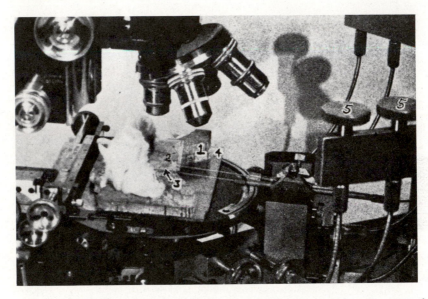

Fig. 1 Equipment for micromanipulation of capillary vessels in mesentery of mouse. 1, cork wall of moist chamber, with glass base (4), open at front for insertion of operating needles. 2, cover slip resting over exposed mesentery loop drawn over a glass ring on top of moist chamber and vaguely discernible (3 with arrow) through roofing cover slip. 5, 5, two of six control screws (others not visible in photograph.

Under normal conditions, no rapid coloring of the tissue about a capillary could be detected, when 1 to 2 cc. of a 2% solution of Congo red in Ringers was injected directly into the blood stream by way of the ventricle of the heart. However, with a change in the permeability of the capillary wall, the dye would seep through more rapidly into the tissue.

Often it was necessary to determine the number of cells that make up the wall of a particular capillary. A 5% to 10% silver nitrate solution was introduced with a micropipette and sprayed directly onto the capillary wall. This stained the cement substance between contiguous endothelial cells without impeding the circulation through that vessel.

I wish to thank Prof. Robert Chambers for his continued interest and cooperation throughout this work.

RESULTS

Because the concept of two types of capillaries is a new and important one, additional data together with photographic evidence is being presented in this paper.

Not all of the capillaries are functionally active at the same time or to the same degree. However, certain of the capillaries continue to convey an active flow of blood, even when the tissues are in a resting or anemic state. These latter vessels are main central highways for the continuous transport of the blood. A vigorous circulation always courses through them because, as direct extensions of the arterial vessels, they offer the least resistance to the forward propulsion of blood. The arteriolar pathway, therefore, not only distributes side branches but also continues through without interruption to the venule. This continuous trunk may be divided for descriptive purposes into three portions, the terminal arteriole or precapillary, the capillary, and the venule (fig. 2). The capillary portion of the trunk, in contrast to the other, less constantly used capillary side channels, at all times connects the arterioles and venules and was designated in a previous article ('37 a), the arteriolo-venular or a-v bridge.

The contractile tunic of the small arterioles, being continued along the a-v bridge as a series of modified muscle elements, the bridge may be regarded as a 'muscular capillary.' The muscle cells progressively thin out and become increasingly branched in the longer a-v bridges so that the cells become

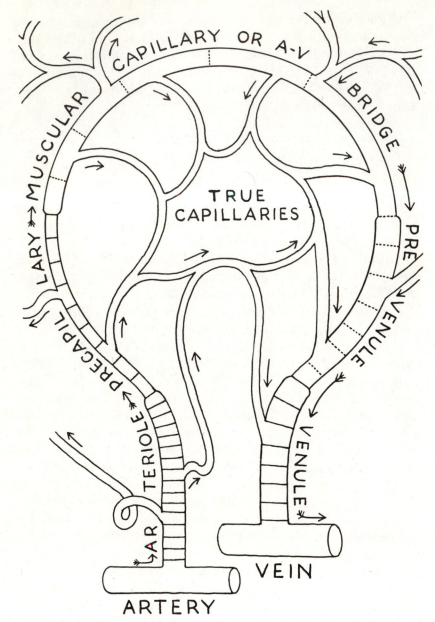

Fig. 2 Diagrammatic representation of capillary bed. Subdivisions of continuous central trunk are labeled and manner of branching of true capillaries is indicated. Typical smooth muscle cells are shown as solid cross lines, branched muscle elements by dotted cross lines.

indistinguishable from other adventitial elements in the distal parts of the vessels. Careful measurements showed that the a-v bridges are somewhat wider than true capillaries, being 12 to 16 μ in diameter.

The a-v capillary is to be considered as a central or focal pathway from which the remander of the capillary vessels are distributed as side channels (fig. 3). These offshoots are purely endothelial in character and may be termed 'non-muscular or true capillaries.' The true capillaries anastomose freely with one another and finally rejoin the distal continuation of the a-v channel as it continues toward the venous end.

The two types of capillaries are more difficult to distinguish in fixed preparations because the most striking feature of identification is a functional one. A-v bridges in fixed normal tissues were characterized by containing a greater accumulation of blood cells than true capillaries.

Pattern in different forms and tissues

The number of permanently open capillaries, the a-v bridges, varies with different tissues according to the basal level of tissue activity. In addition, the ratio between the number of vessels of the muscular type as compared to that of the non-muscular type varies with each tissue. This depends upon the degree of fluctuation in activity which that tissue normally exhibits. In the skin, both in the frog and ear of the mouse, which may be regarded as having a constant level of activity, almost all of the minute vessels extending to the epithelial surface were found to consist of the a-v bridge type. In the nictitating membrane the two types of capillaries were seen in about equal numbers; in the mesentery the true capillaries were several times more numerous than a-v vessels; in striated muscle, where extreme fluctuations in nutritive demands occur, the a-v capillaries were relatively infrequent as compared to their abrupt capillary side branches which made up 75% to 90% of the vessels.

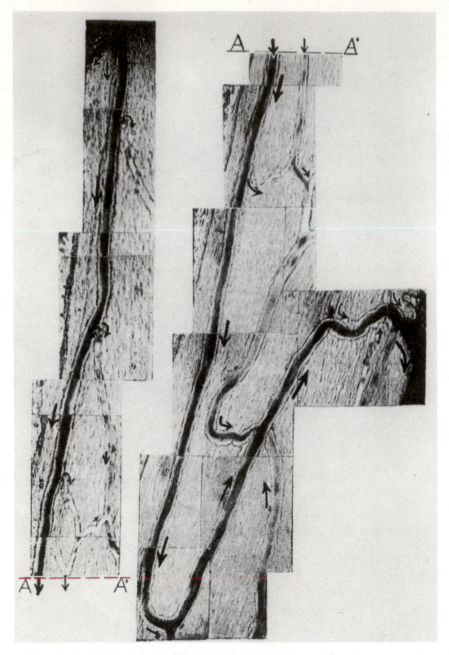

Fig. 3 Arteriole-venular bridge shown through its entire course from its arterial to its venous end. Note offshoots constituting the true capillaries. (Reconstructed by assembling from a motion picture film.) Low power.

480

Angle of capillary branching and its significance

An interesting feature of the capillary pattern is the characteristic manner in which the successive segments of the central vascular trunk distribute their capillary offshoots. There appears to be a direct correlation between the intensity of blood flow in the parent trunk and the manner in which the capillary offshoot leaves the central channel. At the arterial end, the offshoots were found to come off abruptly, curve sharply backward and continue for some distance in a contorted or spiral course (fig. 4 a). Further downstream, where the muscular coat begins to be scattered, the capillary offshoots come off at right angles and then take a sharp backward course (fig. 4 b). The flow of blood in the above-mentioned offshoots is suddenly and markedly slowed. This slowing can readily be ascribed to the peculiar angle of branching. As the blood continued through the central trunk toward the venous outlet, a gradual diminution in the rate of flow develops and is paralleled by the less and less acute angles at which the successive capillary branches leave the a-v vessel (fig. 4 c, d). The most distal portions became progressively a receiving channel and are joined by tributaries that approach the vessel at a gentle slope and drain into it (fig. 4 e).

The abrupt side branches of the arterioles possessed muscle cells about their proximal curved portion, but not elsewhere along the offshoot. This portion, therefore, can be considered as a precapillary, the muscle elements of which are in direct continuity with those of the parent arteriole. At the point of exit of the capillary branch, the wall of the arteriole was usually reenforced by a grouping of muscle cells about that side of the vessel where the branch leaves it.

*Endothelial valves at capillary exit on arterial portion
of a-v trunk*

A valve-like fold of endothelium is present at the point of capillary exit in those regions where the capillary offshoot leaves the arteriole and a-v vessels in a sharp backward angle.

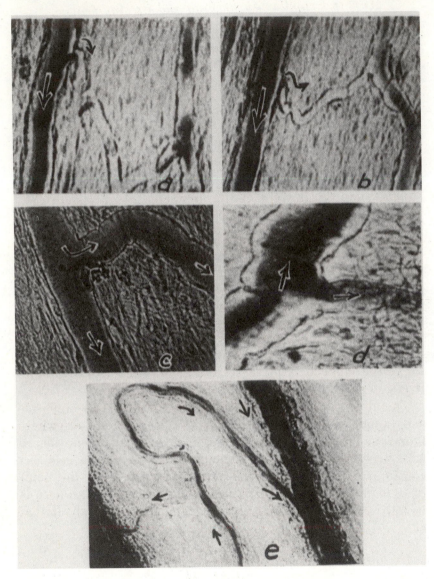

Fig. 4 Capillary offshoots from successive portions of the a-v bridge to
illustrate the progressive change in angle of branching from (a, b) close to
arteriolar source, through (c, d) in mid a-v region, to (e) where vessels fuse
at a gentle slope to form a venule. a, b, e, low power; c, d, medium power.
Mesentery of frog.

Two semi-rigid folds protrude into the lumen so that red cells, as they are swept by, are caught on the obstruction (fig. 5). The folds behave as an 'endothelial sphincter.' Movements of the a-v wall occur during periods of extended increase or decrease in blood flow through the vessel, and alter the degree to which the endothelial folds obstruct the orifice into the capillary offshoot. During a-v dilatation, the apposed, free edges of the endothelial folds were drawn further apart. This effected a wider passage for the entrance of blood into the capillary offshoot. The folds of the endothelial sphincter become more closely approximated when the parent trunk

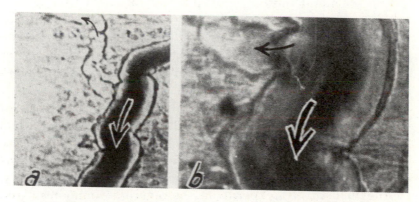

Fig. 5 Endothelial valves at point of exit of capillary offshoot on arterial end of a-v channel. a, low power; b, high power. Mesentery of mouse.

partially contracts and often the passage of blood cells into the capillary branch is completely prevented. In arterioles the partial closure was aided by muscle cells about the point of capillary exit.

Blood flow through capillaries

Freshly exposed tissues which have been disturbed as little as possible by handling tend to have a pale anemic color. Under such conditions, which may be considered as representative of the resting or basal level of the tissue, the circulation through the capillary bed occurred chiefly through the a-v bridges. The true capillaries were either collapsed or simply devoid of circulating blood cells.

No active increase in capillary caliber was seen in anemic tissues so long as no blood circulated through that vessel. Expansion of the a-v circulation into the empty true capillaries was effected experimentally in a number of ways. The flow of blood was diverted from the a-v vessel into the capillary branch by pinching off the parent vessel just below the point of exit of a capillary offshoot. A similar effect was obtained by repeated compression of the a-v bridge at the point where it was joined by an empty capillary. Alternate compression and release invoked a suction effect that drew a pulsating column of blood in from the arterial end. Thirdly, when the tissue adjacent to an empty capillary was mechanically irritated for 1 to 2 minutes with a microneedle, a slow trickle of fluid and subsequently of blood cells was initiated into the capillary.

The lumen of the narrowed capillary opens in a series of stages. A partial increase in width appeared first with a seepage of fluid into the capillary. No further opening of the lumen occurred if at this stage the connected arteriole was compressed so that no blood could enter into the capillary. In the undisturbed experiment, however, a number of red cells were deformed and squeezed into the contracted capillary. The distorted cells bobbed back and forth and, as they did so, the portion of the capillary tube, with which they had made direct contact during each pulsation, gradually opened up. This type of sporadic flow continued until the vessel as a whole was wide enough for the red cells to pass through without being excessively deformed.

Capillary diameter

Capillaries differ in width not only through variations in distension, but by consisting of a different number of endothelial cells in cross section. One vessel observed in a completely dilated state may actually be narrower than a neighboring undistended capillary simply because the wall of the first has fewer cells about its circumference. This was demonstrated by bringing the endothelial cell outlines into evidence with silver nitrate (10%), sprayed directly onto the vessel with a micropipette (fig. 6).

The most frequently used pathways, the a-v bridges, are the widest of the capillary vessels, with five to seven cells in cross section. The accessory side channels, the true capillaries, have but two to five cells about their circumference. Because of this discrepancy between two and five cells, the true capillaries show wide extremes in their normal width. After continued hyperemic blood flow, the larger of the true capillaries distend and approximate the diameter of the a-v vessels.

The true capillaries differ greatly in length. Short vessels, during the period in which they convey blood, have a nearly uniform diameter throughout their extent. In contrast, long capillaries become considerably wider on their venous side.

Long continued observations of undisturbed capillaries disclosed no sudden marked alterations in caliber. On the other hand, mechanical stimulation of the naked endothelial wall elicited, in both mammals and Amphibia, a definite localized thickening, wrinkling and indentation. The greatest endothelial response was obtained in the true naked capillaries. Responses were found to be more marked in capillaries of the frog than in the mouse. The indentation response becomes less and less evident as the endothelial tube is explored along its course toward the venous channels. A similar gradation in the magnitude of response is found in the various smooth muscle elements along the a-v channels. Perivascular smooth muscle cells in the arteriolar portions were most effective as contractile units. With a progressive loss in the typical spindle shape of these muscle cells along the a-v vessels, there was a corresponding decrease in their contractile effects. Contractile perivascular elements were conspicuously absent on true capillaries. With the transition to the small venule type (prevenule), fusiform smooth muscle ele-

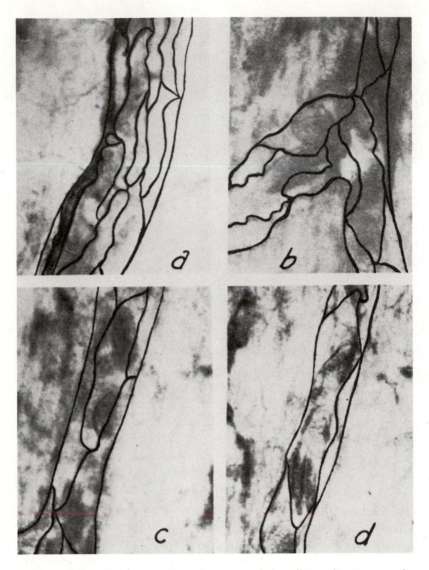

Fig. 6 Endothelial cell outlines demonstrated by silver nitrate sprayed on living capillary wall with micropipette. b, c, d are true capillaries; a is an a-v bridge. Medium power, mesentery of frog.

ments appeared again and were capable of indenting the underlying wall.

Influence of capillary tone

The normal true capillary possesses tone in that it behaves as a reversibly distensible tube. The presence of the tone must be ascribed to the endothelial cells that comprise its wall. Alterations in the tone (turgor) of the endothelium is one of the factors that influence capillary diameter. It was found that when the tissue was repeatedly irritated by mechanical prodding, the nearby capillary dilated although the blood pressure had not been changed. A similar dilatation was produced by re-routing venous blood so that it flowed in an opposite direction through the capillaries. This was done by compressing a venule with the side of a micro-needle just below the point of junction with a capillary vessel. Under this condition of temporary dilatation, the endothelium was found to be more pliable and less rigid than normal, and offered little resistance to distortion by the needle.

During the resting stage of activity, the true capillaries, both in the mouse and frog, maintained a relatively fixed diameter so long as blood continued to flow through them. Increased blood flow alone had little effect on capillary diameter. Likewise, loss of tone in vessels with no flow through them had no influence on capillary caliber. Vascular distension occurred only in capillaries which had blood circulating through them. Such evidence indicates that before the blood pressure had an effect on diameter, the endothelial wall previously must have been weakened by loss of its normal tone.

The removal of the factor responsible for the hyperemic flow was followed by a gradual slowing of the circulation through the a-v bridges and a slight narrowing of the vessel. In turn, the flow of blood through the capillary offshoots became sporadic and then gradually ceased. Those true capillaries, in which no blood was circulating and which were in good tone, narrowed over an extended period and were completely contracted within 15 to 40 minutes. Vessels whose tone was less marked remained open but, due to a change in the color of the lumen and vessel wall, gradually faded from view. It should be emphasized that capillaries with an active circulation were never seen to contract down so as to interrupt the flow of blood through them.

Local anemic and hyperemic states

The change from a resting to a more active vascular condition occurred spontaneously in a mesentery that had been exposed for about 30 to 80 minutes, and in the intact skin which had been unduly handled or warmed. Similar changes were induced by mild, prolonged local manipulation of the capillary bed and its surrounding tissue. In such cases a filling of the stagnant, true capillaries and a dilatation of those in the immediate vicinity of the focus of irritation occurred even when the pericapillary tissue alone was manipulated (fig. 7).

The outstanding vascular phenomena, that were involved in the change from an anemic to a hyperemic condition, occurred in the following sequence:

1. The blood cells became more closely packed and concentrated as they traversed the length of the a-v capillary and approached the venous end. The increased viscosity of the blood presented a higher venous resistance.

2. The normal capillary wall did not permit Congo red to pass out of the blood stream in quantities sufficient to stain the perivascular tissue. At this point, however, an increased outward passage of the dye was visible.

3. The circulation was temporarily slowed through the open a-v channels.

4. The pericapillary tissue became heavily stained by a more noticeable egression of Congo red from the blood stream.

5. The venous portion of the a-v bridges and small venules were the first to become somewhat distended.

6. Those arterioles that distributed blood to the capillaries in this area are dilated and, due to an increased propelling force, the capillaries became flushed and filled with blood.

7. Many new capillary side channels began to be opened.

8. Continued distension of the a-v wall widened the orifice between the endothelial folds interposed at the point of capillary exit, so that blood more easily entered the capillary side channels.

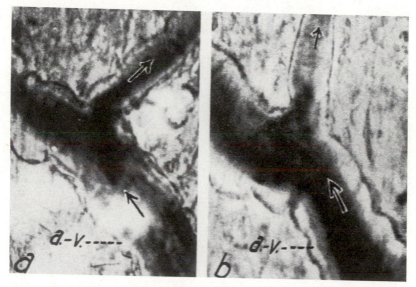

Fig. 7 Dilatation of a-v bridge and filling of true capillary branch following irritation of pericapillary tissue further distally along same vessel. a, before b, after manipulation. Medium power, mesentery of frog.

9. Finally, the continued rapid arteriolar flow introduced blood into all of the capillary channels.

An interesting detail here is the method whereby a circulation of blood was diverted into stagnant capillaries. When such a capillary was irritated, Congo red seeped through its wall indicating an increase in its permeability. This was followed by a slow movement of the entire column of blood until there was an active circulation through that vessel. One might therefore assume that, under normal conditions, an accumulation of metabolites about a stagnant capillary acts on the vessel wall by increasing its permeability. This in turn will be reflected by a movement of blood toward the region of increased permeability.

DISCUSSION

When the capillary bed is considered from an embryological viewpoint, the subdivision into two types of capillaries becomes apparent. Thoma (1893), Clark ('18), Chapman ('18), and Hughes ('35) have shown that in the embryo only those capillaries which had a vigorous flow of blood through them differentiated into arteries and veins. The other vessels either disappeared or persisted as capillaries. It is suggested that a similar type of differentiation may also occur in the capillary bed during its development. The extent of the transformation of the pericapillary elements would depend upon the intensity, type and duration of blood flow to which the vessel has been exposed. Vessels which were subjected to an active flow of long duration now possess specialized perivascular elements. Furthest advanced are the a-v bridges which are capable of acting as capillary vessels but are structurally more advanced than the undifferentiated true capillaries.

It is probable that even the adult capillary bed is not a fixed entity, its constituents being very labile structures. The nature of the perivascular elements may change with extended variations in the circulation through these small vessels. Clark and Clark ('35) followed in the rabbit's ear the development of muscular vessels out of undifferentiated endothelial tubes and described reversible changes in their distribution with variations in the blood flow through that tissue. The preponderance of a-v capillaries in tissues like the skin further demonstrates the effect of a blood flow, that is maintained at a certain level of intensity, upon the nature of the capillaries in that tissue.

The experiments of L. Hill ('21) can be offered as indirect evidence for the classification of capillaries into two groups.

He used the Roy and Graham-Brown apparatus for capillary pressure and found two groups of results. The gradual application of pressure interrupted the flow first through the side channels "but it continued through the most direct pathway connecting arterioles with venules, wherein the velocity was greatest to start with." Evidence like that of Kahn and Pollack ('31) and Fields ('36), in which two kinds of contractile response were obtained following electrical stimulation, likewise substantiates the existence of two types of capillaries.

Hughes ('37) found a direct relationship between the intensity of blood flow and the diameter of the embryonic capillaries. The stimulus of the blood flow acted to increase the number of endothelial cells that formed the capillary. It was therefore not surprising to find that the so-called normal diameter of adult true capillaries varied with different vessels, because of this fact alone. This makes it difficult to evaluate the comparative degree of dilatation of contraction of neighboring capillaries by simple observation.

The rate of blood flow also has a direct influence on the manner in which the side branches leave the central trunk. Roux (1895) and Thoma (1893) found that the angle at which branches leave the main trunk can be related to the fluid friction generated in such a system. Such a relationship was found along the central trunk from arteriole to venule in both the frog and mouse. The progressive slowing of blood flow is accompanied by a change in the manner and angle at which the capillary offshoots leave the arteriole and a-v vessels.

Most of the true capillaries are abrupt side branches and as such can be effectively isolated from the circulation through the true capillaries. Jacobi ('20) also found that a majority of the capillaries are at acute angles and contain no blood most of the time. The abrupt manner of branching introduces a set of endothelial obstructions or folds at the point of junction. These also act to cut off the true capillaries from the circulation. Klemensiewcz ('21) pointed out the sphincter-like closure of the capillary junction with the pre-capillary during partial contraction of the parent trunk.

The central vascular trunk is featured by two possible contractile elements, endothelium and smooth muscle, whose distribution counterbalances one against the other. The terminal arterioles are narrower than the succeeding capillaries because of the presence of well-developed muscle cells in their walls. In this portion of the vascular tree, the contractile effect of the endothelium is relatively unimportant. Endothelium is contractile but this is effective only within certain limits. Where the blood pressure is high, as in small arterioles and precapillaries, endothelium is supplemented by well-developed smooth muscle cells. Further distally, with a diminution in intensity of blood flow and a decline in the number and character of the pericapillary smooth muscle elements, the endothelium becomes a more potent factor. Finally, in the true capillary side branches the endothelium remains as the sole contractile element.

The changes in capillary diameter that do occur are slow and passive. What is the mechanism underlying these gradual changes in diameter? It appears that three factors, acting separately or together are concerned: tone of endothelium, inherent elasticity of endothelium, and intercapillary pressure. The relative amount of tone was interpreted and measured by the reaction of the endothelium to prodding and manipulation. It was thus shown that endothelial tone fluctuates with alterations in the activity of the tissues and the resulting accumulation of metabolites in that area. Clark and Clark ('35) found a similar change in endothelial 'elasticity' with dilatation of the capillaries.

The interplay of two opposing factors, intracapillary pressure and endothelial tone, produced varying results depending upon changes in either or both of these factors. Dilatation was the result of poor tone accompanied by an increased or maintained intracapillary pressure. Closure of the capillary lumen was a result of ischemia following a period of active circulation. The a-v blood flow is sufficient to nourish the

tissues during the ischemic state. The presence of good tone
and diminished intracapillary pressure in the empty true
capillaries resulted in a gradual narrowing of these vessels
over a period of 15 to 30 minutes. Similar, drawn out contractions are reported by Sandison ('32), and Clark and
Clark ('35) in the rabbit's ear. A somewhat analogous situation is reported by Rous and Gilding ('29) who found that
after ischemia induced by bleeding, the deprivation of blood
invokes a local vaso-constriction.

Interpretation of mechanism of hyperemic capillary flow

When blood is pumped under low pressure into the
elastic capillary, the blood will be propelled in a forward
direction so long as the resistance ahead of the tube is not
excessively high. When the pressure is raised and an increased amount of blood is pumped into that vessel, there will
be a distinct tendency for the circulating fluid to distend that
tube. Normally, the pressure in the small arterioles is maintained at a level just sufficient to overcome the resistance of
the vascular tree ahead (in the venous end of a-v vessels and
prevenules). This main channel is used exclusively so long
as the traffic ahead is not too congested. With increased
venous congestion, the side pathways are opened and the flow
is redistributed.

Two effects of local disturbances, such as arise through
mechanical irritation, were seen during the change into a
hyperemic circulation. An increased capillary permeability
develops soon after the onset of the irritation and results in
a concentration of the blood elements as they traverse the
vessel toward the venous end. Within 3 to 5 seconds a 'reflex'
dilatation of the feeding arteriole ensues. Whether the increased venous resistance or the tissue irritation act separately or together to produce the arteriolar dilatation is not
clear.

The blood, which now enters the a-v bridge under an increased propelling force, fills the vessel to capacity and not
only distends it, but, in addition, spurts out through the weak

points in its wall, the numerous orifices into the capillary offshoots. These factors, combined with the concurrent movement apart of the endothelial folds at the entrance into the capillary offshoots, enhance the flow of blood into the hitherto stagnant, subsidiary channels, the true capillaries.

The reverse occurred as follows: With a diminution in the resistance of the venous vessels, the arterial pressure was again free to be translated into the forward propulsion of the blood. The removal of the cause of irritation was rapidly followed by a diminished arteriolar flow. In turn, the distended elastic endothelium of the a-v vessels slowly thickened and, as the vessel became narrowed, the endothelial folds at the entrance to the capillary side channels were more closely approximated. The closure of these points of exit cut off the circulation from the true capillaries. Within 5 to 6 minutes only the a-v bridges contain a continuous flow of blood and the circulation is again of the basal or resting type.

LITERATURE CITED

CHAPMAN, W. B. 1918 Effect of the heart beat upon development of the vascular system in the chick. Am. J. Anat., vol. 23, p. 175.

CLARK, E. R. 1918 Studies on growth of blood vessels in the tail of frog larva by observation and experiment on living animals. Am. J. Anat., vol. 23, p. 37.

CLARK, E. R., AND E. L. CLARK 1935 Observations on changes in blood vascular endothelium in the living animal. Am. J. Anat., vol. 57, p. 385.

FIELDS, M. E. 1936 Reaction of the blood capillaries of frog and rat to mechanical and electrical stimulation. Skand. Arch. f. Physiol., Bd. 72, S. 175.

HILL, L. 1921 Capillary pressure. II. Proc. Physiol. Soc., J. Physiol., vol. 54, p. XCIII.

HUGHES, A. F. W. 1935 Studies on area vasculosa of embryo chick. I. Differentiation of vitelline arteries. J. Anat., vol. 70, p. 76.

———— 1937 II. The influence of the circulation on the diameter of the vessels. J. Anat., vol. 72, p. 1.

JACOBI, W. 1920 Beobachtungen am peripheren Gefässaparat unter lokaler Beeinflussung desselben durch pharmokologische Agentien. Arch. f. exp. Path. u. Pharm., Bd. 86, S. 49.

KAHN, R. H., AND F. POLLACK 1931 Die aktive Verengerung des lumens der Capillaren Blutgefässe. Pfluger's Arch. ges. Physiol., Bd. 226, S. 799.

KLEMENSIEWCZ, R. 1921 Verfahren und Einrichtungen zur Beobachtung des Blutstromes am Kaltblütern, in E. Abderhalden's Handbuch der biologischen Arbeitsmethoden. Abth. 5, Teil 4, S. 1.

ROUS, P., AND H. P. GILDING 1929 Studies on tissue maintenance. III. Persisting bloodlessness after functional ischemia. J. Exp. Med., vol. 50, p. 471.

ROUX, W. 1895 Die Bedeutung der Ablenkung des Arterien systems bei der Astabgabe. Jena. Zeit. f. Naturwiss., Bd. 13, S. 321.

SANDISON, J. C. 1932 Contraction of blood vessels and observations on circulation in the traparent chamber in the rabbit's ear. Anat. Rec., vol. 54, p. 105.

THOMA, R. 1893 Untersuchungen über die Histogenese und Histomechanik des Gefässesystems, Stuttgart, F. Enke.

ZWEIFACH, B. W. 1937 a The structure and reactions of the small blood vessels in amphibia. Am. J. Anat., vol. 60, p. 473.

ZWEIFACH, B. W., AND C. E. KOSSMANN 1937 b Micromanipulation of small blood vessels in the mouse. Am. J. Physiol., vol. 120, p. 23.

THE ANATOMICAL RECORD, VOL. 73, NO. 4

Reprinted from *Am. J. Anat.*, **66**(1), 1–49 (1940)

MICROSCOPIC OBSERVATIONS ON THE EXTRA-ENDOTHELIAL CELLS OF LIVING MAMMALIAN BLOOD VESSELS [1]

ELIOT R. CLARK AND ELEANOR LINTON CLARK

Department of Anatomy, University of Pennsylvania, Philadelphia

TWENTY FIGURES

INTRODUCTION

The growth of new blood vessels in the living mammal, as observed in transparent chambers installed in the ears of rabbits, has been studied microscopically and described in detail (Sandison, '28; Clark et al., '31; Clark and Clark, '39). Briefly, it was found that new capillaries arose as endothelial outgrowths from preexisting vascular endothelium, which advanced as blindly ending sprouts, anastomosed with neighboring sprouts to form loops and continued to advance as a plexus with a growing edge of new sprouts. Although the pattern of the new vascular network in each chamber, like that of the intact ear, was different, in standard round table chambers of uniform size and controlled thickness, the tempo at which new capillaries entered the observation space (average of 7 days after the operation) and the rate at which they advanced across it (0.2 to 0.65 mm. per diem) were relatively uniform.

The primitive form of the growing vascular network was at first that of an indifferent capillary plexus but as it continued to advance the older portions of the plexus near the table edge soon showed differentiation of vessels receiving a greater supply and drainage into arterioles and venules. Simultaneously, many of the intervening capillaries retracted and disappeared. Vascularization of the table space was usually complete at 2 to 3 weeks after the operation when the sprouts from opposite sides of the table met and anastomosed.

[1] With the support of grants from the Rockefeller Foundation and (later) from the Penrose Fund of the American Philosophical Society.

1

THE AMERICAN JOURNAL OF ANATOMY, VOL. 66, NO. 1
JANUARY, 1940

Further differentiation continued for a few days through enlargement of those new arterioles and venules more favorably placed as to blood flow into arteries and veins and through the further reduction of surplus capillaries by retraction, after which the 'adult' plexus remained relatively stable provided the chamber was kept free from mechanical insults, irritation and excessive temperature changes. However, the blood vascular endothelium was found to be extremely labile and relatively slight mechanical and thermal stimuli were observed to result in the sending out of new capillary sprouts and the subsequent remodelling of completely vascularized areas.

The process by which new blood vessels invade a small hole artificially made in the ear of an adult rabbit by the sending out of endothelial sprouts which anastomose to form a capillary plexus and the subsequent differentiation of arteries and veins from the indifferent capillary network with the simultaneous reduction of surplus capillaries is essentially the same as that observed for the growth of capillaries in the transparent tails of amphibian larvae (Clark, '18), in injected embryos and in the yolk sac of the chick (Evans, '09; Thoma, 1893). The same process of blood vessel growth was also observed to take place in transparent chambers installed in the ears of dogs (Moore, '36). Moreover, microscopic studies of regenerating blood vessels in living mammals showed them to resemble the growing vessels of amphibian larvae in their specificity, cytological appearance, and in the behavior of their endothelium (Clark and Clark, '39).

The chief differences noted between the developing blood vessels of amphibian larvae and the regenerating mammalian vessels were: the greater richness of the new vascular network in the mammal and the greater specialization of mammalian arteries both in regard to the nature and number of their extra-endothelial cells and in their contractile powers. The observations reported here embody chiefly the results of microscopic studies in the living rabbit of the development of extra-endothelial cells on the walls of peripheral blood vessels and of the behavior and changes of these cells on arteries, veins and capillaries in response to circulatory conditions.

METHOD

The 'round table' chamber was used in the present study. This is the type in which a celluloid table 0.65 cm. in diameter is inserted in a hole cut clear through the ear at the time of operation, leaving a space of known and controlled thickness, enclosed between the celluloid base and mica cover slip, into which the new blood vessels advance as outgrowths from preformed vessels around the periphery in the manner already described (Clark et al., '31). The four small celluloid buffers glued to the table which determine the depth of the observation space varied from 40 μ to 75 μ in the various chambers studied. The thinner chambers (40 μ to 50 μ) were best adapted for observing fine details of individual cells with the oil immersion lens while the thicker ones proved to be more favorable for the formation of larger arteries and for the regeneration of nerves resulting in the development of contractility in regenerated arteries (Clark, Clark and Williams, '34). The details of the construction of the chambers have already been given (Clark et al., '30; Varian, '31) as well as the method of handling the rabbits during and between observations (Clark, Sandison and Hou, '31). The detached splints, which protect the chambers from injuries and strains were employed in the specimens used for these studies (Clark and Clark, '32 b).

DEVELOPMENT OF EXTRA ENDOTHELIAL CELLS

Although the newly formed capillaries in the transparent chambers consisted at first of simple endothelium, extra-endothelial cells appeared on their walls within 24 hours of their first appearance—more speedily than was the case in the growing vessels of amphibian larvae—frequently even before the onset of circulation through them. During the stage of vascular invasion of the table area, the growing edge of the advancing plexus consisted of a plexus of indifferent capillaries with a border of blindly ending capillary sprouts. In the older regions near the table edge a beginning differentiation into arterioles and venules of capillaries receiving a greater supplying or draining blood flow, was observed after 48 hours. Changes such as straightening of their course, increase in diameter and, on the arterial side, thickening of the endothelial wall were all characteristic of a similar differentiation in the vessels of the tadpole's tail (Clark, '18). In addition, in the regenerating mammalian vessels, an increase in extra-endothelial cells occurred followed by a change in their form and arrangement so that they soon formed a continuous layer indistinguishable from the muscular walls of arteries present in the original ear tissue.

Figure 1 shows the characteristic differences of arterioles, capillaries and venules in a plexus of regenerated vessels 3 months after their first appearance as an indifferent capillary plexus. In this figure and also in the photographs (fig. 2) it will be seen that the venules are wider than the capillaries but that their walls are quite similar, while the arterioles are narrower than venules and as narrow as or even narrower than capillaries but that their walls differ in the number, arrangement and form of the extra-endothelial cells. Arteries in the completely vascularized chambers, which received the main blood supply for the table area enlarged to a wider caliber than the capillaries and venules but remained conspicuously narrower than veins of comparable importance. In the living animal, differences in the circulation are also distinguishing marks for the various types of vessels since the blood flow is steady and rapid in the arteries and arterioles, when they are not contracting, steady but slower in the veins and slow with frequent hesitations and reversals in the capillaries.

The character of the various types of extra-endothelial cells and the manner in which they become attached to the vessel wall have been studied in the transparent tails of amphibian larvae (Clark and Clark, '25), where the origin of the two most common types of extra-endothelial cells present on amphibian vessels was followed by prolonged observation in the living. Cells of the first type—the chromatophores— were seen to wrap themselves around the blood vessels in the same manner observed in the vessels of Fundulus (Loeb, 1893; Stockard, '15). The other type of adventitial cell, which

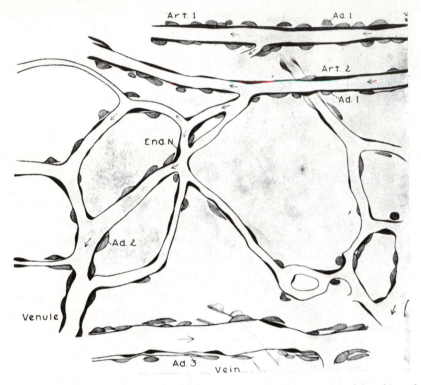

Fig. 1   Newly formed plexus of living vessels showing two arterioles (Art. 1, Art. 2), capillaries, venule and vein with types of extra-endothelial cells on each. Ad. 1, rounded cells (muscle) on wall of arteriole. Ad. 2, longitudinally arranged adventitial cells on capillary and venule. Ad. 3, secondary longitudinal layer of cells outside vein. Leitz drawing eye-piece. × 315.

appears to be identical with the adventitial cells on capillaries and venules of mammals, was found to be derived from stellate connective tissue cells which were seen to come in contact with growing and actively circulating capillaries and to adhere to their outer walls. In a number of cases, mitosis of a connective tissue cell was observed following which one of the daughter cells became attached to a capillary, with its long axis parallel with the vessel wall where it remained as an adventitial cell, while the other cell moved away and persisted as a typical stellate cell. In larvae of Hyla pickeringii the formation, character and behavior of this second type of adventitial cell, which has been called the 'Rouget cell' by Vimtrup ('22) could be followed with great ease owing to the sparsity of chromatophores and the absence of the melanophores which wrapped around the vessels of other amphibian forms and of Fundulus.

In the case of the regenerating mammalian vessels as seen in the transparent chambers, although the endothelial nuclei, the capillary walls and the adventitial cells on the sides of the walls could all be clearly seen, the mode of development of the latter was more difficult to follow, owing to the relative density of the intervascular tissue than was the case in the tadpole's tail. However, in the case of the thinner chambers (40 μ to 50 μ in depth) immobilized by detached splints, migration of connective tissue cells and formation of fibers was delayed and the new capillaries grew out into a region of fibrin and sparsely distributed blood cells in which their tips and the cytological details of their walls were clearly visible. In such specimens it was possible on many different occasions to observe individual wandering cells of various types continuously and to see fibroblasts approach the exterior of a new capillary, become attached to its wall where they remained as advantitial cells, which could be identified

Fig. 2 Photomicrographs of newly formed living blood vessels showing appearance and distribution of extra-endothelial cells on capillaries, veins and arterioles. a. Capillary plexus with scanty flow, a few longitudinal adventitial cells (Ad.). E.N., endothelial nucleus. b. Newly formed arteriole with continuous wall of extra-endothelial cells, chiefly rounded muscle cells (Mus.). c. Capillary and terminal portion of arteriole showing similarity of caliber and difference in wall. Mus., muscle cell on arteriole—transition to longitudinal adventitial cells at distal (upper) end. d. Capillaries with fast flow in larger vessel. Ad., typical adventitial cell. e. Venule. Wide caliber as compared with capillaries and arterioles—longitudinally arranged adventitial cells. f. Venule with sparsely distributed adventitial cells, Ad. E. N., endothelial nucleus; M., macrophage. a.c.d. × 480. b. × 333. e. f. × 491.

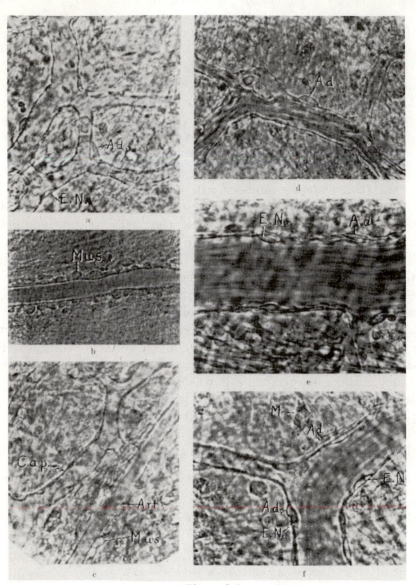

Figure 2

for many hours and frequently for days. This process has been described and illustrated in a recent publication (Clark and Clark, '39).

A fibroblast which formed an adventitial cell in this manner was observed to line up with its long axis parallel to the vessel wall and with its cell processes extending longitudinally along the wall (fig. 1, Ad. 2). For the first few hours it retained its original form and appeared to adhere to the capillary mainly by means of its two processes, since a space was usually present between the cell body and the vessel wall. On succeeding days it became flatter and more closely applied to the endothelium while its processes became shorter (fig. 1, Ad. 1 and fig. 12). Such cells, for the first few days were capable of slow amoeboid motion. The process of attachment of fibroblasts to the outer walls of blood vessels occurred most rapidly in the stage of active formation of capillaries.

The numbers of adventitial cells and the speed with which they became attached to new blood vessels varied with the numbers of fibroblasts present in the intervascular tissue. In chambers in which a large number of connective tissue cells migrated into the table space simultaneously with the invasion of new capillary sprouts, fibroblasts adhered to the walls of growing vessels soon after their formation, often before circulation in them had started and in greater numbers than was the case in the thin immobilized chambers in which emigration of fibroblasts was delayed and their numbers less. In specimens of the latter kind in which outside fibroblasts were scarce, new capillaries were seen to extend for a considerable distance with the addition of only a few extra-endothelial cells located at infrequent intervals with wide gaps of naked endothelium between them. Later, coincident with the invasion of a larger number of fibroblasts at the table edge the vessels in this region were seen to acquire a great number of extra-endothelial cells within 24 hours. As the 'army' of fibroblasts continued to advance toward the center of the table in the interstices of the vascular plexus, the numbers of adventitial cells increased progressively in the more distal vessels.

In some instances of chambers which were protected from mechanical stresses and in which emigration of fibroblasts and connective tissue formation was especially slow (Clark and Clark, '39), relatively few fibroblasts reached the central area of the table and in this region a number of capillaries with only a very few adventitial cells persisted for several months, during which time some of them increased to the size of veins without showing an appreciable increase in the number of their extra-endothelial cells (fig. 2f and fig. 3).

The extra-endothelial cells, whose formation from fibroblasts which adhered to the walls of young capillaries was observed microscopically in the living mammal, were identical in appearance with the adventitial cells (other than chromatophores) on the vessels of Amphibia whose development from stellate connective tissue cells was watched in living tadpoles (Clark and Clark, '25).

EXTRA-ENDOTHELIAL CELLS ON CAPILLARIES AND VENULES

At first the newly acquired adventitial cells on young mammalian blood vessels were, as a rule, sparsely and somewhat irregularly distributed. As already mentioned their numbers increased during the first month by the adherence of new fibroblasts to the vessel walls in chambers or in regions into which such cells migrated in large numbers. The further development and eventual fate of the extra-endothelial cells depended upon the fate of the individual vessel, which might continue as a capillary, retrogress, or become part of a new vein or artery. Moreover, at a later date the vessel might at times undergo a further change from vein to artery, from artery to vein or from either back to capillary. All of these changes in vascular size and form were accompanied by changes in the extra-endothelial cells and were found to be dependent upon changes in circulation and pressure.

When the same region of blood vessels was followed in daily microscopic observations, the circulation in the capillaries was seen to be remarkably variable, subject to frequent reversals in direction of the current while intervals of relatively steady flow were interspersed with periods of stasis, plasma skimming, or temporary absence of flow with the vessels remaining open and filled with plasma (fig. 2a and c).

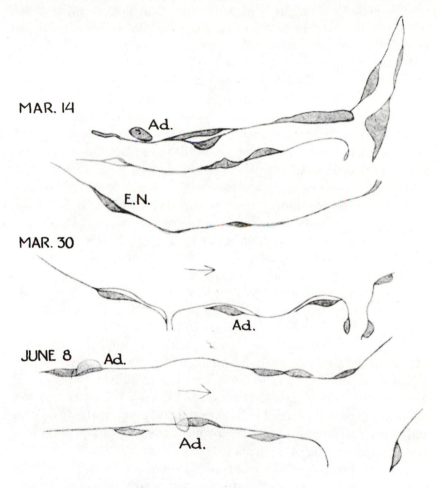

Fig. 3 Series of records of the same blood vessel over a period of months. Vessel which was a growing capillary March 14 enlarged to venule March 30. Ad., longitudinally arranged adventitial cells (lighter shading), changed position on wall but showed little increase in number. E.N., endothelial nuclei (deeper shading). Leitz drawing eye-piece. × 560.

In most of the new vessels which remained as capillaries for months the number of adventitial cells remained fairly constant and, after the first week when the newly acquired extra-endothelial cells were slightly amoeboid, they frequently could be located day after day in the same position on the wall (fig. 4, cells A and B). On capillaries which received a relatively steady supply of blood flow for several succeeding days an occasional increase in the number of adventitial cells by mitotic division was observed (fig. 5). At the beginning of division the previously flattened adventitial cell was seen to withdraw its processes, round up and separate into two cells which remained swollen for varying lengths of time (figs. 5 and 6). Following the division the daughter cells moved apart and again flattened out on the capillary wall where they remained as typical adventitial cells.

In many instances capillaries which were observed to receive a moderate blood supply for days or weeks, during which period their adventitial cells remained unchanged or increased through occasional mitotic division, later remained non-circulating for some time. The absence of circulation was followed by a gradual narrowing of the capillary lumen which was accompanied by a pulling away of the endothelium from the adventitial cells, leaving a space (fig. 5, April 9 and fig. 8, March 30, cell A). If the circulation returned on succeeding days the capillary again widened slightly and the extra-endothelial cells then appeared as typical adventitial cells closely applied to the outside of the capillary wall (fig. 5, May 13). If the circulation remained scanty or absent in the capillary, the adventitial cells were seen to separate from the wall still further and at times to become completely detached and disappear (fig. 4, cell B).

A more prolonged decrease or absence of circulation was followed by further narrowing of the capillary until it became solid, separated into two portions which then retracted in the manner previously described (Clark, '18; Sandison, '28). This was the case in the capillary shown in figure 4, which retracted on the day following the record shown on

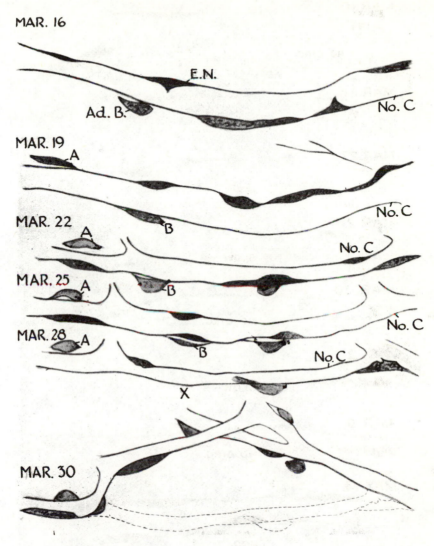

Fig. 4   Series of records of the same capillary over a period of 2 weeks during which circulation diminished. The same adventitial cells (A and B) located in same position on wall on successive days. March 16–March 25. On March 28 cell B became detached and disappeared (X). On March 29 capillary retracted. Following increased circulation, March 30, new capillaries were sent out from two ends. Dotted line marks position of former capillary. Leitz drawing eye-piece. × 560.

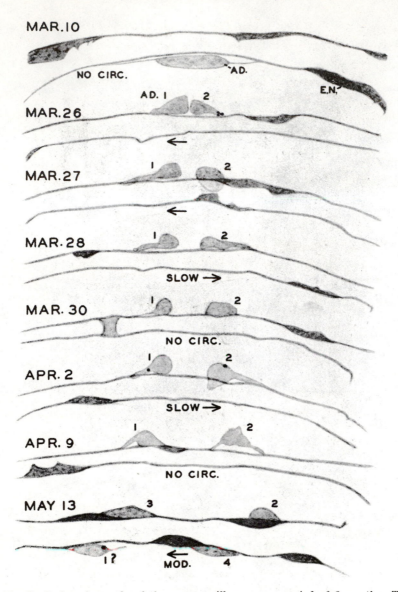

Fig. 5 Series of records of the same capillary over a period of 2 months. The one adventitial cell (Ad.) present on this stretch of vessel March 10 moved to the opposite side of a vessel and divided, after which the daughter cells, 1 and 2, were identified in the same location for a month. Later—May 13—following a slight increase in circulation two new cells (3 and 4) appeared on the wall. Leitz drawing eye-piece. × 672.

March 28. After a period of increased circulation in the two formerly connected vessels, two new capillary sprouts were sent out which anastomosed in a different location from that occupied by the original capillary (fig. 4, March 30). Retraction of capillaries took place more rapidly in growing and in newly formed vascular networks than was the case in more stable plexuses a month or two later. In the former case, the vessel

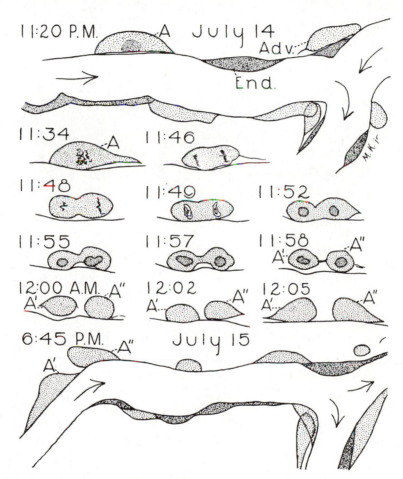

Fig. 6 Mitosis of an adventitial cell (A) on a capillary. Daughter cells a' and a" had moved a short distance on following day (July 15). Leitz drawing eye-piece. × 672.

narrowed and the endothelium was withdrawn into the connecting vessels before the disappearance of adventitial cells present on its wall. Thus in figure 7 the adventitial cell on capillary B could be identified in the tissue on the day after the capillary to which it had been attached, had retracted completely and

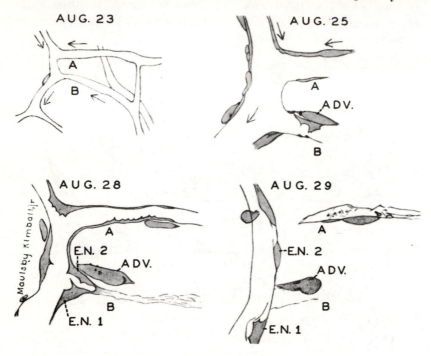

Fig. 7 Series of records showing disappearance of two vessels (A and B) of a capillary plexus. August 23, low power sketch of plexus, × 135. August 28, capillary B retracting, adventitial cell (Adv.) separating from wall. August 29, capillary A separated from former connection. Capillary B retracted—adventitial cell isolated in tissue. Leitz drawing eye-piece. × 630. (August 25–29).

its endothelial nucleus had been reincorporated in the wall of the parent vessel (fig. 7, August 28, 29).

Other capillaries which received an increased blood flow, which continued for several days, were seen to enlarge and become venules or parts of veins, depending upon the amount of flow and upon their location with regard to connecting

THE AMERICAN JOURNAL OF ANATOMY, VOL. 66, NO. 1

paths of drainage. In certain stable chambers, in which the table area was especially protected from mechanical stresses and in which the migration of fibroblasts was delayed and their numbers diminished, certain capillaries were seen to enlarge into veins without any appreciable addition of extra-endothelial cells for weeks or even months (fig. 2f and fig. 3). In most cases, however, the change from capillary to vein or venule which involved a greater and more steady blood flow, an increase in caliber and a straightening of the course was accompanied by an increase in the number of adventitial cells which were derived in part from fibroblasts and in part by division of cells already present (figs. 5, 6). In figure 8 the history of a vessel is recorded from its beginning as a sprout (March 13) for a period of 3 months. During the first 2 months it remained a capillary and in the latter part of this period, following a time of diminished flow, it grew narrower and lost one of its three adventitial cells, while the other two became partially detached from the wall (March 30–April 9). Following a subsequent increase in circulation the capillary enlarged and became part of a vein and soon thereafter acquired a few new adventitial cells (May 3, June 8).

The extra-endothelial cells which developed on venules and veins in the regenerated vascular network retained the same longitudinal arrangement characteristic of the adventitial cells of capillaries. Around some of the larger veins a capsule-like frame-work of connective tissue was seen to form outside the layer of adventitial cells. In one such specimen a large vein, which had acquired a connective tissue capsule, persisted for several months unchanged. Following a mechanical disturbance of the chamber area much of the blood flow was diverted from this vessel into other channels. The vein responded to the circulatory change by shrinking to half its former caliber, while the connective tissue capsule persisted, outlining the former borders of the vessel and leaving a clear 'shrinkage space' outside the narrowed vein (Clark and Clark, '37). Scattered adventitial cells of the typical longitudinal kind remained on the wall of the narrowed vein.

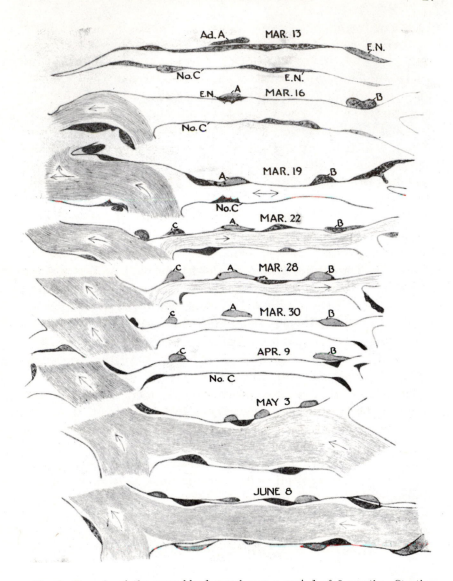

Fig. 8 Records of the same blood vessel over a period of 3 months. Starting as a capillary sprout (March 13) with one adventitial cell (Ad. A.) the vessel remained a capillary for 2 months. During the first week (March 16–March 22) two new adventitial cells (B and C) adhered to the wall. The three cells remained in approximately the same position for 10 days. March 30–April 9, flow through vessel diminished and one of the cells (A) disappeared. Later the circulation through the vessel increased, the capillary enlarged and became a venule and new adventitial cells appeared (May 30–June 8). Leitz drawing eye-piece. × 420.

According to our observations and those of other workers in this laboratory which involved studying the same vessels day after day in many different chambers for the past 10 years, the adventitial cells on capillaries and venules remained inert and were never seen to contract. In the case of capillaries and venules which temporarily narrowed passively, following changes in circulation, or which grew narrower gradually following several hours or days of diminished flow, a space appeared between the endothelium and the adventitial cells. The same thing was true of the adventitial cells present on the original capillaries and venules of the ear as seen in the 'preformed tissue' chambers.

In the original ear vessels, observed in 'preformed tissue' chambers certain of the larger veins which possessed smooth muscle cells in addition to the typical adventitial cells were observed to undergo active spontaneous contractions. They were found to be veins which received a large supply of arterial blood from a number of arterio-venous anastomoses (Clark and Clark, '34 a). Although the formation of new arterio-venous anastomoses has been observed repeatedly in the 'round table' chambers some of which acquired a nerve supply and displayed the same kind of active contractility seen in the preformed vessels (Clark and Clark, '34 b), active contractions of regenerated veins have not yet been seen. The new veins which develop in the limited area of the table are seldom as large as those in which contractility was observed in the case of preformed vessels and although several arterio-venous anastomoses from the same artery have been observed, the clusters of A.V.A.'s which frequently empty into the same vein in the preformed tissue have not developed in the regenerated plexuses up to the present.

EXTRA-ENDOTHELIAL CELLS ON ARTERIOLES AND ARTERIES

In the case of capillaries of the newly formed network which were so located as to receive an increased blood flow continuously, from supplying arteries outside the table area, the changes in the vessel walls were more striking than in the case of vessels which continued as capillaries or which were incorporated into the venous drainage paths. The first changes noted in capillaries of a new plexus so placed as to receive an arterial supply was straightening of their course, visible thickening of the endothelium, increased tonicity and strength of the wall, as evidenced by the maintenance of a uniformly narrower caliber than in vessels receiving the same amount of blood of the return stream and by the greater pressure required to force erythrocytes through their walls as compared with the venous capillaries or with the same vessels before this change had taken place (Sandison, '28; Clark et al., '31). This early change in the walls of arterial capillaries frequently occurred within 24 hours after their formation. The adventitial cells of such capillaries although their numbers increased to some extent, retained their longitudinal arrangement. These differences between the arterial capillaries and the wider thinner walled capillaries and venules which they supply are the same as those noted between the arterial and venous channels in the tadpole's tail.

Following the early changes from an indifferent capillary to an arterial capillary an increasing amount of flow and greater pressure in vessels which became the main pathways of blood supply to the new plexus resulted in still further changes. Such vessels continued to become straighter and to lose more of their branches, while the cells on their walls increased rapidly both by addition of connective tissue cells and by mitotic division of cells already present (figs. 9 and 10). In addition, within a short time (24 to 48 hours) after the increase in flow through such a vessel, the extra-endothelial cells were observed to undergo changes both in form and arrangement. The flattened, elongated adventitial cells, with processes extending parallel with the vessel wall, were seen to become rounder and more compact and to change their cell axis from longitudinal to transverse with their cell processes extending around the vessel wall. Figure 11 illustrates such a transformation in a single cell, watched continuously in the living, from a longitudinally oriented adventitial cell to a

THE AMERICAN JOURNAL OF ANATOMY, VOL. 66, NO. 1

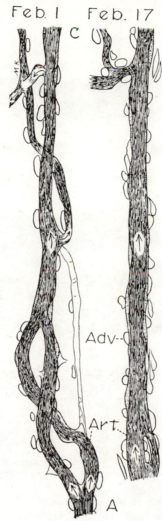

Fig. 9   Records showing development of an arteriole from a capillary plexus. The stretch A–C, February 1, became a single vessel February 17 by straightening of course receiving the greatest flow and retraction or disappearance of branches. Adventitial cells on new arteriole became more numerous. Leitz drawing eye-piece. × 420.

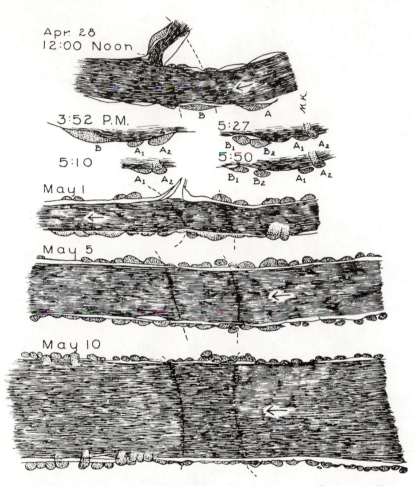

Fig. 10 Series of records of the development of an artery. Shows rounding up and division of two of the longitudinally arranged adventitial cells present on the original arterial capillary (April 28). Later records (May 1–May 10) show increase in caliber of vessel, increase in numbers of adventitial cells and change to rounded form and circular arrangement characteristic of smooth muscle cells. Dotted lines show the same region of the vessel on successive days. Leitz drawing eye-piece. × 285.

round muscle cell. Coincident with the change in cell form and position the extra-endothelial cells on arterioles became more refractile. The process just described, by which new arterioles formed from capillaries, commenced in the older

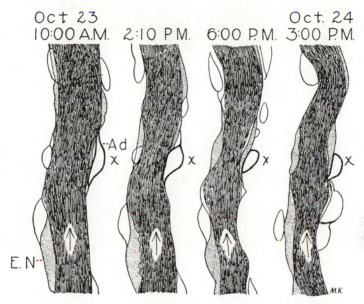

Fig. 11 Successive records of the same stretch of a developing arteriole showing transformation of a single longitudinally arranged adventitial cell (Ad. X) into a rounded circularly arranged cell. E.N., endothelial nucleus (shaded). Leitz drawing eye-piece. × 630.

portions of the new network, near the edge of the table and progressed distally toward the younger regions in the center. The increase in extra-endothelial cells on new arterioles and their change to a more specialized type of cell took place rapidly since a continuous layer of outside cells was usually seen to form within 6 days or less (fig. 12).

Fig. 12 Series of records of the same vessel showing transformation of a capillary into an arteriole with accompanying increase in numbers and change in form of extra-endothelial cells. E.N., endothelial nucleus (solid black). F.B., fibroblasts (dotted) approaching and adhering to vessel wall. Adv. 1, elongated adventitial cells recently formed from fibroblasts. Adv. 2, older adventitial cells, some of them acquiring circular orientation. Adv. 3, circularly arranged adventitial cells characteristic of muscle cells on arterial wall. Leitz drawing eye-piece. × 285.

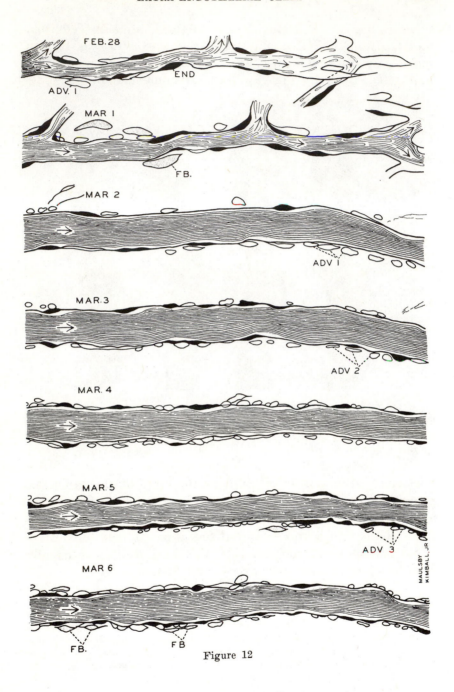

Figure 12

When the same stretch of a developing artery was watched continuously, with camera lucida records of the individual extra-endothelial cells, the increase was seen to take place by the addition of fibroblasts and by mitotic division of some of the cells followed by changes in the form and arrangement of the cells. However, owing to the great number of cells involved, the possibility that some of the new cells might have been derived by migration of muscle cells from connecting preformed arteries at the table edge could not be excluded. Since observations of the region at the table edge were carried out repeatedly without disclosing any such migration it seems probable that most if not all of the new muscle cells on regenerating arterioles are formed in the manner described in the above observations.

In new arteries which followed a straight course the extra-endothelial cells were usually distributed uniformly along the vessel walls while in arteries which curved they showed a tendency to arrange themselves on the convex side of the vessel (fig. 13, compare fig. 10).

In vessels which continued to receive the same amount of blood flow and remained arterioles in respect to their narrow caliber, the cells on their walls formed a single row and remained relatively unchanged in numbers and it was frequently possible to identify the same cells day after day. For example, in one specimen, eight newly formed muscle cells were identified and found to occupy the same position on the wall for over a week, during which time no new cells appeared on this stretch of the arteriole. In another specimen ten individual cells were recorded in daily observations for 14 days.

In other cases, certain arterioles received an increasing blood flow during the period of differentiation of the newly formed vascular network into an 'adult' pattern, whereupon the narrow arterioles grew wider and became arteries and their walls became still thicker.

Conversely, on arterioles through which the circulation diminished the vessel caliber narrowed and a reduction in the number of extra-endothelial cells occurred (fig. 14, Art. 1).

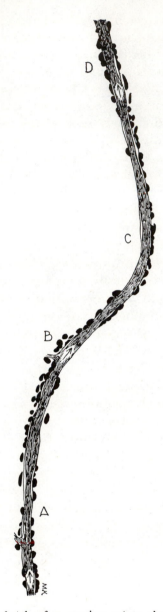

Fig. 13 Low power sketch of a curving artery showing tendency of extra-endothelial cells to become oriented on the convex side. Muscle cells in solid black. On straight stretches A and D, cells on two walls approximately equal. On curved stretches B and C, cells more numerous on convex side. Leitz drawing eye-piece. × 187.

This decrease was seen to be preceded in some cases by a flattening of the rounded cells and a return to their longitudinal arrangement after which the cells became detached from the wall. This process of reversal was observed, so far, only in cases of vessels which had not developed active contractility. In other cases, some of the muscle cells were observed to become opaque with sharply defined outlines and to degenerate and disappear without the preliminary reversal to the longitudinal type of cell. The disappearance of muscle cells from arterioles whose blood supply decreased took place more rapidly than was the case of the adventitial cells on capillaries and venules which received a diminished blood flow (p. 14). Figure 14, November–December shows an arteriole (Art. 1) followed for 3 weeks during which time the circulation decreased and the number of muscle cells diminished. During the next month the blood flow increased and more cells were added to the wall (January 5). A second artery (Art. 2) in the same chamber which received a greater blood flow acquired a larger number of muscle cells which persisted throughout the same period of observation.

In a few instances such as those described in the case of certain arterio-venous anastomoses which persisted for weeks or months, and which acquired the same contractility observed in the original vessels of the ear and then were obliterated (Clark and Clark, '34 b), the thick wall was visible up until the time of disappearance. The vessels in these cases were all actively contractile vessels, apparently supplied with nerves and their disappearance was preceded either by diversion of blood flow for some time to a new capillary plexus supplied by the same artery or, in one instance, to spasm of a small vessel which remained persistently contracted with its lumen obliterated during many hours of observation on several successive days. In the latter case the thick wall of the contracted vessel was the last thing visible.

During the period of vascular invasion in which both sprouting of new capillaries and retraction of surplus capillaries takes place most rapidly, the reduction of branches was greater

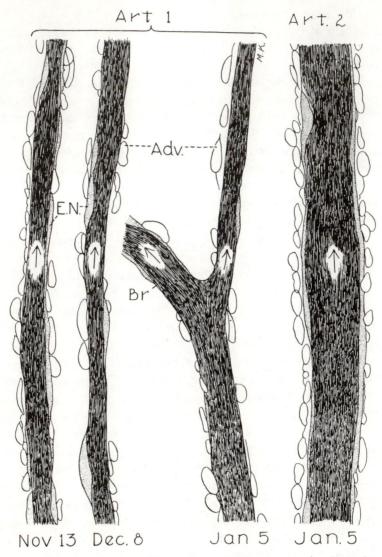

Fig. 14   Artery 1—three records of same arteriole on successive dates showing decrease in number of extra-endothelial cells (Adv.)—December 8, following decrease in blood flow, and increase, January 5, following increased flow. En., endothelial nucleus. Art. 2 another arteriole in the same chamber area which received a greater flow during the same period, showing continuous layer of extra-endothelial cells. Leitz drawing eye-piece. × 630.

on the arterial than on the venous side. In the stable plexus after the formation of a continuous layer of muscle cells on the newly differentiated arterioles, sending out of new sprouts from such vessels, such as was observed to occur repeatedly from capillaries, venules and veins following periods of increased circulation accompanied by an exudate, was rarely observed. An exception to this is described on page 37. Following the development of the layer of muscle cells on arterioles, haemorrhages in the chamber area, due to pressure over the cover slip or due to inflammatory conditions which injured the endothelium (Clark and Clark, '35), were found to occur chiefly through the walls of veins and capillaries and rarely from arteries or arterioles unless the trauma was excessive.

In addition to the obvious strengthening of the wall of the new arteries following the development of extra-endothelial cells, the thicker wall showed increased tonicity. This was evidenced by the maintenance of an arterial caliber which was persistently narrower than that of veins of equal relative importance in the same area and by the tendency of the new arteries to narrow down and constrict the lumen, when the whole circulation of the ear was reduced by the narrowing of the arterial supply in response to cold and to various local mechanical stimuli, to a degree which was either absent or much less marked in the case of other vessels in the same area which were subjected to the same stimuli.

The development of active spontaneous rhythmic contractility of the regenerated arteries and arterioles in the round table chambers as well as of their active contractile response to mechanical or auditory stimulation of the rabbit so that their behavior was indistinguishable from that of the original arteries of the ear as seen in preformed tissue chambers (Clark and Clark, '32) has been observed repeatedly (fig. 15). However although the regenerated arteries and arterioles, following increase in blood flow and pressure, all developed a thick wall of extra-endothelial cells which was indistinguishable in appearance from that of the original arteries of the ear and

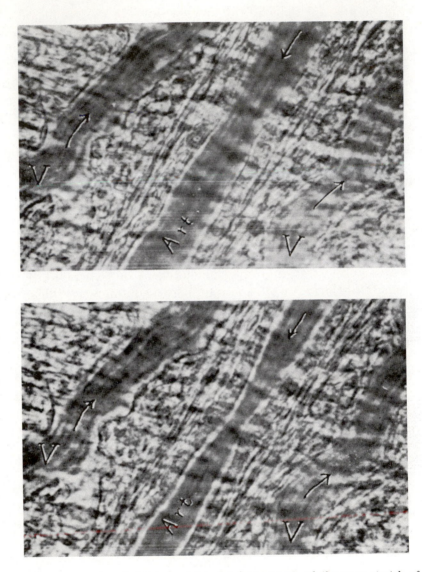

Fig. 15   Two microphotographs, taken 1 minute apart, of the same stretch of a regenerated artery which acquired active contractility (see text, p. 30). The upper photograph shows the artery (Art.) dilated and the lower contracted. The venule (V.) located on either side retained the same caliber throughout the observations. Continuous layer of muscle cells on artery 1. ✕ 500.

which showed the same characteristics of increased strength and tonicity, the acquisition of active contractility of the nature found in the preformed vessels was sporadic.

In the many chambers studied, some of the new arteries showed active spontaneous contractions as well as contractions in response to stimulation of the animal as early as a week after their formation from capillaries, others after weeks or months, while in still other cases such contractions were not seen during the entire observation period of 1 to 2 years. Such differences in the behavior of regenerated arteries were frequently encountered in the same table area. Arteries which contracted rhythmically and in response to stimulation of the rabbit were often located close to other arteries which failed to show such contractions, while in other cases one branch of an artery might display active contractions and another branch of the same artery fail to do so. Again, a stretch of an artery near the table edge has been seen to undergo active contractions while a more distal portion remained inactive for months. In many cases the region of active contractility extended progressively further with the passage of time and a previously non-contracting branch might acquire contractility weeks or months later than other branches or than the main stem of the artery, while in other nearby vessels the extent of active contractility remained unchanged for months. Typical active contractions of regenerated arteries have been observed in vessels 8 days after their first appearance as capillary sprouts and 5 to 6 days after their acquisition of a layer of muscle cells. In other vessels active contractility was first noticed after they were a month old. In one chamber, contractions were first seen in one artery of a chamber $3\frac{1}{2}$ months after the ingrowth of new vessels and in another at $7\frac{1}{2}$ months. In another specimen, containing four main arteries, two developed active contractility at 9 days, the third at 21 days and the fourth at 35 days.

The explanation for the differences in behavior of some of the regenerated arteries and arterioles from those of preformed vessels and from others in the same vascular areas, despite the similarity in the character of the cells on their walls, has been furnished by experiments in which differentiation of arteries from capillaries, formation of a typical muscular wall and gradual extension peripherally of the area of active contractility was followed by daily observations and records, combined with successive intravital injections of methylene blue, in which it was demonstrated that active spontaneous contractions and contractions in response to stimulation of the animal in regenerated arteries were dependent upon the regeneration of supplying sympathetic nerves (Clark, Clark and Williams, '34).

Although regenerated arteries which do not receive a new nerve supply fail to contract spontaneously and in response to mechanical or auditory stimulation of the rabbit, there is evidence that their extra-endothelial cells are capable of contracting under special circumstances. In certain of the chambers, which had remained for some time in the ear, squeezing occurred in the region of the table edge due to excessive development of connective tissue fibers. In such regions, following a temporary decrease in the blood flow due to active contraction of supplying arteries outside the table area, arteries have been seen to constrict until the lumen was obliterated while veins and capillaries in the same area were merely flattened. In other chambers, new arteries which did not exhibit spontaneous rhythmic contractions and which failed to respond when the rabbit was prodded, were occasionally seen to contract actively, even to obliteration of the lumen, following a violent struggle of the rabbit. In such cases, no constriction of capillaries or veins of the same area was seen. This reaction was probably due to a discharge of adrenalin which in this case affected the muscle directly, since no nerve-controlled contractions had been observed during hours of microscopic study for many days before and after such an observation. Again, the extreme contractions lasting for as long as a minute in which the lumen was obliterated, noted by Abell and Schenck ('38) following the administration of horse serum to sensitized rabbits, were observed in 'moat' chambers where

THE AMERICAN JOURNAL OF ANATOMY, VOL. 66, NO. 1

the same regenerated arteries showed no evidence of nerve-controlled contractions either before or after the experiment. In this case too the capillaries and venules in the same chamber area showed no caliber changes during the period of pronounced arterial contraction.

CHANGES IN VESSELS AND EXTRA-ENDOTHELIAL CELLS

Although in splinted chambers free from injuries or mechanical stresses, following the stage of vascularization of the table area and differentiation of arteries and veins, the regenerated plexus assumed a stable pattern in which the same vessels remained relatively unchanged, aside from the minor alterations in caliber already referred to, comparatively slight mechanical and thermal stimuli which produced changes in the circulation through the network resulted frequently in modifications of individual vessels or, in some instances, of the whole vascular pattern of the observation area. The lability of the vascular system in respect to its growth capacity whereby a few days of increased circulation accompanied by an exudate was followed by the sending out of new capillary sprouts, formation of new connections and the subsequent remodelling of the veins draining the new plexus has been described (Clark et al., '31). Conversely, with a diminished circulation continued for some time capillaries were observed to retract resulting again in decreased size of veins or change of veins to capillary caliber. Similar changes have been seen repeatedly in preformed tissue chambers (Clark and Clark, '32). Although the arteries of both preformed and regenerated tissue were found to be more stable than veins and capillaries, circulatory changes which persisted for some time were found to affect the former vessels also, producing in a number of cases, profound modifications in their size, course, and also in the character of their walls.

In a number of specimens, following a sudden increase in circulation the formation of direct connections between arteries and veins have been seen to form (Clark and Clark, '34).

In such cases the extra-endothelial cells increased rapidly on the anastomosis following the increase in the arterial blood flow through it and the new cells quickly changed to a circular arrangement in the manner described for new forming arterioles. Many of the new anastomoses were temporary and with the return of a more subdued circulation reverted to capillary

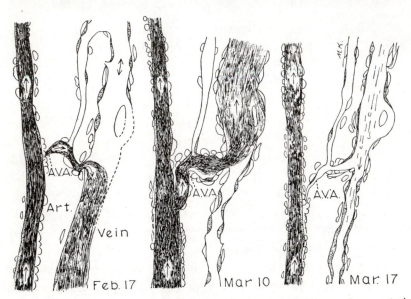

Fig. 16 Series of records showing formation and subsidence of an arterio-venous anastomosis. March 10, increase in caliber and in numbers of cells on wall of A.V.A. with increased flow. Also reversal of flow and increase in caliber of connecting vein. March 17, decrease in numbers of extra-endothelial cells following diminished flow. Leitz drawing eye-piece. × 231.

size and some of the cells on their walls changed back to a longitudinal arrangement while others became detached and disappeared.

Figure 16 illustrates the formation of a new arterio-venous anastomosis from a capillary, which received a suddenly increased flow of blood so strong as to cause reversal of flow in a part of the vein into which it emptied followed by increase in extra-endothelial cells on the walls and by a change in their axis to a circular arrangement (March 10). In the last record the change of the A.V.A. back to a capillary accompanied by loss of extra-endothelial cells, following the return of a quieter circulation, is shown. Another type of disappearance of an arterio-venous anastomosis which had become actively contractile, in which the lumen was obliterated for most if not all of the time for several days before the disappearance of the thick wall of muscle cells, has been referred to (p. 26).

The low power records shown in figure 17 illustrate the radical changes which certain vessels in the chamber area may undergo following alterations in the direction and character of the circulation through them. In this instance a venule which had persisted with steady blood flow for several months, following a mild inflammation in which the bulk of its flow was diverted for part of its course (AB) became part of a capillary plexus, after which an arteriole at one end of the plexus received an increased flow and extended rapidly incorporating some of the capillaries in its path. By this means, an arteriole eventually came to replace a former venule after an intervening period in which the channel became part of a capillary plexus. High power studies of this region showed that the extra-endothelial cells which were sparsely distributed on the original venule and on the vessels of the capillary plexus increased rapidly on the extending arteriole and at the date of the last record (fig. 17, February 18) had formed a continuous wall of circularly arranged muscle cells. Figure 18 shows the transformation of a vein into an artery with accompanying rapid increase in the cells on the wall.

In another specimen, a vein differentiated in the new vascular network which extended across the table and remained for 8 months as one of the conspicuous vessels in the observation area. At the end of this time, following a period of more active blood flow, the region near the table edge in the vicinity of one end of this vein received an increasing supply of arterial blood flow through a connection outside the table area. Within a few days a new artery differentiated in the region at the table edge by enlargement and straightening of capillary channels already present, accompanied by increase and change in

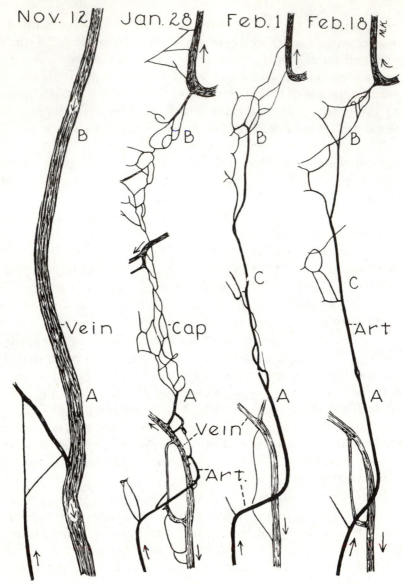

Fig. 17 Series of low power records showing transformation of a vein (November 12) into a capillary plexus (January 28), following period of diminished flow, and subsequent formation of an arteriole from the plexus, following an increase in flow entering the plexus from right branch of artery supplying one end of plexus (February 1 and February 18). A, B and C indicate the same region on successive dates. Leitz drawing eye-piece. × 72.

orientation of the extra-endothelial cells. A short distance from the table edge the new arterial channel extended through a formerly small connection into the path of the vein and in a short time the former vein throughout most of its course became transformed into an artery both with respect to the character of its blood flow and the character of its wall. The new artery retained the same curvings of the former vein but had a narrower caliber. In this case, as in those of the new

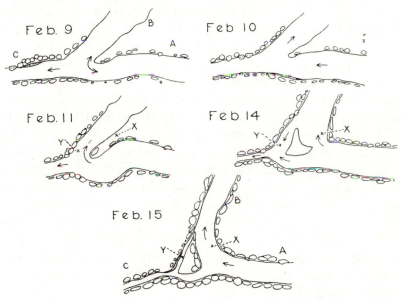

Fig. 18 Series of records showing transformation of a vein into an artery with accompanying rapid increase in cells on the wall. February 9 artery (A–C) formed a connection with a neighboring vein (B). Y, first connection with vein (February 11). X, secondary connection (February 14) which became the main channel (February 15). × 184.

arteries derived from capillaries in the stage of primary differentiation (p. 19), the rapid addition of extra-endothelial cells and their change in axis from a longitudinal to a circular position on the wall were followed in the living. This artery whose transformation from a vein was observed in the living persisted as one of the more permanent arteries as long as the chamber was under observation.

Although for the greater part of its course the new artery which replaced the former vein developed a characteristic wall composed of a continuous layer of muscle cells, in its more distal portion it was found that despite its abundant flow the cells on the walls were more sparsely distributed than was the case in vessels of comparable size and pressure conditions. In this distal region the new artery circulated inside a capsule of connective tissue fibers which outlined the limits of the former vein and a clear shrinkage space remained between the artery wall and the capsule (p. 16). The cells which were present on this portion of the artery were oriented in the circular position characteristic of muscle cells. In the distal portion of the new artery which replaced the vein in the region in which muscle cells were separated by a gap of naked endothelium interesting growth phenomena were observed to occur in response to changes in the circulation. These are illustrated in figure 19 and show the formation of numerous new branches and short connections between this portion of the artery and accompanying vessels following increased blood flow due to a slight mechanical injury, resulting in a new capillary plexus (February 18), with subsequent loss of connections and reduction of vessels when the circulation again subsided. The absence of sprout formation in the case of most arteries in which the layer of muscle cells was continuous has been mentioned (p. 28).

The opposite course of events is illustrated in figure 20. The newly formed arteriole under observation consisted of two branches for a short stretch which reunited to form a single vessel. For several days the two branches received an equal supply of blood, were uniform in size and had approximately the same numbers of extra-endothelial cells. On the day shown in the first record in the figure (October 24) a greater proportion of the blood stream started to circulate through one of the branches (the upper one in the figure) which then increased in diameter while the other branch (A-B) narrowed. This condition continued for several days during which the branch receiving the lesser flow became smaller and the cells

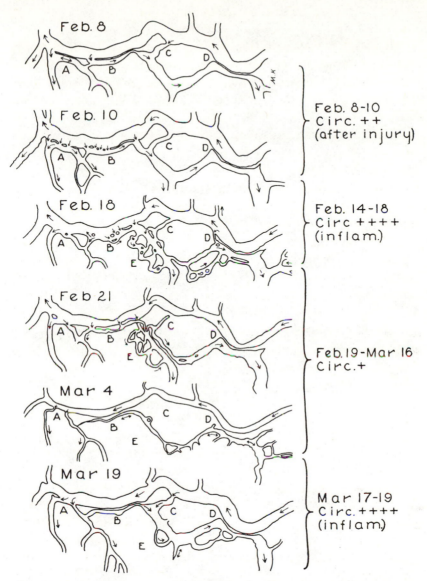

Fig. 19 Series of low power records of the terminal portion of an arteriole in which the continuous layer of muscle cells had not developed (see text). Shows formation of numerous new connections with a neighboring vein and of secondary loops after a period of increased blood flow due to inflammation (February 8–18), followed by retraction of new vessels and return of the capillary plexus to a small venule after subsidence of inflammation (February 19–March 6)— repetition of the process following a new period of increased flow March 17–19. Leitz drawing eye-piece. × 66.

38

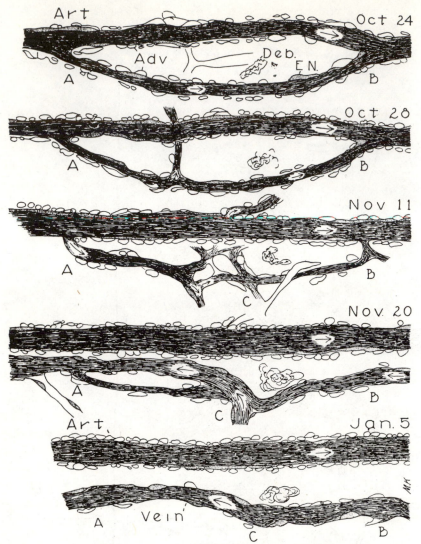

Fig. 20 Series of records of the same arteriole over a period of months showing changes in form and size of vessel and in numbers and character of the extra-endothelial cells in response to circulatory changes. October 24, branching artery soon after its differentiation—two branches approximately equal in respect to blood flow and numbers of cells on wall. Following this, bulk of arterial flow was carried by the upper branch and the lower one (A–B) became smaller. Rounded extra-endothelial cells reverted to longitudinal form (October 28) after which they became detached and disappeared (see text, p. 40). The vessel A–B became part of a capillary plexus (November 11) after which it became detached from the artery and transformed into a vein (November 20–January 5). Leitz drawing eye-piece. × 280.

39

on its walls reverted from a circular to a longitudinal arrangement. Later the vessel subsided still further to capillary size and formed part of a capillary plexus (November 11). A few days later a return flow through this plexus increased in amount and the former arteriole became transformed into a venule while the other branches of the capillary plexus retracted (November 20–January 5).

In this instance the individual extra-endothelial cells on the two branches of the artery were followed in daily camera lucida records during the period in which the branch receiving the decreased flow reverted from an artery to a capillary. Within 3 days after the shifting of the bulk of the arterial flow to the upper branch, the cells on the other branch (A-B) with diminished flow had nearly all lost their circular arrangement and six of them had disappeared, while on the same date the extra-endothelial cells on the larger branch with increased flow were circular in arrangement and eighteen additional ones were present. Three days later, the cells remaining on the smaller branch were arranged longitudinally and resembled the typical adventitial cells on capillaries and venules while seven more had disappeared. In the meantime, eight more circular cells had appeared on the wall of the larger branch which now possessed a continuous layer of muscle cells. Five days later, the branch receiving the lessened flow had become a typical capillary and only thirteen of the original forty cells present on its wall remained. The larger branch had approximately the same number of muscle cells arranged in a continuous layer.

DISCUSSION

Interest in the nature and behavior of the extra-endothelial cells of blood capillaries dates chiefly from 1922 when Krogh, basing his theory largely on the work of Vimtrup ('22) on amphibian vessels, brought out the view that much of the peripheral control of circulation is carried out by localized contraction of capillaries inaugurated by contractions of extra-endothelial cells which he termed 'Rouget' cells. Up until this time no serious question of the view that peripheral control of circulation in the mammal resided in the arteries and arterioles, mediated through smooth muscle cells chiefly under the control of the nervous system, had been offered. Although previous to this time the work of Stricker (1868), Tarchanoff (1874), Steinach and Kahn ('03) and others had yielded evidence that capillaries were contractile as well as elastic, the effect of such contractions on control of peripheral circulation was considered to be relatively unimportant.

Rouget (1873) described certain cells outside the endothelium of blood capillaries which he called 'cellules adventices.' In the hyaloid membrane of the adult frog he pictured them as forming a continuous layer of cells with many branched processes encircling the capillaries. In the tadpole's tail he found no such cells, only chromatophores. In mammals he found widely separated extra-endothelial cells. In a later publication, Rouget (1879) described cells on the vessels of the hyaloid membrane as contractile, responding to various types of stimulation, and considered them to be a form of smooth muscle cell. With no further evidence he inferred that there was everywhere a complete, contractile layer extending over arterioles, capillaries and venules which acted in the same manner as in the hyaloid membrane.

Vimtrup ('22) studied the behavior of capillaries in amphibian larvae and described the presence of scattered cells outside the endothelium which Rouget had failed to see and observed narrowing of capillaries which he thought was initiated by contraction of the outside cells. In the nictitating membrane Bensley and Vimtrup ('28) described cells with branched processes, similar to those described by Rouget in the hyaloid membrane, encircling the capillaries, which contracted when stimulated electrically. These extra-endothelial cells were named by Krogh 'Rouget' cells and, like Rouget, Krogh extended his view of their behavior to cover all capillaries in mammals as well as Amphibia.

The authors (Clark and Clark, '25) watched the development of extra-endothelial cells from connective tissue cells on the walls of capillaries in the transparent tails of living amphibian larvae and the behavior of the capillaries both before and after acquisition of the so-called 'Rouget' cells. It was found that definite active spontaneous contractions of capillary endothelium occurred in the tadpole's tail and that endothelial contractions could also be induced experimentally. However, no indication was found that the scattered longitudinally arranged adventitial cells played any part in such contractions since young capillaries were observed to contract in the same manner before the acquisition of any outside cells while after such cells were present contractions were seen to start more frequently at a distance from them than in their immediate vicinity, while at the time of a capillary contraction which chanced to occur near a 'Rouget' cell, a space appeared between the outside cell and the vessel wall. Recently, Zweifach ('34) has carried out studies on the capillaries of the frog's mesentery in which the inertness of the adventitial (Rouget) cells and the contractility of the capillary endothelium were demonstrated by micro-manipulation.

From all these observations it appears that the capillary endothelium of Amphibia is contractile, that spontaneous contractions of capillaries and contraction in response to stimulation, in such forms, may exert a sporadic control of the peripheral circulation and that these contractions occur independently of the scattered, longitudinally arranged adventitial cells which may or may not be present on their walls.

With regard to the contractility of mammalian capillaries the story appears to be somewhat different. Much of the evidence for capillary contractility has been obtained, for lack of suitable transparent regions in the living animal, by indirect evidence such as blanching or reddening of areas observed through the skin or by carrying over interpretations derived from observations on lower forms. Studies of the vessels of rabbits' and dogs' ears in transparent chambers where the finest cytological details could be studied by prolonged observation in unanaesthetized animals, carried out by a number of observers in this laboratory during the past 10 years have yielded no evidence for any significant powers of contractility of either the endothelial cells or the longitudinally arranged adventitial cells of mammalian capillaries (Clark, '36; Clark and Clark, '32, '35; Sandison, '32; Moore, '36). To be sure, Beecher ('36) working in Krogh's laboratory with this method has reported that 10% of the adventitial cells of rabbits' capillaries undergo contractions which cause the endothelial nuclei to protrude into the vessel lumen. However, his records show only short stretches of vessels with no description of the circulatory conditions in communicating veins and arteries at the time of the apparent contraction so that passive narrowings due to sudden decrease in blood flow, suction, or squeezing are not excluded (Clark and Clark, '32).

Hartmann and Evans ('29) studied microscopically the effect of a variety of drugs on the vessels of the sartorius muscle of the cat, using a straight glass rod as a conductor of light, and failed to find any definite contractility of capillaries. Florey and Carleton ('26) concluded from their studies of the mammalian vessels in the mesentery and omentum that the adventitial cells were not concerned with capillary contractions. Rogers ('32, '34) carried out extensive studies of the vessels of the mesentery and omentum in living mammals with the micro-manipulator and failed to find definite contractility of either the endothelial or the adventitial cells of the capillaries.

It would appear that in mammalian vessels there is considerable doubt as to whether true active contractions of capillary endothelium occur spontaneously or in response to most types of stimulation and that in any case contractions if present are so sporadic and slight as to be negligible as a factor in the control of peripheral circulation. The bulk of the evidence derived from prolonged microscopic observations in the living mammal and from micro-manipulation shows that the longitudinally arranged adventitial cells on mammalian capillaries, like those on amphibian vessels, are inert and not concerned with vascular contractility. The real factors responsible for control of peripheral circulation in the mammal have been shown to be the smooth muscle cells on arteries, arterioles, arterio-venous anastomoses and a few of the larger veins mediated through the sympathetic nerves (Clark, Clark and Williams, '34). The active spontaneous rhythmic contractions of such vessels as observed in transparent chambers in the ears of unanesthetized rabbits (Clark and Clark, '32) and demonstrated by cinematographic records (Clark, Clark and Swenson, '33) are so positive and violent as to eclipse the slight, infrequent and apparently passive changes in caliber of the thin-walled capillaries and venules.

The observations reported here, that the longitudinally arranged adventitial cells, derived from fibroblasts, may increase in number and become transformed into circularly arranged smooth muscle cells following increased pressure in the vessel and that, conversely, muscle cells may revert to the longitudinal arrangement or degenerate following a return to a slower type of circulation with reduced blood pressure, confirm the histomechanical principle proposed by Thoma (1893) that the thickness of the vessel wall is dependent upon the blood pressure.

From the descriptions given by the workers who have studied the extra-endothelial cells on the vessels of the nictitating and hyaloid membranes, of the arrangement of these cells with prongs extending around the vessel walls and of their apparent response to electrical stimulation, it appears possible that these cells, as Rouget (1879) originally suggested, may represent a form of primitive smooth muscle cell which is transitional between the longitudinally arranged, sparsely distributed and apparently non-contractile cells present on the vessels of the tadpole's tail, frog's mesentery, and on the capillaries and venules of mammals, and the more highly specialized contractile smooth muscle cells on the mammalian arteries and arterioles. It is in these two regions, namely, the nictitating and hyaloid membranes of the frog, that the bulk of the evidence for the contractility of the extra-endothelial cells of Amphibia was obtained (Rouget, Vimtrup, Bensley,

Krogh) and which was applied without sufficient additional evidence to the adventitial cells of capillaries in other forms and other regions. The staining of myofibrils in the 'Rouget' cells in these regions by Bensley and Vimtrup ('28) which could not be obtained by Florey and Carleton or by Rogers in the case of mammalian adventitial cells, would favor this explanation for the difference in the two cell types. The recent study of Zweifach ('37) in which he finds a myofibrillar arrangement in the extra-endothelial cells on arterial capillaries of the frog's mesentery and no such structure in the adventitial cells of capillaries and venules also supports this view of the existence of a non-contractile and a contractile type of extra-endothelial cells.

SUMMARY

It has been possible, in transparent chambers introduced into the rabbit's ear, to make microscopic observations on the mode of formation, subsequent fate and behavior of extra-endothelial cells on living mammalian blood vessels, with the following results:

Adventitial cells on regenerating mammalian capillaries develop, like those on amphibian vessels, from connective tissue cells. Fibroblast-like cells were observed to flatten out on the walls of new blood vessels at an early stage—often during sprout formation—where they assumed a longitudinal arrangement with processes extending parallel with the vessel wall. The numbers of new adventitial cells which formed in this fashion on growing capillaries appeared to vary with the numbers of fibroblasts present in the region outside.

The subsequent fate of the newly formed extra-endothelial cells depended upon the fate of the vessel to which they were attached. If the vessel remained a capillary, they might increase slightly in number by mitotic division or there might be no increase or even a decrease in the original number. The cells remained permanently as sparsely distributed, inert cells. In capillaries which retrogressed, adventitial cells were observed to remain behind in the tissue.

In the case of capillaries which became parts of venules or small veins the number of adventitial cells increased slightly, while they retained their longitudinal arrangement and remained inert as regards contractility. Around some of the larger veins a capsular arrangement of fine connective tissue fibrillae or reticulum formed outside the layer of adventitial cells.

In the case of new vessels so situated as to receive an increased flow from supplying arteries the changes in form of the capillary and in the character of its wall were more extensive and rapid. The change from capillary to new arteriole consisted in straightening of the vessel course, loss of many of the side branches, narrowing of the caliber and increase in thickness and strength of the endothelium. These changes were accompanied by a rapid increase in the number of extra-endothelial cells, in part at least by mitotic division, until by the end of 6 days there might be a continuous layer of outside cells. At the same time a change in the axis of the outside cells from a longitudinal to a transverse position was observed to take place.

Although the newly formed blood vessels, after the stage of ingrowth and differentiation, frequently remained relatively unchanged, slight mechanical and thermal stimuli which produced circulatory changes through the network resulted frequently in modifications of individual vessels and in some instances of much of the vascular pattern. Occasionally vessels which had functioned for weeks or months as veins were observed to change into arteries, while arteries were seen to change into veins following such modifications in the vascular pattern. Both arterioles and venules were seen to revert and become parts of a capillary plexus following diminished flow, while, as reported previously, in response to increased circulation accompanied by a mild inflammatory exudate, new capillary networks have repeatedly been observed to form, with subsequent differentiation of new arterioles and venules.

The longitudinally arranged adventitial cells on capillaries and small venules showed no evidence of contractility. On arteries and arterioles definite active contractility was seen to develop in the transversely arranged cells which became smooth muscle cells, providing they were reached by a regenerating vasomotor nerve.

LITERATURE CITED

ABELL, R. G., AND H. P. SCHENCK 1938 Microscopic observations on the behavior of living blood vessels of the rabbit during the reaction of anaphylaxis. J. Immun., vol. 34, p. 195.

BEECHER, H. K. 1936 The independent control of the capillary circulation in the mammal. Skand. Arch. f. Physiol., vol. 73, p. 1.

BENSLEY, R. R., AND B. VIMTRUP 1928 On the nature of the Rouget cells of capillaries. Anat. Rec., vol. 39, p. 37.

CLARK, E. R. 1918 Studies on the growth of blood vessels in the tail of the frog larva by observation and experiment on the living animal. Am. J. Anat., vol. 23, p. 37.

———— 1936 Growth and development of function in blood vessels and lymphatics. Ann. of Int. Med., vol. 9, p. 1043.

CLARK, E. R., AND E. L. CLARK 1925 a The development of adventitial (Rouget) cells on the blood capillaries of amphibian larvae. Am. J. Anat., vol. 35, p. 239.

———— 1925 b The relation of Rouget cells to capillary contractility. Am. J. Anat., vol. 35, p. 265.

———— 1932 a Observations on living preformed blood vessels as seen in a transparent chamber inserted into the rabbit's ear. Am. J. Anat., vol. 49, p. 441.

———— 1932 b Observations on the new growth of lymphatic vessels as seen in transparent chambers introduced into the rabbit's ear. Am. J. Anat., vol. 51, p. 49.

———— 1934 a Observations on living arterio-venous anastomoses as seen in transparent chambers introduced into the rabbit's ear. Am. J. Anat., vol. 54, p. 229.

———— 1934 b The new formation of arterio-venous anastomoses in the rabbit's ear. Am. J. Anat., vol. 55, p. 407.

———— 1935 Observations on changes in blood vascular endothelium in the living animal. Am. J. Anat., vol. 57, p. 385.

———— 1937 Observations on living mammalian lymphatic capillaries—their relation to the blood vessels. Am. J. Anat., vol. 60, p. 253.

———— 1939 Microscopic observations on the growth of blood capillaries in the living mammal. Am. J. Anat. vol. 64, p. 251.

CLARK, E. R., E. L. CLARK AND E. A. SWENSON 1933 Studies on contraction of arterioles. Am. J. Med. Sci., vol. 185, p. 399.

CLARK, E. R., E. L. CLARK AND R. G. WILLIAMS 1934 Microscopic observations in the living rabbit of the new growth of nerves and the establishment of nerve-controlled contractions of newly formed arterioles. Am. J. Anat., vol. 55, p. 47.

THE AMERICAN JOURNAL OF ANATOMY, VOL. 66, NO. 1

CLARK, E. R., H. T. KIRBY-SMITH, R. O. REX AND R. G. WILLIAMS 1930 Recent modifications in the method of studying living cells and tissues in transparent chambers inserted in the rabbit's ear. Anat. Rec., vol. 47, p. 187.

CLARK, E. R., W. J. HITSCHLER, H. T. KIRBY-SMITH, R. O. REX AND J. H. SMITH 1931 General observations on the ingrowth of new blood vessels into standardized chambers in the rabbit's ear, and the subsequent changes in the newly grown vessels over a period of months. Anat. Rec., vol. 50, p. 129.

CLARK, E. R., J. C. SANDISON AND H. C. HOU 1931 A new rabbit board for use in studying living vessels in transparent chambers introduced into the ear. Anat. Rec., vol. 50, p. 169.

EVANS, H. M. 1909 On the development of the aortal, cardinal, and umbilical veins and the other blood vessels of vertebrate embryos from capillaries. Anat. Rec., vol. 3, p. 498.

FLOREY, H. W., AND H. M. CARLETON 1926 The Rouget cells and their function. Proc. Royal Soc., vol. 100, p. 23.

HARTMANN, F., AND J. L. EVANS 1929 Control of capillaries of skeletal muscles. Am. J. Physiol., vol. 90, p. 668.

KROGH, A. 1922 The anatomy and physiology of capillaries. Yale Univ Press.

LOEB, J. 1893 Ueber die Entwicklung von Fischenbryonen ohne Kreislauf. Pflüg. Arch., vol. 54, p. 525.

MOORE, R. L. 1936 Adaptation of the transparent chamber technique to the ear of the dog. Anat. Rec., vol. 64, p. 387.

ROGERS, J. B. 1932 Observations on pericapillary cells in the mesenteries of rabbits. Anat. Rec., vol. 55, p. 1.

——— 1935 Observations in vivo on the capillaries in the greater omentum of cats. Anat. Rec., vol. 61, Suppl., p. 42.

ROUGET, C. 1873 Mémoire sur le développement, la structure et les propriétés physiologiques des capillaires sanguins et lymphatiques. Arch. de Phys., vol. 5, p. 603.

——— 1879 Sur la contractilité des capillaires sanguins. C. R. de l'Acad. de Sc., vol. 88, p. 916.

SANDISON, J. C. 1928 Observations on the growth of blood vessels as seen in the transparent chamber introduced into the rabbit's ear. Am. J. Anat., vol. 41, p. 475.

——— 1932 Contraction of blood vessels and observations on the circulation in the transparent chamber in the rabbit's ear. Anat. Rec., vol. 54, p. 105.

STEINACH, E., AND R. H. KAHN 1903 Echte Contractilität und motorische Innervation der Blutcapillären. Pflüg. Arch., vol. 97, p. 105.

STOCKARD, C. R. 1915 A study of wandering mesenchymal cells on the living yolk sac and their developmental products: chromatophores, vascular endothelium and blood cells. Am. J. Anat., vol. 18, p. 525.

STRICKER, S. 1868 Untersuchungen über die capillaren Blutgefässe der Nickhaut des Frosches. Sitzungsb. d. Wien. Akad. d. Wiss., vol. 51, p. 16.

TARCHANOFF, J. F. 1874 Beobachtungen über contraktile Elemente in den Blut und Lymphcapillaren. Pflüg. Arch., vol. 9, p. 407.

THOMA, R. 1893 Untersuchungen über die Histogenese und Histomechanik des Gefässsystems. Stuttgart.

VARIAN, B. B. 1931 A transparent elastic glue, used in making chambers for insertion in the rabbit's ear. Science, vol. 73, p. 678.

VIMTRUP, B. 1922 Beiträge zur Anatomie der Capillären: Über contractile Elemente in der Gefässwand der Blutcapillaren. Zeitschr. f. Anat. u. Entw., vol. 65, p. 150.

ZWEIFACH, B. W. 1934 A micro-manipulative study of blood capillaries. Anat. Rec., vol. 59, p. 83.

————— 1937 The structure and reactions of the small blood vessels in Amphibia. Am. J. Anat., vol. 60, p. 473.

13

Copyright © 1954 by The Wistar Institute Press

Reprinted from *Anat. Rec.*, **120**, 293–307 (1954)

THE USE OF THE HAMSTER CHEEK POUCH FOR THE STUDY OF VASCULAR CHANGES AT THE MICROSCOPIC LEVEL [1]

BRENTON R. LUTZ AND GEORGE P. FULTON
Department of Biology, Boston University

EIGHTEEN FIGURES

INTRODUCTION

Precise microscopic study of the peripheral circulation in the living animal requires the use of a thin, non-pigmented tissue which can be transilluminated to reveal at high power, the structure of the smallest vessels, the conditions of flow and the activity of the formed elements. Such a tissue is found in the membranous cheek pouch of both the golden hamster, *Mesocricetus auratus* (Fulton, Jackson and Lutz, '46) and the Chinese hamster, *Cricetulus griseus* (Fulton, Lutz, Patt and Yerganian, '54). In this laboratory we have used the former for the study of blood pressure, inflammation, hemostasis, petechial formation, thromboembolism, immuno-thrombocytopenic purpura, the function of mast cells, the effects of anticoagulants, ionizing radiations, adrenalectomy and cortisone, bacterial and parasitic infections, drugs, x-ray opaque substances, tumor growth, and the vascularization of tumor transplants.

MORPHOLOGY OF THE CHEEK POUCH

The cheek pouch of the hamster is a paired structure located in the buccal wall, with a slit-like entrance just inside

[1] The work on the hamster cheek pouch in the Department of Biology at Boston University has been supported in part by research grants from the Atomic Energy Commission, the National Heart Institute and the National Cancer Institute of the U. S. Public Health Service, and the American Cancer Society (Mass. Division).

293

the corner of the mouth. *In situ* the pouch wall has many longitudinal folds allowing distension, thus providing a large flat area for the study of blood vessels when the pouch is everted. The normal pouch is one and one-half inches long and extends posteriorly to the region of the shoulder (Priddy and Brodie, '48).

The histology of the pouch of the golden hamster has been described by Fulton, Jackson and Lutz in 1947 (fig. 3). They found it to be 0.4 mm thick. The cheek pouch of the Chinese hamster is about 0.07 mm thick (fig. 4). No glands, vascular papillae or hairs are present in either pouch. Blood vessels are numerous in the connective tissue and among the striated muscle fibers, which are few at the blind end leaving a large area suitable for transillumination. The muscle fibers terminate in branching elongated processes in the connective tissue or on other muscle cells (fig. 5). A wide meshed nonmyelinated nerve plexus in the connective tissue gives rise to a perivascular nerve plexus (fig. 6). Large numbers of mast cells appear crowded along the blood vessels and scattered in the tissues (Maynard, Battit, Lutz, Patt and Fulton, '52).

METHODS AND TECHNIQUE OF CINEPHOTOMICROSCOPY

The cheek pouch of either the golden hamster or the Chinese hamster may be prepared according to the method described originally by Fulton, Jackson and Lutz ('47). The golden hamster is anesthetized by an intraperitoneal injection of 10 mg of Nembutal (pentobarbital sodium, Abbot) per 100 gm of body weight. Fortification by 1.5 to 2.5 mg increments may be needed if the animal is worked on for an hour or more. Because the Chinese hamster weighs only about 35 gm as compared with 100–120 gm for the golden hamster, anesthetization must be carefully controlled. In practice 1.0 mg per 12 gm of body weight is adequate. The anesthetized animal is placed on a warm plastic operating dish (5.5 by 6 inches) equipped with a transilluminating block ($1 \times 1 \times \frac{3}{8}$ inch) cemented over an aperture in the bottom. The block and the adjacent pinning material (cork or rubber) are located in a shallow moat (1.5×5 inches) separating the rest of the operating dish which is supporting the hamster. The moat is kept filled with Ringer's solution at 37°C. Either pouch is everted by gentle traction with forceps. The thin white portion of the pouch at the blind tip is extended in the Ringer bath, spread over the transilluminating block and pinned with "bank" pins to the adjacent cork, forming a flat double-layered preparation, excellent for low power work (fig. 2).

When superior cinephotography at 200 to 1200 $\times$ is desired a single membrane preparation is used. A semicircular cut is made through the upper layer forming a small flap, which is then extended. The operating dish is transferred to an electrically heated microscope stage. A light-splitting prism permits simultaneous viewing and motion picture recording. By means of a micromanipulator, minute instruments such as microelectrodes, micropipettes, microneedles, microprobes, and microknives may be applied to the small blood vessels. Kodachrome (16 mm) film, a 100 watt zirconium lamp and a "Cinekodak Special" motion picture camera have been used successfully in this laboratory, with a device for positioning the camera and an arrangement for "time lapse" recording (fig. 1).

The cheek pouch is ideally suited for direct microscopic investigations on living blood vessels (fig. 11), because the thin stratified squamous epithelium presents a normal physiological surface and the blood vessels are adult, surrounded by their usual tissue environment. The same pouch may be used on successive days, weeks or months, and a particular spot may be marked with a minute glass bead. The thinness of the cheek pouch of the Chinese hamster (fig. 4) gives it a greater transparency and makes it almost the equal of the retrolingual membrane of the frog, originally described by Pratt and Reid ('30).

Cheek pouches are exceedingly vascular (fig. 9). The vascularity exceeds that of comparable mammalian preparations such as the mesentery or mesoappendix of rodents, or membranes within transparent chambers. The vascular pattern differs somewhat from that described by Chambers and Zweifach ('44) for the mesentery in that preferential channels are not obvious. A rich network of vein to vein anastomoses, some arteriovenous anastomoses and many arteriolar anastomoses are found.

Spontaneous intermittency of flow is of two kinds (1) that produced by the action of sphincters at the arterial end of capillaries, originally described in the frog by Fulton and Lutz ('40); and (2) that produced by changes in blood pressure differentials. Arterioles occasionally exhibit spontaneous vasomotion which can be recorded without "time lapse." They rarely contract completely, and independently acting sphincters deprive small areas only temporarily of moving blood.

The extreme vascularity of the cheek pouch, its position as an "end organ," and its freedom from pressure and ease of manipulation, make tumor transplantation extremely successful and advantageous (figs. 7 and 8). Tumors grow freely and symmetrically, and can be measured and observed at successive periods during their growth, so that growth curves of a given tumor in the same animal may be made. The early inflammatory reaction and the subsequent revascularization of a transplant can be followed (fig. 10) by an injection technique (Williams, '48).

USES FOR THE CHEEK POUCH PREPARATION

Lutz, Fulton and Akers ('51) have reported the presence of platelet thromboembolic conditions in the hamster after trauma (fig. 17), stimulation of the blood vessel wall with a microelectrode, generalized infection, and malignant neoplasia. A red thrombus was photographed forming in the lee of a white thrombus. When the preventive properties of heparin, Dicumarol, Tromexan and phenylindanedione were tested, the difference between coagulation and agglutination became apparent, since in hypocoagulable blood, platelet agglutination and hemostatic plug formation were enhanced

(Fulton, Akers and Lutz, '53). Red corpuscles tend at times to circulate in groups (Fahraeus, '29), but the "basic" sludged blood of Knisely and coworkers ('47) has not been observed in our laboratory with staphylococcus infection, either general or local, trauma, including massive limb crushing, visceral manipulation, production of small burns, and chronic malignant neoplasia (Lutz, '51). As a terminal phenomenon, after lethal total body x-irradiation and cortisone poisoning, red corpuscles gather in loose clumps (fig. 12), a condition called "chunky flow" (Fulton, Lutz, Joftes and Maynard, '52). The corpuscles separate easily with microprobing, pass singly through capillaries, but reform clumps in the slower venous flow.

Since endothelial damage may be a factor in thromboembolism we have tested for thrombus susceptibility in two ways: first, by the use of electrical stimulation, and second, by topical application of thrombin. In normal hamsters a threshold stimulus for thrombus formation is a shock of 5 to 7 volts of 10 milliseconds duration applied with a microelectrode; while in the various conditions mentioned above, thrombi are formed at definitely lower thresholds (Fulton, Akers and Lutz, '53). When thrombin is applied topically (Berman, Lutz and Fulton, '54) doses ranging from 2.5 to 5% are necessary to produce thrombi. With cortisone treated hamsters (5–10 mg per day), 21 out of 28 developed thrombi with as low as 1.25%, and with total body x-irradiated (1500 r) hamsters, 19 out of 25 developed thrombi with 5% or greater. Thrombi were formed only in the venules and small veins and never on the arterial side or in the capillaries.

Whereas generalized bacterial infection was accompanied by embolization (Lutz, Fulton and Akers, '51), the local inflammation accompanying abscess formation (Young, '54), or invasion with *Trichinella spiralis* (Humes and Akers, '52) prevented thrombus formation. With local bacterial infection petechiae appeared spontaneously in large numbers at venous junctions in from 5 to 24 hours (fig. 16), but disappeared as the first inflammatory response subsided. Apparently increased blood flow was important in preventing white thrombus formation and the subsequent red clot, and conversely, venous stagnation favored thrombus formation.

Petechial formation appeared to be of non-specific origin. Petechiae were seen (90–1200 ×) under the following conditions: (a) inflammation produced by topical application of filtrates of *Streptococcus hemolyticus* (N Y 5) and other cultures, and local infections with *Staphylococcus aureus;* (b) nonbacterial inflammation with formaldehyde, turpentine, croton oil and mustard oil; (c) anticoagulants *in vivo,* such as heparin Dicumarol, Tromexan and phenylindanedione, (d) partial cheek pouch x-irradiation ($\frac{3}{8}$ inch diameter) of 15,000 to 25,000 r, and (fig. 15) implanted beta-emitting Sr^{90} glass beads (140 µc, after 24 hours); (e) implantation of DCA pellets; (f) implantation of tumor transplants; (g) positive pressure used in determining blood pressure in cheek pouch vessels; and (h) trauma produced by physical means as bruising by falling weights, standardized minute burns, pin holes, and drying (Lutz, Fulton, Young, Shulman and Berman, '53).

The anticoagulants heparin, Dicumarol, Tromexan and phenylindanedione not only increased the adhesiveness of platelets and leukocytes, but also increased the fragility of the walls of the venules as indicated by the weak stimulation with a microelectrode needed to produce perivascular bleeding (figs. 13 and 14), and by petechial formation, either spontaneous or by production with a low negative pressure. Total body x-irradiation (1000–1500 r) also increased the fragility of the blood vessels.

The mechanism of petechial formation was studied by motion picture recording at 900 × during actual production in the hamster cheek pouch and frog retrolingual membrane (Arendt, Shulman, Fulton and Lutz, '53). For convenience petechiae were produced by topical application of moccasin venom dissolved in mammalian Ringer's solution. At two to 5 minutes prior to stasis, petechiae developed extensively primarily at venous junctions. Erythrocytes "popped out" one by one through a single hole, in spurts related to blood pressure without a permanent opening and without platelet plug formation. Since there is no valid evidence for involvement of the capillaries under ordinary conditions the term "capillary fragility" should be abandoned.

Adrenalectomy of 60 hamsters (Wyman, Fulton and Shulman, '53) did not alter the blood vessels until 24 hours before death at 5–7 days, when a decreased rate of flow associated with bradycardia occurred. Minute burns (fig. 18) were prevented from healing by 10 mg of cortisone acetate (Shulman, Fulton and Moront, '53). In 168 untreated hamsters petechiae appeared in 50%, and in 48 hours a "rosette" of new vessels developed, followed by scarless healing. With cortisone pretreatment the pouch remained avascular, and 90% were infected in 120 hours.

BASIC PERIPHERAL VASCULAR FACTORS

The blood pressure in the cheek pouch has been measured by a modification of the "pressure cuff" method (Berman, '53). In 52 normal hamsters (8–12 weeks), under light Nembutal, the mean pressure was 90 mm Hg as compared with 116 mm Hg determined by direct cannulation of the carotid artery. Direct observation of cheek pouch vessels during a rise to 185 mm Hg with subsequent fall to 45 mm Hg (due to 0.15 cm³ of 1:10,000 Noradrenalin) showed almost complete venous stasis during the hypotension, with marked constriction of arterioles. Total body x-irradiation (1500 r) produced only a slight temporary depression during the early post-irradiation period, followed by a continued drop to the terminal period of "chunky" flow and probable tissue anoxia. Kidney encapsulation (latex, silk) produced a permanent rise to 126.4 mm Hg in 16 hamsters. Blood pressure in 32 hamsters over one year old was 78 mm Hg as compared with 90 mm Hg in young hamsters, and no concomitant pathological changes were found in the vessel walls, even on an egg-yolk diet.

The venous side of the circulation appears to be the critical region for petechial formation, leukocyte sticking, permeability changes, and white thrombus formation. Berman ('53) determined the number, diameter, volume, endothelial surface, and cross sectional area of the arteries, capillaries and veins in the cheek pouch of normal living hamsters. By the statistical method the ratio of the endothelial surface in arteries, capillaries, and veins is 1 to 6 to 3; by mapping it is 2 to 2.5 to 4. Similarly the capacity ratios are 2 to 1.8 to 6 and 2.2 to 0.4 to 7.4 respectively. These figures indicate that the small veins (thrombus potentiality) contain 60–75% of the blood at any instant and that their endothelial area may comprise almost 75% of the peripheral surface available for exchange.

We cannot accept the pharmacological and clinical practice of inferring the specific nature of vasomotor responses, and classifying drugs as "vasoconstrictor" or "vasodilator" from the results of indirect methods, such as changes in blood pressure, skin temperature, plethymographically determined volume, or even from gross observations of erythema. The designation of a substance as "vasodilator" or "vasoconstrictor" should be based on direct observation of caliber changes. Furthermore, the use of the terms "capillary dilation" and "capillary constriction" implying an active participation of the capillary wall in a vasomotor response is not in accord with the modern concepts concerning the regulation of blood flow through capillaries (Fulton and Lutz, '40; Clark and Clark, '43; Chambers and Zweifach, '44; Chen and Tsai, '48).

LITERATURE CITED

ARENDT, K. A., M. H. SHULMAN, G. P. FULTON AND B. R. LUTZ 1953 Post irradiation petechiae and the mechanism of formation with snake venom. Anat. Rec., *117*: 595–596.

BERMAN, H. J. 1953 Observations on the blood pressure of the golden hamster (*Mesocricetus auratus*). Ph.D. Thesis, Department of Biology, Boston University.

BERMAN, H. J., B. R. LUTZ AND G. P. FULTON 1954 White and red thrombi produced by thrombin applied to the hamster cheek pouch. Fed. Proc., *13*: 12–13.

CHAMBERS, R., AND B. W. ZWEIFACH 1944 Topography and function of the mesenteric capillary circulation. Am. J. Anat., *75:* 173–205.

CHEN, T. I., AND C. TSAI 1948 The mechanism of hemostasis in peripheral vessels. J. Physiol., *107:* 280–288.

CLARK, E. R., AND E. L. CLARK 1943 Caliber changes in minute blood vessels observed in the living mammal. Am. J. Anat., *73:* 215–250.

FAHRAEUS, R. 1929 The suspension stability of the blood. Physiol. Rev., *9:* 241–274.

FULTON, G. P., AND B. R. LUTZ 1940 The neuromotor mechanism of the small blood vessels of the frog. Science, *92:* 223–224.

FULTON, G. P., B. R. LUTZ, D. L. JOFTES AND F. W. MAYNARD 1952 Effects of beta and x-irradiation on the circulation in the hamster cheek pouch (motion picture). Fed. Proc., *11:* 52.

FULTON, G. P., R. G. JACKSON AND B. R. LUTZ 1946 Cinephotomicroscopy of normal blood circulation in the cheek pouch of the hamster, *Cricetus auratus.* Anat. Rec., *96:* 537.

———— 1947 Cinephotomicroscopy of normal blood circulation in the cheek pouch of the hamster. Science, *105:* 361.

FULTON, G. P., R. P. AKERS AND B. R. LUTZ 1953 White thrombo-embolism and vascular fragility in the hamster cheek pouch after anticoagulants. Blood, *8:* 140–152.

FULTON, G. P., B. R. LUTZ, D. I. PATT AND G. YERGANIAN 1954 The cheek pouch of the Chinese hamster *(Cricetulus griseus)* for cinephotomicroscopy of blood circulation and tumor growth. J. Lab. Clin. Med., *44:* 145–148.

HUMES, A. G., AND R. P. AKERS 1952 Vascular changes in the cheek pouch of the golden hamster during infection with *Trichinella spiralis* larvae. Anat. Rec., *114:* 103–114.

KNISELY, M. H., E. H. BLOCH, T. S. ELIOT AND L. WARNER 1947 Sludged blood. Science, *106:* 431–440.

LUTZ, B. R. 1951 Intravascular agglutination of formed elements of blood. Physiol. Rev., *31:* 107–130.

LUTZ, B. R., G. P. FULTON AND R. P. AKERS 1951 White thromboembolism in the hamster cheek pouch after trauma, infection and neoplasia. Circulation, *3:* 339–352.

LUTZ, B. R., G. P. FULTON, G. YOUNG, M. H. SHULMAN AND H. J. BERMAN 1953 Petechial formation in the cheek pouch of the hamster *(Mesocricetus auratus).* Fed. Proc., *12:* 92.

MAYNARD, F. W., G. E. BATTIT, B. R. LUTZ, D. I. PATT AND G. P. FULTON 1952 The pattern and innervation of blood vessels in normal, irradiated, and tumor bearing cheek pouches of the hamster. Anat. Rec., *112:* 457–458.

PRATT, F. H., AND M. A. REID 1930 A method for working on the terminal nerve-muscle unit. Science, *72:* 431–433.

PRIDDY, R. B., AND A. F. BRODIE 1948 Facial musculature, nerves and blood vessels of the hamster in relation to the cheek pouch. J. Morph., *83:* 149–180.

SHULMAN, M. H., G. P. FULTON AND G. P. MORONT 1953 Effects of cortisone acetate on the healing of burns in the hamster cheek pouch. Fed. Proc., 12: 132.

WILLIAMS, T. W. 1948 The visualization of vertebrate capillary beds by intravascular precipitation of lead chromate. Anat. Rec., 100: 115–125.

WYMAN, L. C., G. P. FULTON AND M. H. SHULMAN 1953 Direct observations on the circulation in the hamster cheek pouch in adrenal insufficiency and experimental hypercorticalism. Ann. N. Y. Acad. Sci., 56: 643–658.

YOUNG, G. 1954 Experimental staphylococcus infection in the hamster cheek pouch: the process of localization. J. Exp. Med., 99: 299–306.

PLATE 1

EXPLANATION OF FIGURES

1   Apparatus for cinephotomicroscopy of small blood vessels, including 100 watt zirconium lamp for transillumination, beam-splitting prism, micromanipulator, electronic stimulator and motion picture camera.

2   Everted cheek pouch spread over optical block. × 3.

3   Cross section of the cheek pouch of the golden hamster *(Mesocricetus auratus)*, note external stratified squamous epithelial layers with connective tissue and blood vessels between. Hematoxylin and eosin. × 100.

4   Cross section of the cheek pouch of the Chinese hamster *(Cricetulus griseus)*. × 100.

5   Skeletal muscle attachment, anterior portion of pouch. Methylene blue. × 200.

6   Perivascular non-myelinated nerve plexus, and mast cells associated with an arteriole. Methylene blue. × 100.

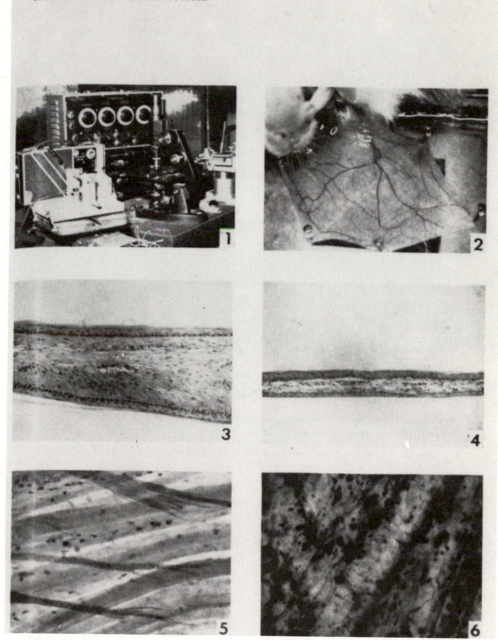

7 Methylcholanthrene tumor transplant growing in the cheek pouch. Twelve days old, 11th generation. × 2.

8 Transilluminated salivary gland tumor growing in the hamster cheek pouch. Sixty six days old. First generation transplant. × 3.

9 Normal vascular pattern in the cheek pouch, as shown by the intravascular precipitation of lead chromate. Transillumined. × 7.

10 Vascular pattern of methylcholanthrene tumor transplant, 9 days old. Reflected light. × 7.

11 Normal blood flow in a vein of the Chinese hamster cheek pouch. Electronic flash photograph. Note peripheral leukocytes. × 900.

12 Blood flow in an arteriole of the cheek pouch of the Chinese hamster, just before death. Twelve days after 900 r, total body x-irradiation. Note red corpuscle aggregates. Electronic flash photograph. × 500.

BRENTON R. LUTZ AND GEORGE P. FULTON

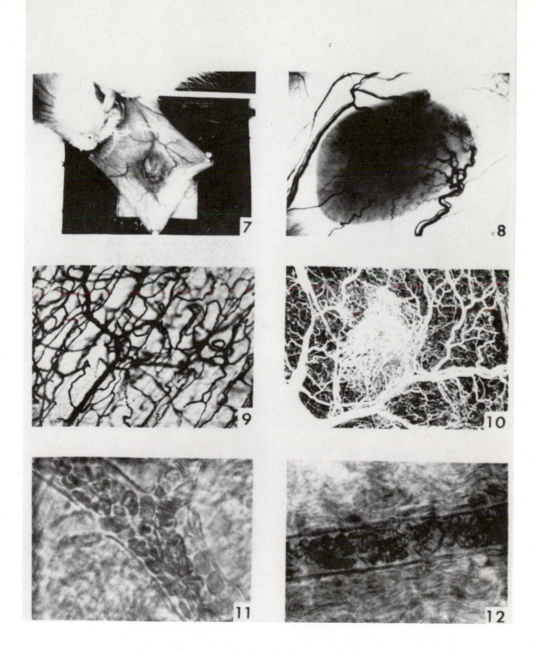

13   Microelectrode in position for venular ''fragility'' test after administration of heparin. Scene taken from a Kodachrome motion picture record. $\times$ 260.

14   Same vein seen in figure 13. One-fourth second after weak electrical stimulation. Note start of bleeding. $\times$ 260.

15   Petechial hemorrhages on venules around beta-emitting strontium 90 glass bead (141 microcuries). Twenty-four hours after implantation. Bead diameter 1.3 mm. $\times$ 7.

16   Petechial hemorrhages at venous junctions 5 hours after injection of 0.05 cm^3 of *S. aureus* culture at a nearby point. $\times$ 10.

17   Platelet thrombus resulting from forceps trauma. $\times$ 520.

18   Standard burn after two days. Animal given daily subcutaneous injections of 5 mg of cortisone acetate beginning one day before burn. $\times$ 7.

306

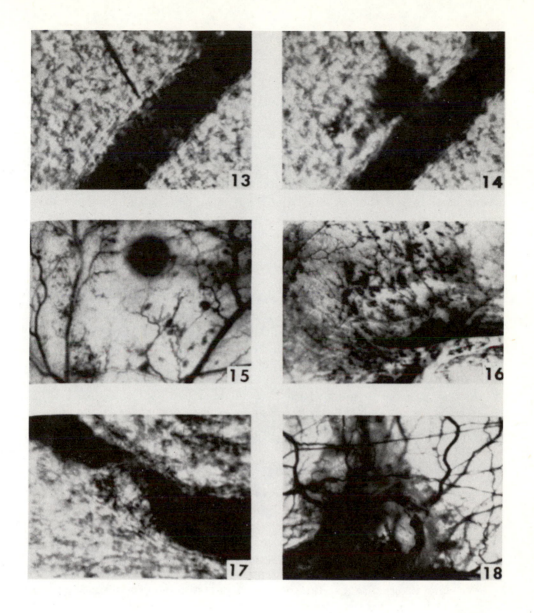

307

Reprinted from *Angiology*, **6**(4), 291–308 (1955)

VASCULAR PATTERNS AND ACTIVE VASOMOTION AS DETERMINERS OF FLOW THROUGH MINUTE VESSELS

PAUL A. NICOLL, Ph.D. and RICHARD L. WEBB, Ph.D.

Of the sites where living cells and tissues may be observed, we feel that the wing membrane of the bat offers a most advantageous arrangement for studies on the vascular system. Shortly before the turn of the century, the advantages of this area were exploited. Since then it has been used only by a few investigators interested in vital studies. For many years the web of the frog's foot was preferred as a natural area for studies on the vascular system. While significant knowledge of the vascular pattern in amphibia has been gained by earlier investigators, certain critical points have been overlooked because of the difference between the amphibian pattern and that of the mammalian vascular system. Probably the most significant error in this respect has been in the conception of the capillaries. Investigations by Clark and Clark indicated such pitfalls and led to the development of a new technique of direct study on the rabbit ear, resulting in a more accurate conception of blood vessels in the mammal.

In scanning the program of the first Microcirculatory Conference held in Galveston, one is impressed by the examples of ingenuity employed in preparing the mammalian tissues so that the vascular system can be observed directly (1). Each has its special advantages in gaining an insight into the behavior of the vessels under study.

In formulating the present paper, we have omitted a detailed description of technique and special methods, since they were described exhaustively in the first conference (2). When the central theme of a vascular study is the analysis of a fundamental mechanism of capillary behavior, the advantages of the bat wing technique are most evident. Specific adaptations of the circulation following long term subjection to altered physiological or pathological states are not suitable problems for this particular approach.

We claim no originality in the selection of the bat as an experimental animal. We do wish, however, to emphasize that because of the simplicity and accessibility of its blood and nerve supply, the necessity for devising complicated methods is minimized. As an example, studies on the normal activity of these structures can be made without resorting to surgical procedure involving the use of anesthesia. These data are invaluable when comparisons are to be made with other experiments.

OBSERVATIONS AND RESULTS

Vascular arcuate systems

The arcuate configurations on the arterial side begin with arteriolar vessels (2). Each system consists of anastomotic vessels of approximately equal diameter. Since 2 or sometimes 3 distinct arteriolar arcuate systems can be identified in

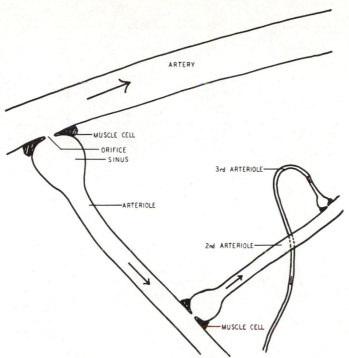

Fig. 1. Indian Club origins of arteriolar vessels. Many instances where origins of all three arcuate systems may be found in close proximity are seen in these wing membranes.

these vascular beds, the parent vessel can be either an artery or a large arteriole. All origins of an arcuate system show 2 characteristic features. One is their angle of origin from the parent vessel which is always 90° or less in reference to the forward direction of flow in the parent vessel. The second feature is the appearance at the origin where the vessel exhibits a dilatation as compared to its average diameter elsewhere, while the actual orifice from the parent vessel is smaller than its average diameter. This formation has been aptly termed "Indian Club" (fig. 1) and is a functional configuration dependent on the tonus exhibited by the muscle cells in the wall. The relative diameters of the orifice, dilated bulb and vessel may show considerable difference when tonus varies in the muscle cells or as they contract actively. Within any arcuate system, no sinuses are found at the junctional points, and angles of branching have no specific relation to flow patterns. Terminal arterioles are vessels of varying length and complexity that feed the extensive capillary net. They may arise from any of the arcuate arterioles or occasionally from a small artery. The majority of them, of course, originate from the smallest arcuate vessels.

Capillaries form extensive nets with numerous terminal arteriolar feeders and equally numerous drainage channels (fig. 2). Thus, specific or preferential flow paths within the capillaries are not observed in these subcutaneous minute vascular beds. Such conditions, if they exist in other minute vascular fields, must

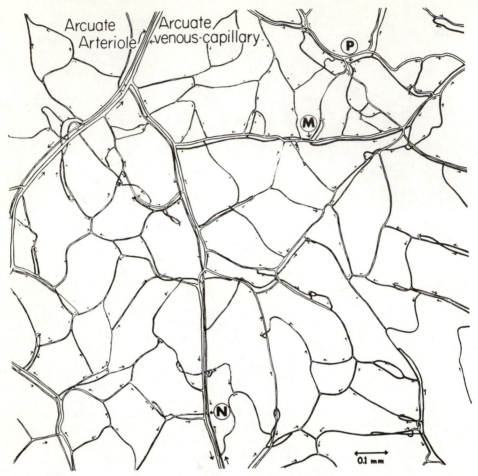

FIG. 2. Arcuate patterns of arterioles and venous capillaries and the connection of terminal arterioles with the capillaries. Arrows indicate flow direction at time sketch was made. Note points N, M and P where flow from two directions meet in the arcuate arterioles.

represent specialized relationships in those sites. They should not be ascribed to a fundamental organization of capillary structure (3). The distribution of flow from any particular terminal arteriole within the capillary net usually is not extensive. Local conditions within the minute vessels determine the actual flow path and are changing constantly.

The drainage channels are formed by the joining of the capillary structures and show frequent anastomotic connections. This leads to the development of an arcuate pattern of venous capillaries, which roughly parallels the arcuate arteriolar vessels (fig. 3). They differ from the smaller capillaries only in size and probably show the same permeability. Claims have been made that their permeability is greater than that of the smaller capillaries (4). Vasoreactive agents

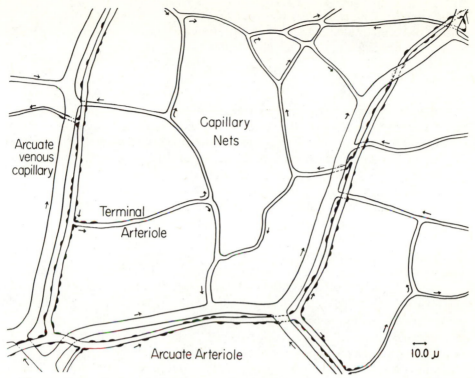

Fig. 3. Capillaries and arcuate patterns in arteriole and venous-capillary. Note close proximity of the arteriole and venous-capillary vessels.

brought in by the blood stream and metabolic by-products picked up by the capillaries that affect smooth muscle tonus could reach the arterioles by this route. The orifice at the confluence of these venous capillaries with the venules is protected by either a well developed valve or a protruding cusp, although occasionally no such structure is evident. Since the muscular coat of the venule appears in the immediate vicinity of the valve, this site may be considered as the true junctional point between capillary and venule.

Flow characteristics and patterns within the smaller capillaries are determined chiefly by the behavior of the terminal arterioles. If they are dilated, flow is rapid and continuous within the smaller capillaries. Since the diameter of the terminal arterioles is smaller than that of the capillaries which they supply, arteriolar flow is more rapid than capillary flow. If the terminal arteriole or any of its branches is closed, flow stops in the capillary branches. With the many supplying terminal arterioles closed intermittently and aphasically, flow into the arcuate net of the venous capillaries becomes continuous.

If a junction of a venous capillary and a venule is protected by an adequate valve, blood leaves only when the valve is relaxed. This causes the movement out of the venous capillary to be intermittent. On the other hand, if the junction has no valve or an imperfect one, pressure changes within the venule are reflected in the venous capillaries. Then blood moves sluggishly with frequent changes in path and direction along the anastomotic branches of the net. Obviously this results in inefficient emptying of the involved capillary bed.

Active vasomotion

Active vasomotion is the outstanding motor phenomenon observed in peripheral vascular structures. It refers to changes in lumen diameter that result from activity of the muscle cells in the vessel wall. The action may be dependent either on changes in tonus of the smooth muscle cells or on their active contraction at any initial tonus level. Depending on the nature of the response, the modification in diameter may be either an increase or decrease, and either slow or fast in its development. In the subcutaneous sites studied here, it is exhibited by all vessels having muscles in their walls, but is not seen in the capillaries.

Arteries and occasionally the largest arterioles exhibit active vasomotion in two distinct ways. One is a slowly developing caliber change that appears to be dependent on the tonus level in the muscular coat. This is not perceived usually and probably represents minor fluctuations of the mechanism that keeps these vessels only partially dilated. The second manifestation of active vasomotion in these vessels is a rapid caliber change that represents contraction of the muscle cells. Such a response is observed typically following either direct excitation of the nerves to the area or as a reflex response to noxious stimuli. Its dependence on neurological connections with the central nervous system is shown also by its sudden loss following acute section of the appropriate nerves. When time is allowed for complete degeneration of the nerve fibers, no reappearance of the rapid type of active vasomotion is seen although gradual recovery of tonus and slow tonus changes occur.

Active vasomotion in the arterioles, especially the smaller arcuate and terminal arterioles, appears to be an independent effector mechanism of the muscle cells without any direct dependency on nerve connections. This factor makes analysis into tonus changes and contractile responses almost impossible. All types of responses both as to magnitude and frequency may be observed without any clear separation into specific types. However, two patterns of response are recognizable in these vessels depending on the anatomical arrangements of the muscle cells that wind spirally around the vessels. An individual cell makes four to six complete turns around a vessel. These coils are closely wound and usually overlap along the stem of the terminal arterioles. This permits activity to spread by direct muscular transmission. Peristaltic waves which are a common occurrence move from the origins of the arcuate arterioles toward terminal arterioles. The second pattern is one of localized contraction infrequently observed in arcuate vessels, but found normally as the response of the final cells of the terminal arteriole. These precapillary sphincters exhibit the greatest degree of independent action of any vascular site.

The result of active vasomotion on flow in capillaries is directly correlated with the degree and duration of arteriolar patency. If the degree of constriction is not great enough to obliterate completely the lumen, only certain components of blood may be held back. This produces, for example, the phenomenon of "plasma skimming" where only the cellular components are held back while plasma and platelets continue into and through the capillaries ahead. When the degree of constriction is sufficient to close the arteriolar lumen, flow in affected capillaries ceases for the duration of the activity. This may last for several minutes in certain cases of localized contractions of capillary sphincters, but is transient with the peristaltic type. The latter results in rhythmical opening and closing of the arterial supply to the capillary beds, creating intermittent flow in the capillaries beyond.

Capillaries, simple tubes of endothelial cells, are never observed to make active changes in their caliber. Since they possess distensible qualities they may show deformation under variable conditions. These responses are usually slow in their development and given no indication of active participation by the endothelial cells.

Venules, starting at the sites of the first valves, and all veins exhibit marked active vasomotion. The action is a sharp contraction that sweeps centripetally as a peristaltic wave. The segment of any vessel between two valves forms a responsive unit. Contraction is initiated at the sinus of the peripheral valve and moves centrally to the next valve where it dies out. Since the majority of the valves are located at the confluence of two or more tributaries, the activities of which are independent, valve action and blood flow often appear unrelated to active vasomotion. This is complicated by the fact that the segment central to the valve also responds independently of the tributaries concerned. Thus, the pressure wave in any responding segment that precedes and usually opens the cusps of the central valve, may arrive when the pressure in that valve sinus is too high for it to open. This can occur either because another tributary is actively discharging or the segment ahead is contracting. Failure to recognize these relationships misled Carrier (5) into minimizing the significance of active vasomotion in the regulation of venous flow in these vascular fields.

In most cases two major tributaries form the next vessel and are observed to contract alternately. One empties into the segment ahead while the other tributary is relaxed. The central segment then contracts. The frequency of the action in the segments involved is usually too rapid for perfect coordination of the activities and some flow distortion results. Single tributaries entering any segment, whether exhibiting active vasomotion of their own or not, empty into the central segment during its period of relaxation. As the larger veins are formed, the distance between valves becomes greater which increases the storage volume of the segment. Thus, contraction frequencies need not increase to insure adequate forward flow of blood in these veins.

Regulation of active vasomotion

With active vasomotion in arteries, arterioles and veins serving as the main functional determiner of capillary flow and probably of capillary pressures, the manner of regulation in the various structures is of paramount importance. No observations on the vascular fields considered here are contrary to the thesis that the smooth muscle cells function as independent effectors. This concept assumes these active units to possess an inherent property of either changing their tonus or exhibiting sudden contraction in response to changes in their immediate environment. Argument, as to whether or not they need some type of stimulus or environmental change to call forth a response, is scientifically fruitless. The real meaning behind the term "independent effector" resides in the idea that such structures require no specific stimulus to call forth a response such as usually needed with striated muscle. The problem then in the analysis of the regulation of active vasomotion is one of determination of what environmental changes actually affect the smooth muscle cells.

Three types of environmental changes have been investigated as to the manner in which they modify active vasomotion at the various sites where it is observed normally. The broad classes of stimuli are those associated with nerve impulses, specific or general chemical substances, and physical phenomena such as temperature and pressure. While the ultimate stimulus in all cases might prove to be some common distortion of equilibrium between the reacting cell and its immediate environment, it is more profitable for the present to consider each class of stimulus as a separate entity and present the evidence in that manner.

It is convenient, in the analysis of the regulation of active vasomotion by nerve impulses, to separate the possible sources of the impulse into central and peripheral. The role of impulses of central origin can be evaluated by observing the sites and characteristics of active vasomotion following either direct excitation of the nerves, or reflex responses in the area after some non-specific stimulus is given the animal. In addition, specific changes in the patterns and form of activity following acute or chronic section of the nerves may also indicate the role of impulses of central origin.

Three methods have been employed in study of this problem in these subcutaneous fields. The simplicity of the structures involved and the accessibility of the nerve supply make the technique easy and the results clear cut. Direct excitation of the nerve or reflexly induced active vasomotion is limited strictly to the arteries and some of the larger arterioles. The smaller arcuate and terminal arterioles, pre-capillary sphincters, venules and veins never exhibit initiation or modification of active vasomotion as the direct response to central impulses (6). In the arteries and larger arterioles, where activity is induced by impulses of central origin, the action is one of intense constriction. The duration of the response may vary, but is usually of considerable length—and especially with direct excitation of the nerve is maintained for, and may outlast, the duration of stimulus. Immediately following acute section of the nerve to the area, and continuing throughout its complete degeneration period, all central control is lost. Possible recovery following regeneration has not been investigated. It has also proved impossible to determine what nerve fibers are concerned, but the assumption is made that the sympathetic outflow is involved. No evidence of specific inhibition of either tonus or contraction of the muscle cells by impulses of central origin has been obtained.

Study of possible involvement of impulses of peripheral origin is much more difficult to carry out and results are always hard to interpret. The animal used must have all central nerve connections either cut or blocked. In addition, excitation of peripheral nerves offers serious technical problems. Quantitative factors both as to the stimulus and response dominate the analysis, with simple qualitative relationships becoming decreasingly significant. Some observations have been made, however, that seem to indicate that impulses of peripheral origin are little involved in regulation of active vasomotion. The early loss of tonus following acute section of the nerve, coupled with the absence of any active vasomotion for several hours after denervation, indicate that impulses of peripheral origin are not effective. Although positive evidence is lacking there would seem to be no reason why impulses of peripheral origin would not continue to reach these structures for a considerable time after acute section of the main nerve. The independence of active vasomotion of some vascular structures from impulses of central origin and maintenance of their activity with complete nerve degeneration, indicate nerve impulses are insignificant in regulation of the action.

Two results obtained by entirely different approaches are worthy of consideration. If an arteriole or artery is stroked mechanically with or without previous disturbance of its innervation, there occurs frequently a marked dilatation of the vessel as an initial response. Continued stroking invariably results in severe constriction of the site which lasts long after removal of the exciting stimulus. This might indicate that the muscle cells themselves show a response locally to induced environmental change. A similar phenomenon can be demonstrated in another manner. If a constant current of sufficient magnitude passes between a single fluid electrode on the wing surface and an indifferent electrode, there develop, after a short interval, alternate areas of marked constriction and dilation along the arteries and arterioles. The pattern of distribution of the effect depends on the size of the fluid electrode and its spatial relationship to the vessels, but it remains constant, after once established, as long as the current flows. If the current is reversed there is a rapid shift in the effect upon the responding vessels. The areas formerly constricted now dilate while the dilated regions constrict. This can be repeated over and over with each reversal of current direction. This again indicates, without going into the possible mechanism, that small changes in local environment readily affect the response of these muscle cells. This observation must be taken into account when interpreting apparent response obtained by direct excitation of nerves with microelectrodes.

Many modifications of the chemical environment of the muscle cells profoundly change active vasomotion. The real question is what ones are of physiological importance, and how does active vasomotion change under controlled situations. Numerous aspects of this problem remain unstudied and one can anticipate confidently that this will always be the case. Probably the most outstanding of the physiological vasoreactive agents are epinephrine and its close relatives. Investigation of their action has indicated that it is always constrictive on the arteries and larger arterioles (7). Their effect on active vasomotion of other vascular sites is somewhat different. Here 2 types of action are observed.

The magnitude of the constriction is enhanced and frequency of the response is increased. Actually, this is very similar to the well known effect on atrial musculature where epinephrine increases both the frequency and magnitude of its response.

Other vasoreactive agents of physiological importance have not been thoroughly investigated in these fields. Incidental use of acetylcholine and histamine, for example, have given inconsistent results. Some evidence of inhibition with vascular relaxation by acetylcholine, when topically applied to these minute vessels, has been obtained. The reactions, however, have been weak and fleeting. This result was not entirely unanticipated in view of its known rapid destruction by the ubiquitous enzyme choline-esterase. More important has been the consistent failure to demonstrate a significant modification of active vasomotion following topical application of histamine.

A different approach in the study of chemical factors and regulation of active vasomotion has been the use of respiratory gases of known composition. These data have not been reported previously and a brief description of the technique used is necessary to understand and evaluate their possible significance. The basic procedure is similar to that usually employed (8), with two modifications. The portion of the bat holder where the animal's body is confined has been fitted to permit complete control of the composition of the inspired gas. A second change in technique is that all nerves to the entire wing are sectioned previously, not just the nerves to the area under observation.

The activity of terminal arterioles or precapillary sphincters is observed at high magnification and the characteristics of vasomotion are followed. The duration of both the constriction and relaxation phases are timed and the degree of constriction estimated, as the per cent of complete vessel closure. In some experiments this data was recorded by signal magnets on a kymogram. The operator presses the key in one signal magnet circuit during the constriction phase and varies the frequency of activation of a second signal magnet to represent the magnitude of response. Only spontaneously active sites are used. Change in a measured characteristic of active vasomotion is interpreted as a response to the altered conditions that follow exposure to a given gas mixture. Preliminary studies indicated the first effects on active vasomotion in a terminal arteriole or precapillary sphincter could be expected within 30 to 40 seconds after a change in gas composition. Full effects, however, required a longer period to develop. Also since the characteristics of individual responses always show variations, changes in behavior were determined on average values.

Gas mixtures used were made up of accurately measured percentages of oxygen, carbon dioxide and helium. Helium exerts no measurable effect on active vasomotion. Oxygen has 2 types of action. If an adequate stimulus for the contractive phase is present, the duration of that phase is directly dependent on the available oxygen supply. In the absence of specific stimulus to contraction, both the frequency and magnitude of active vasomotion, however, are reduced with increasing availability of oxygen. Carbon dioxide, contrary to the anticipated effect based on its generally accepted dilatory action, proved to be

TABLE 1

Characteristics of active vasomotion in terminal arterioles measured during exposure to respiratory gases of known composition

Test Animal No.	Gas Mixture			No. of Observations	Characteristics of Active Vasomotion			
					Duration		Constriction	Frequency*
	Air	O_2	CO_2		Contraction	Dilation		
	%	%	%		sec.	sec.	% max.	cycles/min.
4912	100			5	3.9	2.5	26	9.2
4912		90	10	15	3.1	3.1	81	9.7
4912		100	10	10	2.7	2.9	8	10.5
4913		100		5	6.0	2.9	50	6.7
4913		90	10	20	4.3	3.0	90	8.2
4914		100		5	2.8	3.3	30	9.8
4914		90	10	10	4.5	2.4	48	8.1
4960		100		5	2.3	1.8	75	14.6
4960		90	10	26	2.9	2.5	82	11.1
4960		80	20	16	2.9	3.2	67	9.8
4970	100			5	3.8	2.5	42	9.5
4970		90	10	20	3.1	2.0	62	11.7
4971		100		15	2.4	1.9	62	13.9
4971		90	10	10	5.4	2.2	100	7.9
4971	100			10	2.4	3.3	19	10.5
4972	100			10	4.1	4.0	49	7.4
4972		90	10	15	2.8	2.4	91	11.5
4972		100		15	2.7	2.7	62	11.1
4974	100			14	7.5	5.6	82	4.6
4974		90	10	26	8.0	5.0	90	4.6

* Calculated values.

a powerful stimulus of the contractive phase of active vasomotion. The percentage range of carbon dioxide that is stimulatory was rather narrow but one that might be assumed to have physiological significance. A 5 per cent mixture produces no measurable effects, while 10 per cent usually shows some stimulation. The most intense and clear-cut action is observed when 15 per cent carbon dioxide is present in the gas. A further increase to 20 per cent carbon dioxide gives a response that appears to be toxic to the reactive cells since active vasomotion is inhibited. The individual cells lose their contractility and become fixed in a partially contracted state. A summary of the results to date on the respiratory gas mixtures and their action on active vasomotion is given in table 1.

The experimental data from two different tests of the effect on active vasomotion in terminal arterioles is presented in figure 4. In both tests time is plotted along the bottom and shows when each series of observations was started. The actual points in each series are plotted as consecutive readings and their position does not represent actual elapsed time. In test A both the strength and, initially, the duration of the contractive phase are increased during the period of breathing the CO_2-O_2 mixture. When pure O_2 replaces the mixture, a notice-

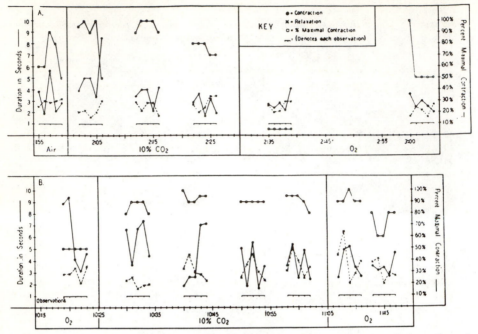

FIG. 4, A and B. Duration of cyclic phases and degree of vascular constriction of terminal arterioles in two tests where CO_2 is added to the inspired gas. For complete description see text.

able loss in the strength of contraction rapidly develops but duration shows little change. Since the animal was never actually deprived of oxygen this might be expected. Test B, where the gas changes were from pure O_2 to CO_2-O_2 mixture and return to pure O_2, confirms the stimulating action of CO_2 on strength of contraction. This demonstrates again that with adequate oxygen present the duration of contraction or relaxation is little if any affected.

The role of oxygen in the regulation of active vasomotion is more clearly evident from the kymogram data shown graphically in figure 5. Only duration of the contraction and relaxation phases are included. Magnitude also increased when CO_2 was used. Both durations are plotted in sequence. The relaxation period plotted with each contraction is the one that followed. Although the total lapsed time differs in each part of figure 5, all represent the data within the first ten minutes after exposure to the gas or gas mixture indicated. Normal variations in phasic duration when the animal is in air are shown in figure 5A. When air is replaced with 15 per cent CO_2-85 per cent O_2 the duration of contraction increases while relaxation becomes uniformly brief. However, when the same stimulus of 15 per cent CO_2 is used, but the oxygen available is severely limited, duration of contraction actually falls below normal and frequent periods of long relaxation are observed (fig. 5B). The tendency of low oxygen to favor relaxation is clearly evident in figure 5D, E and F where the behavior with 100 per cent helium is compared to that in oxygen both before and after the anoxic

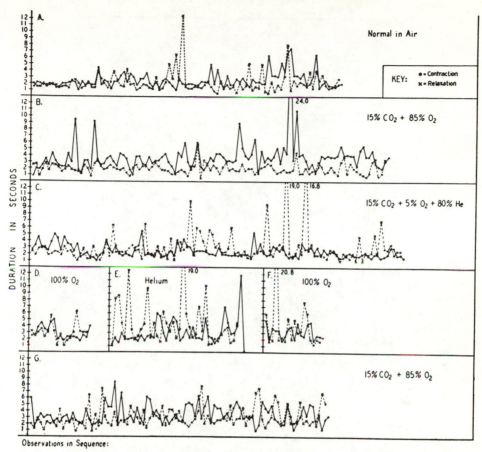

FIG. 5, A–G. Phase duration of consecutive spontaneous active vasomotion cycles in a terminal arteriole as influenced by inspired gas mixtures. Data from kymogram records. For details see text.

period. The increase in duration of contraction as anoxia proceeds is more apparent than real. Actually magnitude of contraction falls sharply and a state of incomplete relaxation or contracture supervenes. If anoxia is maintained for still longer periods all activity ceases, and the vessels remain in this state of incomplete relaxation. Under these conditions re-establishment of adequate oxygen does not lead to rapid recovery of vasomotion. This is partially demonstrated in figure 5G when, after a brief time in oxygen following the anoxic period, the animal is again subjected to the 15 per cent CO_2-85 per cent O_2 mixture. Here duration of the contraction phase tends to lengthen but relaxation does not shorten and the frequency of the cyclic action decreases.

The influence on active vasomotion of 2 physical characteristics of the environment of these minute vessels has been studied. Temperature effects were analyzed quantitatively in terms of the frequency of active vasomotion in veins and venules. These structures were selected as test sites in preference to other components of the vascular bed because of their independence from nerve

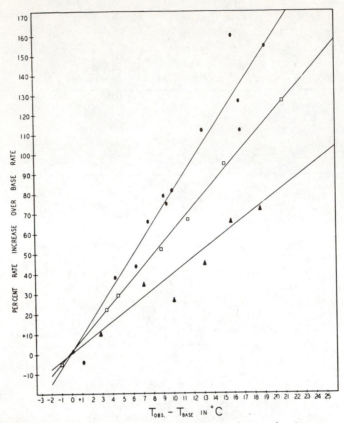

FIG. 6. Frequency change of active vasomotion cycles in venules (upper curve) and two small veins (lower curves) as a function of environmental temperature. Ordinate: per cent rate increase over base rate. Abscissa: temperature difference between observation value and base temperature.

control and their stable base frequencies. Qualitative comparisons indicate arteriolar structures behave in a similar manner. A second physical characteristic, that of changes in internal pressure, has been analyzed qualitatively with observations made on all vessel types.

Temperatures were varied locally in the denervated wing while the animal's body was kept at room temperature. A thin film of mineral oil of the desired temperature flowed continuously over the observation site. The multiple warm junctions of thermocouples placed on the surface to surround the site under observation permitted continuous readings of environmental temperatures to 0.1°C. The extreme thinness of the wing membrane is assumed to allow rapid equilibrium of internal environmental and oil film temperatures. An interesting side observation showed the Zirconium light had no effect on environmental temperatures under these conditions.

Three examples of the change in frequency of active vasomotion with increasing temperatures are given in figure 6. The two lower curves are data from two small venous branches. The upper curve is compiled from data on four different sites among the larger venules. It is apparent from these data that the frequency of active vasomotion varies directly with temperatures within the physiological range. The Q_{10} values are approximately two in all cases despite the different absolute slopes which probably indicate lower responsiveness in the larger vessels.

Changes in the internal pressure of vessels produce marked effects on active vasomotion. If the change is relatively slow in its development the vessel responds by a gradual adjustment of its tone. This probably results from changes in tonus of the smooth muscle cells and involves either increase or decrease in tonus depending on whether the pressure rises or falls. Sudden increase in internal pressure produces a different response. The vessel initially is distended mechanically with resulting stretch of the muscle cells in the wall. They immediately respond with a powerful contraction that may close the vessel if the initial stimulus is strong enough. The action may then spread as a peristaltic wave along the vessel.

This phenomenon can be demonstrated by suitable cannulation of the small arterioles or venules. A syringe, filled with balanced salt solution, is attached to the cannula and normal blood flow through the vessel is allowed to be reestablished. If one now taps the barrel of the syringe a small volume of fluid is forced into the vessel producing a sudden distension. There is an immediate reaction at the site of the stretch. The muscle cells contract and the activity spreads rapidly as a peristaltic wave for considerable distances. In the arterioles it spreads more readily towards the periphery while in the venules and veins it is localized to the segment involved. Although quantitative data is not available there is a possibility that the rhythmical patterns of peristaltic waves frequently observed in the arteriolar vessels may be originated by sudden changes in internal pressures at their origins.

Numerous examples of spontaneous changes in vascular tone resulting from tonus adjustments of the muscle cells following a rise or fall of internal pressure have been observed. If one occludes a small arterial branch with a probe placed on the surface of the wing, flow stops in the majority of vessels normally supplied by that source. If the block is maintained for several minutes and then released, flow is resumed, but initially shows a distinctive pattern. The vessels distend, indicating a loss of tone during the period of occlusion, and flow is first resumed in the branches close to the occlusion site. As they fill and distend they react and contract, increasing their resistance and thus shunt blood along to the next branches. This reaction rapidly spreads over the entire distribution of the occluded vessel until normal behavior patterns of flow are re-established.

Another probable example of this same mechanism is seen in the unusually high tone of the arteriolar vessels that develops when the main arteries have been denervated with their resultant dilation. Since only a small portion of the arterial system has been affected by the denervation and dilatation, it is reasonable to suppose the actual pressure within the arteriole has been raised above the normal values. The resulting increase in pressure in these arterioles could account for increased tone. This often proceeds to the extent that flow through arterioles and capillary beds is reduced.

DISCUSSION

The arcuate arrangements of arterioles establishes a vascular pattern that provides structural characteristics of importance for an intrinsic regulation of both flow and pressure within the capillaries. The roughly concentric organizations of the arcuate systems, each of which comprises vessels of approximately the same size that anastomose among themselves, serve as a series of volume reservoirs for the capillaries they supply. This not only assures adequate blood for the capillary beds at reasonable pressures, but also offers considerable protection to this supply from flow fluctuations in the arterial vessels. Such an arrangement is essential in any distributing system that supplies numerous outlets of variable demand where one component, here the distensible conduits, varies its quantitive relationship to the system as a function of pressure.

The mode of origin of each arteriole from its parent vessel, along with their uniformity and free anastomosis, provide a simple structural basis that permits step-wise pressure reductions. At the same time this type of organization assures adequate and nearly equal pressure heads for each outlet from a given system. These conditions, in conjunction with the numerous terminal arterioles that feed the capillary beds, would yield approximately the same pressure in all capillaries regardless of their proximity to the arterial supply. They also permit capillary pressures to be sufficient for their functional requirements at minimal arterial values and so increase cardiac efficiency. The most important part of this intrinsic pressure regulating mechanism is the Indian Club formation at arteriolar origins. While the angle of origin of each arteriole insures a more or less abrupt lowering of pressure from artery to arteriole and from one arteriolar system to the next, the actual size of the orifice of each arteriole governs the magnitude of each reduction step. This size is variable and may be readily changed depending on the tonus or contraction of the muscle cells that cause its formation. It is even possible that internal pressure within the arteries is the principal determiner of the tonus level, providing still another intrinsic mechanism for regulation of flow and pressure in the capillaries.

The efficiently engineered vascular patterns in coordination with the autonomous behavior of the terminal arterioles and precapillary sphincters raise the question of neural control of arterial size. The studies reported here strongly indicate that neural control of arteries is not fundamental for regulation of adequate capillary conditions. Therefore it must be primarily associated with adjustments of volume of the arterial reservoir. The adjustments, if the entire arterial system is involved, might be associated with modification of arterial volume to conform to variations in cardiac function, or with increased demands of particular outflow sites. Whether or not specific adjustments within the arterial system, as a result of increased needs in particular regions, are possible has never been adequately shown. Much indirect evidence argues against any mechanism of neural control for a specific artery. It is difficult to conceive of a condition where sudden reduction of its blood supply would be beneficial to an organ or region of the body. All such adjustments are rather of a compensatory nature to protect the limited blood volume for distribution to areas where the demand has increased.

Active vasomotion in the arcuate arteriole, which is predominantly of the peristaltic wave type, poses a puzzling problem as to its functional significance. It could be related to adjustments of volume or pressure within each arcuate system, but such a suggestion is not very satisfying. There is always the possibility that it serves as a localized adjunctive mechanism to cardiac contraction in providing adequate pressure for the terminal arterioles. However, no positive evidence for such a suggestion actually exists though studies now under way are directed to this problem. Peristaltic waves in the final arcuate and terminal arterioles could serve as a means of increasing slightly the total duration of the contraction phase and thus the period of reduced flow and pressure in the capillaries, without requiring maintained contraction of any individual muscle cell. When local conditions warrant reduction in capillary flow and pressure, the frequently observed maintained contraction of precapillary sphincters would be more efficient.

The ultimate result of active vasomotion in terminal arterioles establishes alternate periods of vigorous flow and reduced or no flow in the capillaries. This flow and pressure pattern in the capillaries no doubt serves capillary function more efficiently than any other. Directly or indirectly it has been detected in a variety of sites in many species (9). Maintenance of this pattern may then be the common goal of all mechanisms that determine capillary flow. Granted adequate pressure and volume at the heads of the terminal arterioles, local conditions must regulate the final expression of the capillary flow and pressure pattern in order to fulfill the immediate requirements of the tissues involved. The principal targets of these local conditions must be the muscle cells of the terminal arterioles. Although adequate data on pressure fluctuations in capillaries are not yet available, all observations of flow support this concept.

The data obtained with respiratory gas mixtures can serve to show how regulation of arteriolar vasomotion affects capillary function. The assumption is made that loss of diffusible capillary constituents to the interstitial fluid occurs more efficiently when capillary flow is vigorous and capillary pressure high. This would be true during the relaxation phase of arteriolar vasomotion. Conversely the return of diffusible substance from interstitial space to capillary would take place principally when arteriolar contraction has stopped flow and lowered pressure in the capillaries. Actual fluid exchange would follow this rule, which is only a slight modification of the principles originally advanced by Starling. Accurate data on movement of diffusible substance across individual capillaries has still to be obtained. There is no evidence, however, to warrant the above assumption as untenable.

With patent arteriole and vigorous capillary flow, metabolic by-products in the interstitial fluid could increase and act as stimuli for contraction of arteriolar muscles. The action of increased CO_2 supports this idea. The duration of the ensuing contraction could be a function of the available oxygen. If this were low or lacking the contraction phase would be brief despite an adequate stimulus. If sufficient oxygen were present the duration of contraction would depend on the strength of the stimulus and the sensitivity of the muscle cells. Under resting conditions, oxygen is probably not a limiting factor and the observed variability of duration of contraction and relaxation phases of active vasomotion follows fluctuations of stimuli strength and sensitivity. During activity oxygen utilization by the tissue rapidly lowers its availability and duration of the contraction phase is shortened. This would result in more ample blood flow for the active tissue. However, contraction still occurs and although brief it is powerful. This permits maintenance of metabolic by-products within physiological concentration by allowing limited periods for their escape.

It is significant that epinephrine increases the frequency of response of active vasomotion under normal conditions, thus indicating its action as largely one of increasing sensitivity of the muscle cells. This might be a protective measure against toxic action of excessive accumulations of metabolic by-products that could occur because of the low available oxygen and resultant suppression of arteriole closure. It is generally assumed that circulating epinephrine increases with activity or anticipated effort. Acetylcholine, on the other hand, may decrease the sensitivity of the arteriolar muscles to local stimuli and thus favor the relaxation phase without abolishing the obligatory periods of arteriolar closure. It is even possible that the very impulses to skeletal muscle that drive their activity may help insure increased blood by lengthening the relaxation phase. The nerves passing to the skeletal muscles in their final distribution lie in close proximity to the arteriolar vessels that supply the muscle capillaries. Numerous observations have indicated the release of acetylcholine as an associated phenomenon of impulse passage all along the nerve fiber.

Active vasomotion in venules and veins probably represents adaptation of an inherent property of the muscle cells in their walls to aid venous return. While it may be more widespread in vascular systems than is usually recognized, peculiar conditions of the expansive thin membranes of the bat may accentuate the need for such an aid in venous return. Pressure within the vessels seems to be the principal stimulus for the action. Chemical and other physical changes have only a basic function in this activity and do not appear to be significant in modifying the behavior in particular situations.

CONCLUSIONS

1. Vasomotor responses dominantly controlled by neural mechanism are limited to regulation of volume of the arterial reservoir. They primarily serve to adapt this volume to changes in cardiac output but may also protect it from excessive loss at outflow sites.

2. Arterioles form concentric arcuate patterns that by their structure and functional adaptation insure nearly equal and adequate pressure and volume conditions at the heads of the terminal arterioles.

3. Active vasomotion of terminal arterioles finally determines flow and pressure patterns within capillaries. Local chemical and physical conditions in their environment regulate the frequency and characteristics of vasomotor activity. Carbon dioxide excites the smooth muscle cells. The duration of the contraction and relaxation phases of each activity depends in part on the avail-

able oxygen supply. Anoxia favors relaxation but other chemical agents such as epinephrine and acetylcholine determine the sensitivity to environmental conditions.

4. The basic tone of all vessels is regulated by tonus adjustments of the smooth muscle cells in their walls. Tonus changes vary directly with the stretch or applied tension on the cells. This amounts to an inherent protective mechanism of the vessels where intravascular pressure modifies vascular size and helps regulate flow and pressure in the system. Capillaries having no muscle cells in their walls show only passive responses to internal pressure changes. In venules and veins this mechanism becomes the dominant regulator of active vasomotion which here aids venous return.

5. Consideration of the probable way these various factors achieve regulation of capillary flow and pressure, suggests that a basic condition for capillary function is the alternation of periods of vigorous flow and elevated pressure with periods of reduced or no flow and low pressure.

Depts. of Physiology and Anatomy
School of Medicine
Indiana University
Bloomington, Ind.

BIBLIOGRAPHY

1. BLOCH, E. F.: First Conference on Microcirculatory Physiology and Pathology. Anat. Rec., **120**: 241, 1954.
2. WEBB, R. L., AND NICOLL, P. A.: The bat wing as a subject for studies in homeostasis of capillary beds. Anat. Rec., **120**: 253, 1954.
3. ZWEIFACH, B. E.: The character and distribution of the blood capillaries. Anat. Rec., **73**: 475, 1939.
4. KAWANO, K.: A new fact and problem concerning the permeability of venules (II). Acta. Path. Jap., **1**: 72, 1951.
5. CARRIER, E. B.: Observation of living cells in the bat's wing. Physiological Papers: 1–9. Copenhagen, Levin and Munkgaard, 1926.
6. WEBB, R. L., AND NICOLL, P. A.: Persistence of active vasomotion after denervation (motion picture). Fed. Proc., **11**: 169, 1952.
7. NICOLL, P. A.: Responses of blood vessels of the bat's wing to epinephrine and nor-epinephrine. Fed. Proc., **9**: 94, 1950.
8. NICOLL, P. A., AND WEBB, R. L.: Blood circulation in the subcutaneous tissue of the living bat's wing. Ann. New York Acad. Sc., **46**: 697, 1946.
9. NICOLL, P. A.: The anatomy and behavior of the vascular systems in *Nereis virens* and *Nereis limbata*. Biol. Bul., **106**: 69, 1954.

V

In the Last Decade

Editor's Comments on Papers 15 Through 20

By 1960, the limitations, liabilities, and advantages of extant *in vivo* techniques had been established. Less time was being devoted to purely descriptive anatomical information (although more was to come), and more time was being spent on the functional aspects of microcirculation. Electron micrographs appeared, and the studies by Majno et al. (which combined the sophistication of electron microscopy and responses of the vascular bed to endogenous materials) exemplify the trend toward developing an understanding of how the system worked. Electron micrographs revealed the endothelial leaks that had been postulated, and these investigators were impressed with the fact that the greatest degree of permeability was found in the venous vessels. The studies by Majno also introduced a new site for microscopic observation of blood vessels, the cremaster muscle of the rat. Majno and his coworkers deplored the fact that a real delineation between capillaries and venous vessels had not been made, but they believed that many of the dimensions and diameter changes previously attributed to the capillaries occurred, in fact, in venous vessels.

The equally sophisticated use of high-speed cinephotography by Bloch added a new dimension in studies of blood flow in minute vessels. Bloch discusses axial flow, the plasma layer, and the shape as well as the velocity, of cellular components in a rapidly moving stream. His high-speed movies were innovative and thrilling to see.

Paper 17 by Björn Folkow on regulatory mechanisms does not contain the results of a single experimental study. It is, rather, an assortment of findings that was gathered by Folkow from the works of numerous authors to support the theory of autoregulation by myogenic activity of vascular smooth muscle cells that he was developing. He questions the concept that intraluminal pressure changes can regulate blood flow to capillary networks, but he finally concludes that, within limits, the myogenic response is regulatory, that it is self-limiting, and that it can be overridden, when necessary, by specific cardiovascular reflexes.

Although Folkow does not deal exclusively with microcirculation, his ability to correlate information from a number of different disciplines and sources and to present an overview has been helpful in unraveling some of the intricacies of regulatory mechanisms.

Paper 18, by Mary P. Wiedeman, demonstrates the necessity for collecting data from the living animal, as opposed to fixed tissue. Until the early 1960s, references to values used in calculations of cross-sectional areas, velocity changes, and other aspects of hemodynamics came from studies done in 1888 by Hall, who used fixed tissue from dog mesentery and who relied on many speculations regarding vascular ramifications.

In the measurements *in vivo* by Wiedeman in 1963 of lengths, diameters, and branches of blood vessels from a distributing artery to a collecting vein, it was found that mammalian capillary diameters averaged 3.7 μ rather than the more generally accepted 8 μ, and a literature search showed that the larger diameter was based on estimation rather than direct observation. It had been reasoned that capillaries must be large enough to permit the passage of a red blood cell (which was about 8 μ in most mammals studied) and that, therefore, capillaries must be 8 μ. In instances of actual measurement of capillaries in mice, rabbits, and dogs by other investigators, the diameters were seen to be between 3–5 μ. Calculations of the total cross-sectional area at different vascular levels showed the greatest total cross-sectional area to be in the venules rather than in the capillaries; they also showed that there was a linear increment in total cross-sectional area from arteries to capillaries. The new values have proved to be more compatible with concurrent rheological studies.

P.-I. Brånemark (Paper 19) took a giant step forward with the introduction of a chamber for viewing the microvasculature in man. Microscopic observations of capillary circulation in the human arm have erased the necessity for pondering over the applicability of experimental findings to problems in man. Brånemark touches on many aspects of microcirculation related to reduced or blocked blood flow and clarifies long-standing problems regarding rouleaux formations, the effect of stasis on the endothelial cells that line blood vessels, and the response of red and white cells and platelets to static conditions. The student interested in microcirculation is encouraged to read other contributions of this talented Swedish investigator.

The final paper, on capillary fluid exchange by C. A. Wiederhielm, produced a better understanding of the complexities of the mechanisms involved in fluid exchange at the capillary level and the maintenance of a proper equilibrium between the fluid contained in the closed vascular system and that in the open interstitial space. The concept of negative interstitial pressure also is investigated and discussed. Comparison of experimental data with computer data confirms some previous assumptions and negates others.

15

Reprinted from *J. Biophys. Biochem. Cytol.*, **11**(3), 607–626 (1961)

STUDIES ON INFLAMMATION

II. The Site of Action of Histamine and Serotonin along the Vascular Tree: A Topographic Study

G. MAJNO, M.D., G. E. PALADE, M.D., and GUTTA I. SCHOEFL

From the Department of Pathology, Harvard Medical School, Boston, and The Rockefeller Institute

ABSTRACT

While it is an established fact that histamine and serotonin increase the permeability of blood vessels, the exact portion of the vascular tree which is so affected has not been conclusively demonstrated. The present study was undertaken to clarify this point.

Our experiments were based on a method to which we refer as "vascular labeling," and which permits one to identify leaking vessels by means of visible accumulations of foreign particles within their walls. The mechanism of the labeling, elucidated by previous electron microscopic studies, is the following. Histamine and serotonin cause the endothelial cells of certain vessels to separate, and thus to create discrete intercellular gaps. Plasma escapes through these gaps, and filters through the basement membrane. If the plasma has been previously loaded (by intravenous injection) with colloidal particles of a black material such as carbon or mercuric sulfide, these particles—too large to pass through the basement membrane—will be retained and accumulate in visible amounts within the wall of the leaking vessel. This method is used to maximal advantage if the tissue is cleared and examined by transillumination *in toto*, so that leaking vessels can be accurately identified in their relationship to the vascular tree.

As a test tissue we used the rat cremaster, a laminar striated muscle which can be easily excised with its vascular supply virtually intact. The rats were prepared with an intravenous injection of carbon or HgS, and a subcutaneous injection into the scrotum of histamine, serotonin, or NaCl (as a control). The injected drug diffused into the underlying cremaster and the vessels became labeled. One hour later, when the carbon had been cleared from the blood stream, the animal was killed. The cremaster was excised, stretched, fixed in formalin, cleared in glycerin, and examined by transillumination under a light microscope.

The lesions induced by histamine and serotonin were identical. The leaking vessels, as indicated by the carbon deposits, always belonged to the venous side of the circulation. The heaviest deposits were found in venules 20 to 30 micra in diameter. The deposits decreased towards larger venules up to a maximum diameter of 75 to 80 micra, and towards the finer vessels until the caliber reached approximately 7 micra. Essentially spared by the deposits were the finest vessels, 4 to 7 micra in diameter, and constituting an extensive network oriented along the muscular fibers.

By killing animals at varying intervals after the injections, it was found that the carbon particles were slowly removed from the vascular walls by the action of phagocytic cells. After 10 months there was still enough carbon locally to be recognized by the naked eye.

607

The process of acute inflammation, according to one of the basic principles of general pathology, is in large measure the result of an increased permeability of blood capillaries (1, 2). This concept is so fundamental that it may appear to lie beyond the range of challenge. To be sure, it would scarcely be reasonable to question the existence of an increased permeability of the blood vessels, an obvious fact which was firmly established by Cohnheim as early as 1873 (3). On the other hand, the actual site of the leak has never been exactly identified. It could conceivably appear in the capillaries, in the arterioles, in the venules, or in a combination of these; perhaps it could even vary according to the injurious agent. Surprising as it may seem, the current belief that the *capillaries* become more permeable is founded not on direct evidence, but rather on tradition born of cursory observations. This is true not only for the process of acute inflammation, but also for the mechanism of action of histamine, serotonin, and the other substances known to affect the permeability of blood vessels.

The lack of precise information on this point is easily explained by three major technical difficulties which are encountered, at the level of the light microscope, when a change as subtle as increased permeability is to be recognized and correctly located in the maze of the vascular network. In the first place, the primary alteration of the endothelium lies beyond the resolution of the light microscope (4, 5), as Cohnheim himself implied when he speculated about a "molecular change" (6). Furthermore, histological sections are singularly unsuited for a study of this kind; the terminal ramifications of the arterial and venous trees, and the capillary network, are difficult or impossible to distinguish from each other when seen in cross-section, and even more so, of course, when the vessels have become abnormal in structure and caliber. Finally, the traditional experiment, currently used to demonstrate an increased vascular permeability, does not lend itself to detailed observations. A dye such as trypan blue is injected into the blood stream; the dye will leak out more readily at the site of vascular damage (1, 2). This procedure is very demonstrative to the naked eye, but disappointing under the microscope; colored plasma escapes freely out of the damaged vessels, and the result is a diffuse blue haze. Hence there is little hope to pinpoint the actual site of the lesion along any single type of vessel.

The first of these difficulties has been overcome by means of the electron microscope: it is now clear that histamine and serotonin cause leaks to appear between endothelial cells, whereas the basement membrane remains intact and literally filters the plasma which escapes through the opening (4, 5). On the basis of this observation it becomes a simple matter to label leaking vessels in such a manner that they may be identified with the light microscope. Instead of a dye, a suspension of suitable particulate matter, such as carbon black, should be injected into the blood stream. Then, wherever a leak is present in the endothelium, plasma will flow out; but the suspended particles, if of appropriate size, should be held back by the filtering effect of the basement membrane, and soon accumulate in amounts large enough to be visible with the light microscope. This effect should be put to maximal advantage by examining the tissue as a whole—with its vascular tree intact—rather than in tissue sections.

We have applied this procedure to the study of two agents which are typical representatives of the compounds known to increase "capillary" permeability: histamine and serotonin. These are the best known chemical mediators of vascular injury in acute inflammation (7, 8). Topographically the result was quite unexpected: both mediators, when studied in this manner, appear to exert their specific effect on the venous side of the vascular tree.

MATERIAL AND METHODS

Most of our observations were made on a laminar muscle of the albino rat, the cremaster. Briefly, the animal first received an intravenous injection of black colloidal particles, and immediately thereafter a local injection of the injurious agent into the subcutaneous tissue of the scrotum. Thus the agent diffused into the underlying muscle, which had not been subjected to direct mechanical trauma. After an appropriate time interval the animal was sacrificed, and the cremaster was excised, fixed, cleared and examined by transillumination.

The anatomical relationships of the cremaster muscle, and some of the reasons for selecting it, were dealt with in the first paper of this series (4). For the purpose of the studies presented herein, it will suffice to recall that each cremaster forms a pouch containing one testis; and that this pouch can be easily isolated and stretched, to become a membrane 2 to 3 cm in diameter and 0.25 mm in thickness which can be mounted on a glass slide in the same fashion as a tissue section. The cremaster is almost ideally suited for topographic studies of the vascular tree; not only because of its thinness, but also and more especially because it can be isolated with its vascular system virtually intact. On the visceral side it presents a natural surface (the serosa) which need not be traumatized by dissection; and the overlying skin has a vascular supply which is relatively independent, as indicated by the fact that it can be cleaved off with very little hemorrhage even in the live anesthetized animal. The muscle itself consists of two very thin layers of striated fibers, and "sandwiched" between these layers run the major arteries and veins: an arrangement which makes it even easier to dissect out the muscle without injury to its main blood vessels.

The rats were of the Sprague-Dawley (Holtzman) strain and weighed 200 to 350 gm; within each experiment, uniform age and weight were maintained. *Preparation of the Cremaster for Microscopic Examination:* Under ether anesthesia the thoracic cage is opened; the ensuing pneumothorax will kill the animal in about 1 minute. Before cardiac arrest, the root of the scrotum is rapidly clamped—on either side—with a large hemostat, applied deeply enough to include the vascular peduncle which leads from the abdominal cavity to the upper pole of the testis. The scrotal skin is rapidly removed, the testes with their envelopes are excised *in toto* and dipped for a few minutes, with the clamps still applied, in 10 per cent formalin. This procedure helps to minimize the loss of blood in subsequent handling and hence to preserve, as much as possible, the natural pattern of vascular injection (if the animal is killed by bleeding the number of visible vessels is sharply decreased). Thereafter the cremasters are dissected off under formalin, gently stretched, and pinned onto dental plate wax. After formalin fixation for 24 hours, the thin fascia on the subcutaneous side is carefully stripped off under the binocular microscope. The muscle is briefly rinsed in water and then cleared in two changes of glycerin (48 and 24 hours). Finally the preparation is trimmed, floated in two changes of warm glycerin jelly for a few minutes, and mounted under coverslips (a modification of the usual formula for glycerin jelly, which was found most suitable for these preparations, consists of a mixture of equal parts of glycerin and 10 per cent gelatin solution, with a few crystals of phenol). In this state the preparation is as permanent as a tissue section, and can be examined by transmitted light with good resolution at magnifications as high as 500. *Local and Intravenous Injections:* With the animal under ether anesthesia, the hair covering the proximal part of the scrotum was gently removed with an electric

clipper, and the colloidal suspension was injected intravenously. Immediately thereafter, one injection either of test substance or of a saline control was administered subcutaneously over the mid-ventral aspect of each cremaster, great care being taken to avoid stretching of the skin and all unnecessary trauma. The order of the intravenous and subcutaneous injections could be reversed with no apparent difference, as long as the two injections were administered in immediate sequence. The labeling of the vessels occurred very rapidly, but 1 hour was allowed for the particulate matter to be removed from the blood stream. After this time the animal was killed and the cremaster prepared as described. Variations in the timing of injections and death of the animal are indicated under Results.

Colloidal Suspensions: We used primarily carbon black especially prepared for experimental use by the Guenther-Wagner Pelikan-Werke, Hannover, Germany (Batch ≠ C11/1431a). This preparation contains about 100 mg/cc of carbon with an indicated average particle size of 200 A; it is stabilized with 4.5 per cent fish glue and contains 1.3 per cent phenol as a preserving agent. This solution was injected into the saphenous vein in a dose of 0.1 cc/100 gm body weight (10 mg carbon/100 gm body weight). Doses five times greater are tolerated by the animals without apparent harm, but require a longer period to be cleared from the blood stream.

In some experiments we used a preparation of colloidal mercuric sulfide (black) prepared by Hille and Co., Chicago, and containing HgS, a stabilizer, and 0.2 per cent cresol. This preparation is supplied as a 2 per cent suspension ("Mersulfol") and also in the form of a dry material which contains approximately 25 per cent of HgS; this was dissolved in saline to a concentration of 4 per cent HgS, and injected intravenously in the dose of 0.5 cc/100 gm. Larger doses sometimes caused the animal to die with pulmonary edema.

Test Solutions: Subcutaneous injections in the skin of the scrotum were all administered in the same volume, 0.05 cc. This was accomplished with the use of a Hamilton microsyringe (made to deliver 0.05 cc with an accuracy of ± 0.1 per cent) fitted with a gauge 30 needle. *Histamine* diphosphate (Abbott Laboratories, North Chicago, Illinois, and Eli Lilly & Co., Indianapolis) was used in a concentration of 1 mg/cc; the dose hereafter referred to as standard, amounted to 18 μg of histamine base in 0.05 cc. *Serotonin* (5-hydroxy-tryptamine creatinine sulfate, Nutritional Biochemicals Corp., Cleveland) was employed as a solution of 0.0126 mg/cc freshly prepared before use. In this concentration, 0.05 cc (0.27 μg of serotonin base) produded a lesion approximately matching that of the histamine standard.

EXPERIMENTAL PROCEDURE AND RESULTS

A. CONTROLS

Effect of the Colloidal Suspension Alone

As soon as the suspension of carbon or HgS had been injected intravenously, the skin and visible mucosae of the rats took on a definite grey hue. Microscopically, preparations of cremaster taken during the first 10 minutes (in the absence of any local injection) were scarcely distinguishable from those of normal animals; there was a faint greyish discoloration of the plasma, together with a dust-like scattering of fine black particles, particularly with the carbon suspension. Whether these particles were all suspended in the blood stream, or sometimes adherent to the endothelial lining, could not be established in our fixed preparations; however, the grains appeared to be randomly and uniformly distributed in all the vessels of the cremaster, and the relevant point for our experiments is that larger aggregates or deposits did not form anywhere.

Controls for the Local Injection of Histamine and Serotonin

In most rats, the test substance (histamine or serotonin) was injected on one side of the scrotum, while the other side was injected with an equal amount of 0.85 per cent NaCl. On this control side, the cremaster usually developed a small lesion often scarcely visible (Fig. 2), but occasionally as large as 5 mm. Microscopically the pattern was identical with that induced by histamine or serotonin: that is, the blackening was limited to the venules (see below). In other animals saline only was injected on both sides, with no concomitant histamine administered to the same animal; the result was the same as with the previous series. The simple introduction of the needle, or the injection of 0.05 cc of air, caused no lesion at all.

B. EFFECT OF HISTAMINE

If histamine is injected locally, and the carbon suspension intravenously, a blackening of the

---

Explanation of Plates

All figures represent rat cremaster muscles, excised, stretched, fixed in formalin, cleared in glycerin (see Methods), and mounted between a glass slide and a coverslip. No histological stains were applied. All figures except Figs. 1 and 2 were taken with a light microscope (Zeiss Ultraphot) at magnifications of 30 to 200. An opal glass 3 mm thick was interposed between the microscope stage and the preparation, as a diffusing filter. Figs. 1 and 2 were taken with a Leitz Aristophot assembly, by a combination of epi- and transillumination.

FIGURE 1

Topographic view of a histamine-induced lesion: a demonstration of the vascular labeling method, whereby leaking vessels are blackened with carbon deposits.

One hour prior to sacrifice, this rat received an i.v. injection of carbon suspension and a local injection of histamine (18 μg). The circulating carbon has now been cleared from the blood stream. *Double arrow:* arteriole. No blackened branches stem from this vessel. *Single arrows:* venules, about 100 micra in caliber. These larger venules appear to be unaffected, but inserted along them are black tree-like structures which represent leaking tributaries, with branches 2 or 3 orders. Scale = 1 mm.

FIGURE 2

Control, in which 0.05 cc of 0.85 per cent NaCl was substituted for histamine (all other conditions as in Fig. 1). There is no indication of vascular leakage, except for a very small region (right center) in which faint carbon deposits have appeared, again only in branches of a venule (*arrow*). Scale = 1 mm.

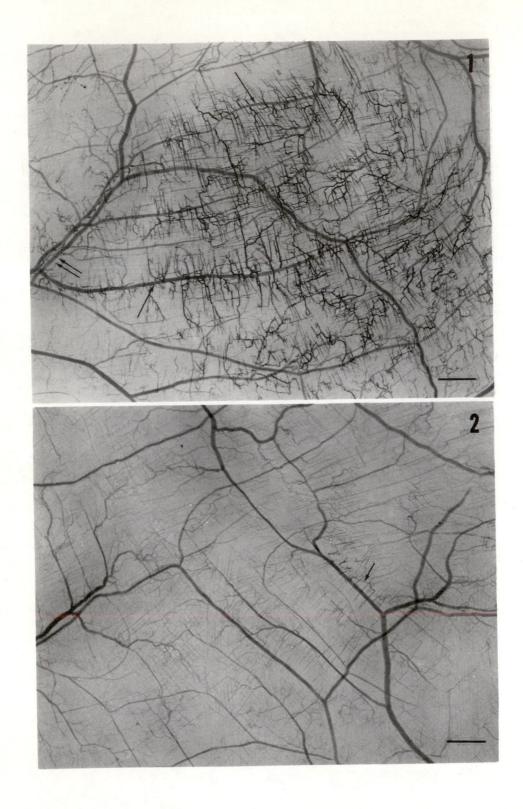

vessels within the cremaster occurs very rapidly. The characteristic effect, which will be referred to hereafter as *vascular labeling*, shows quantitative variations with the dose of histamine; the following description corresponds to the dose which we found to give optimal results (0.05 cc of 0.1 per cent histamine phosphate). If the animal is killed after 2 to 7 minutes, at the site of the subcutaneous injection the cremaster shows a dark patch 15 to 20 mm in diameter in which a faint black network can be detected grossly. In subsequent stages this network becomes more pronounced, and after 10 to 15 minutes it appears to have reached maximum intensity. On closer inspection this area shows a pattern which is sometimes more obvious but always apparent, even to the naked eye, particularly in the preparations cleared with glycerin: the blackened vessels are not uniformly distributed, but mostly grouped in many small, tree-like or feather-like arrangements, separated by narrow clear spaces (Fig. 1). Under a low-power enlargement it is easy to observe that this pattern corresponds to a definite portion of the vascular tree: each discrete unit represents a venule surrounded by its system of converging tributaries. Proximally and distally to this segment of the venous tree, the vessels (capillaries and larger veins) are not blackened (Figs. 3, 5, 6).

The blackening of the venous system is sharply restricted to the terminal portion of the tree, and within a relatively narrow range of calibers. In general, it is heaviest in the venules with an outer diameter of 20 to 30 micra, which at low enlargements appear as black cylinders (Fig. 3). Proceeding in the direction of the blood flow, the carbon deposit ends often very abruptly where the venule opens into a larger vessel (Fig. 7); other times it tapers off along the course of the vessel, and the last traces can be found up to a maximum caliber of 75 to 80 micra. Proceeding towards the capillary, the deposit breaks up into uneven patches, and ceases often quite abruptly where the lumen has narrowed to the point of allowing the passage of a single red blood cell (Figs. 8, 5, 6). Beyond this point there is a vast system of very fine vessels, 4 to 5 micra in diameter, which remain quite free of carbon deposits. These vessels form a three-dimensional network, with long meshes oriented along the muscular fibers (Fig. 8). Some of the meshes are visible because they contain red blood cells; however, the true extent of this network which remains free of deposits is better appreciated if the whole vascular system is injected with an opaque mass[1] (Fig. 4).

At enlargements of 100 to 400 times the mor-

---

[1] We used a mixture of our carbon suspension with a cold gelatin mass which has the advantage of being fluid at room temperature (5 gm of gelatin are dissolved in 100 cc of warm distilled water, then 5 gm of potassium iodide are added). Further details may be found in E. A. Bean, Animal Micrology, University of Chicago Press, 5th edition, 1953, 98.

FIGURES 3 AND 4

Two cremasters prepared in different ways and shown at the same enlargement ($\times$ 45) to demonstrate the fact that a vast number of very fine vessels are not caused to "leak" by the action of histamine or serotonin.

FIGURE 3

Typical example of vascular labeling induced, in this case, by serotonin. The black, branching structures are venules. Experimental procedures as indicated for Fig. 1. Scale = 100 micra.

FIGURE 4

Cremaster of a normal rat, in which the entire vascular system has been injected with a mixture of carbon and gelatin (see Methods). This preparation shows a large number of very fine vessels (capillaries, in the strictest sense) superimposed in different planes. By comparing this photograph with the one above, it becomes obvious that the great majority of these fine vessels are not blackened by the method of vascular labeling. Scale = 100 micra.

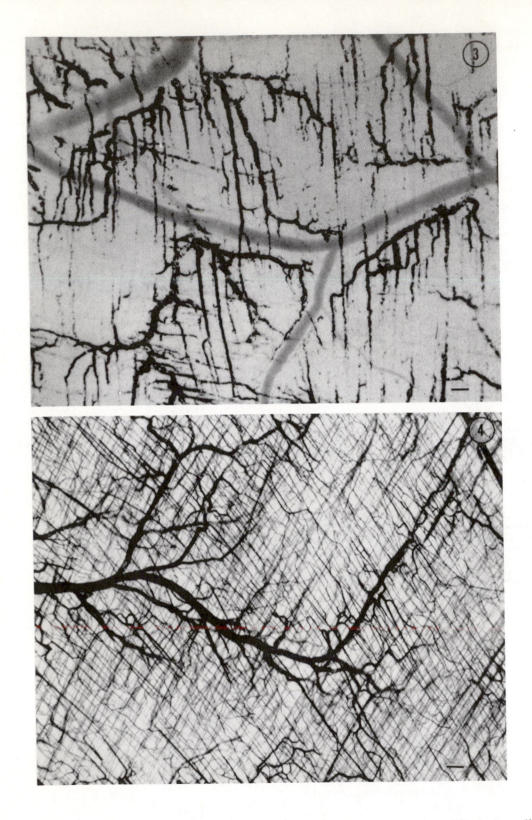

phology of the carbon deposit can be studied in considerable detail. Even where the layer of deposit is heaviest it shows very fine fenestrations, and a ragged, moth-eaten aspect which indicates that the carbon is seeping into a very uneven system of clefts (4). The outer surface, corresponding to the adventitia, is relatively smooth, but occasional leaks can be found where groups of granules have reached as far as 10 to 15 micra into the extravascular spaces (Fig. 9). In the larger venules the deposit is occasionally broken up into irregular rings encircling the vessel, an orientation probably determined by the presence of smooth muscle cells (Fig. 12). More often, where the deposit is slight, it appears in the form of short, straight lines parallel to the axis of the vessel; Fig. 10 shows this pattern, which is frequently repeated along a segment of the venule. A complete flagstone pattern reminiscent of that obtained by perfusion with $AgNO_3$ was never observed.

The amount of carbon injected intravenously can be increased or decreased by a factor of 3 without any recognizable difference in the intensity of the blackening. The smallest dose of histamine phosphate which can bring about a significant blackening is 0.05 cc of a 0.01 per cent solution (1.8 μg of histamine base); with a 0.1 per cent solution which we adopted as a standard dose, the lesion has an average diameter of about 15 mm.

In rats injected with colloidal HgS rather than carbon, the black deposits have the same topographic distribution (Fig. 6) but they are more transparent, and smoother in appearance (Fig. 11), perhaps on account of the smaller dimension of the particles.

Individual variations in the intensity of the response were frequently observed. The variability affected the diameter of the over-all lesion, not the selective location of the carbon deposits along the venular tree. With a given standard dose of histamine the diameter of the blackened patch could vary between 10 and 20 mm. On the other hand, there was much less variation in the response of the two cremasters of a single rat.

Perfusions of the whole animal with horse serum were also accomplished, in order to remove the red blood cells and obtain an even sharper definition of the carbon deposits. Rats were given a local injection of histamine and an intravenous injection of carbon or HgS in the usual fashion. After 10 to 15 min. they were etherized, perfusion was started into the saphenous vein, and a jugular was cut (fluid: 50 to 90 cc. of warm heparinized horse serum, containing 0.3 per cent of trypan blue for a gross control of the success of the perfusion). The heart kept beating for a prolonged period. The preparations of cremaster appeared almost completely devoid of red blood cells. None of the carbon or HgS deposit appeared to have been removed; the blackened vessels stood out in sharper contrast against an almost empty background, but there was otherwise little to be learned from these preparations.

Later Fate of the Carbon Deposits

In a series of rats, a lesion was produced in the cremaster with the combined injections of histamine and carbon black, as usual. The cremasters from these animals were then examined after periods varying between 30 minutes and 10 months. It was found that the particles of carbon tend to emigrate rather rapidly across the wall of the vessel. After 3 hours (Fig. 14) the outer surface of the deposits is noticeably more ragged, and many fine granules appear which at 6 hours

---

FIGURES 5 AND 6

Cremasters after a local injection of histamine; the leaking vessels have been labeled with carbon (Fig. 5) or colloidal HgS (Fig. 6). The deposits of carbon are somewhat coarser than those of HgS, but the distribution is very similar.

The fields have been selected to demonstrate the sequence arteriole → capillary → venule, and thus the elective deposition of tracer particles on the venous side. A = arteriole, V = venule. Note that considerable lengths of the finest capillary segments (C) are spared. The relative number of these unlabeled capillaries is actually much greater than can be judged from these photographs, because many of these vessels lie above and below the plane of focus. Scale = 100 micra. Fig. 5, $\times$ 160. Fig. 6, $\times$ 140.

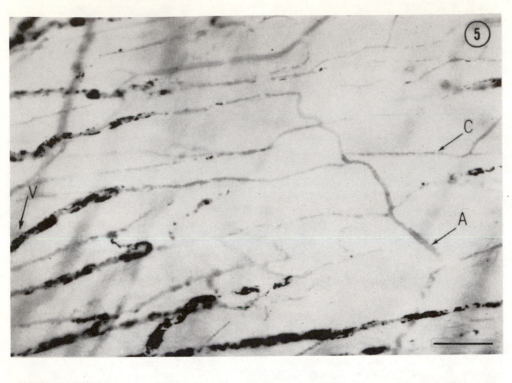

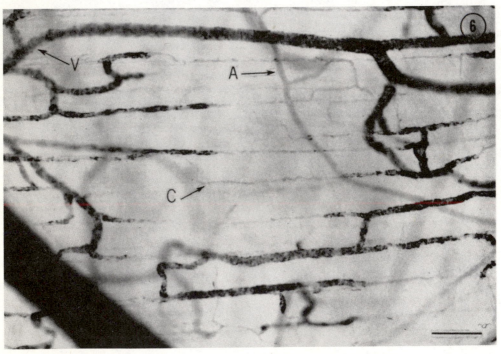

G. Majno, G. E. Palade, and Schoefl, G. I. *Site of Action of Histamine and Serotonin* 615

form an almost continuous sprinkling along the adventitia. At 12 hours many of the granules are collected into lumps, suggestive of single macrophages, and at 24 hours (Fig. 15) even the continuous black layer which obscured the medium-sized venules begins to break up into lumps, probably because it becomes condensed within cells. At 7 days (Fig. 16) the black patch grossly visible on the cremaster begins to fade slightly, indicating that some of the carbon has been carried away; microscopically, the carbon now appears to be collected in macrophages, mostly aligned in rows along the vessels, while others are scattered around the tissue. The larger venules, rather oddly, have a distinct row of macrophages on two opposite sides, as if these cells avoided that portion of the circumference of the vessel which faces the peritoneal or the cutaneous surface. After 1 month (Fig. 17) the black deposits still suggest a vascular pattern, but now the venules are simply outlined by a succession of black, elongated macrophages seemingly flattened against the adventitia; at low powers it appears as if a black pencil had drawn a broken line along the venules. After 3 and 10 months (Figs. 18 and 19) the pattern is the same: a grey patch is still visible, though faintly, to the naked eye; microscopically only the larger venules are outlined, most of the carbon having by now disappeared. A progressive blackening of the lumbar lymph nodes was noticed from the 7th day onwards.

C. EFFECT OF SEROTONIN

When carbon was injected intravenously, and serotonin locally, carbon labeling developed in the venules in a manner identical to that already described for histamine. Quantitatively, however, serotonin was much more powerful on a mole-to-mole basis; a dose calculated to be equimolar with that of the standard amount of histamine (0.05 cc of a 0.126 per cent solution of serotonin creatinine sulfate) induced a lesion so large as to include one whole cremaster and half of that on the opposite side. Judging from the diameter of the lesion, an effect comparable to that of histamine was obtained with a dose approximately one hundredth as great on a molar basis.

DISCUSSION

A. THE PHENOMENON OF VASCULAR LABELING: EARLIER INTERPRETATIONS

All the experiments described in this paper represent an application of the phenomenon to which we referred earlier as vascular labeling. In short, if histamine or serotonin is injected locally, and a carbon suspension intravenously, there develops a blackening of certain vessels in the area of the local injection. On the strength of electron microscopic evidence (4, 5) it is safe to interpret this blackening as follows: the endothelium develops discrete leaks, and as plasma filters through the basement membrane, the suspended tracer particles are retained.

While this interpretation may be new, the actual phenomenon of vascular blackening in injured tissues, after an intravenous injection of India ink or carbon, has been described a number of times in the literature. These earlier studies

---

FIGURES 7 AND 8

Vessels labeled with carbon after local injection of histamine. Examples of the largest (Fig. 7) and the smallest (Fig. 8) vessels which are affected.

FIGURE 7

The deposits cease sharply as the tributaries join the main venule. Scale = 100 micra. × 130.

FIGURE 8

Note the absence of deposits along the finest vessels. The caliber of these vessels (arrows) is indicated by the single row of red blood cells contained in thel umen. As soon as these vessels begin to enlarge (towards the venous end), granular deposits begin to appear. Scale = 100 micra. × 440.

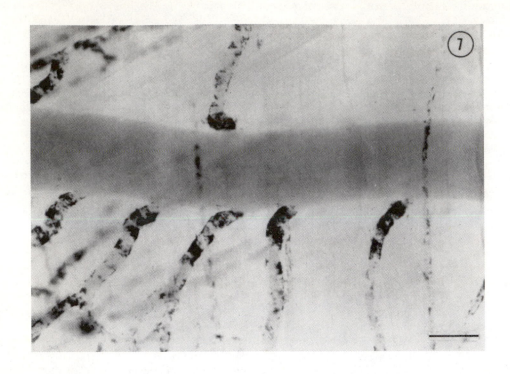

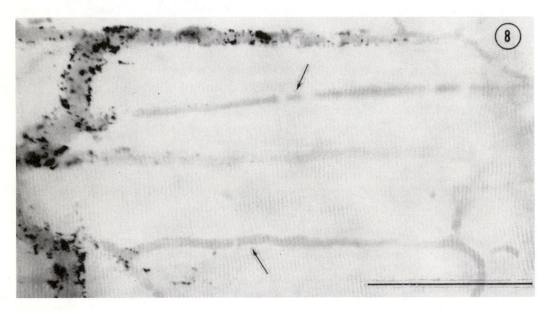

G. Majno, G. E. Palade, and Schoefl, G. I. *Site of Action of Histamine and Serotonin* 617

were made on living tissues or on histological sections, techniques which did not allow one to distinguish clearly between intravascular, intramural and intracellular deposits of the carbon; hence many of the conclusions drawn by these authors can no longer be accepted.

Thus Herzog (9), Stilwell (10) and Schopper (11) who studied the tongue of the living frog after intravenous injection of India ink, interpreted the black deposit as a *superficial coating of the endothelium*, which slowly penetrates and crosses the vascular wall by phagocytosis and cellular transport. In point of fact, these papers include careful descriptions of early *reversible* deposits which leave little doubt that some superficial coating of the endothelium did actually occur. This should be expected, because the material injected was India ink; the latter contains shellac, which promotes intravascular clotting (12). This may well explain the intravascular "filaments" described by Schopper (11). The carbon suspension used in our experiments did not contain shellac. In our previous study we did observe occasional superficial deposits (4); this mechanism, however, may account for only a minor part of the blackening.

The case of Krogh (13) is rather unique, in that he formulated the correct hypothesis, performed our same experiment, and obtained our same results but considered them a failure. Krogh had actually entertained the idea that when the permeability of a blood vessel is increased, this might occur by the formation of "fissures between the endothelial cells, . . . especially at the points where the borders of three or more cells meet." He therefore injected dialyzed India ink intravenously into frogs, and expected that at a site of injury (by urethane) grey plasma would escape: ". . . but the result of the actual experiment was that the indian ink was held back quantitatively, while the clear plasma disappeared as before. . . ." Krogh did not consider the presence of a basement membrane, though it had been described previously (14). Hence, "discarding [the original hypothesis, he] came to the conclusion that mechanical stretching of the capillary wall must be responsible for the increase in permeability. . . ."

Chambers and Zweifach have repeatedly described the deposits of carbon in injured vessels, particularly in venules, and along the intercellular junctions (15, 16). They deduced from these observations that injury brings about a *swelling and stickiness of the intercellular cement* (15, 16).

FIGURES 9 TO 12

Carbon- or HgS-labeled venules after a local injection of histamine: structural details of the deposits. Scale = 100 micra.

FIGURE 9

One hour after the injection of carbon, a few particles (arrow) have found their way as far out as the adventitia. × 490.

FIGURE 10

Carbon deposits in the pattern of regular parallel lines (arrow). This image is interpreted as indicating—in all likelihood (4)—clefts between endothelial cells. × 340.

FIGURE 11

Venule labeled with colloidal HgS. The deposit appears less coarse than with carbon. × 460.

FIGURE 12

Carbon deposits in the pattern of incomplete rings surrounding a venule (*V*). This arrangement may be determined by smooth muscle cells wrapped around the vessel, perpendicular to its axis. *A* = an arteriole, devoid—as usual— of deposits. × 170.

FIGURE 13

Normal rat cremaster, in which the vessels have been injected with a mixture of carbon and gelatin (same preparation as for Fig. 4). Note the characteristic ladder pattern of the finest vessels, which run between the muscle fibers. Scale = 100 micra. × 170.

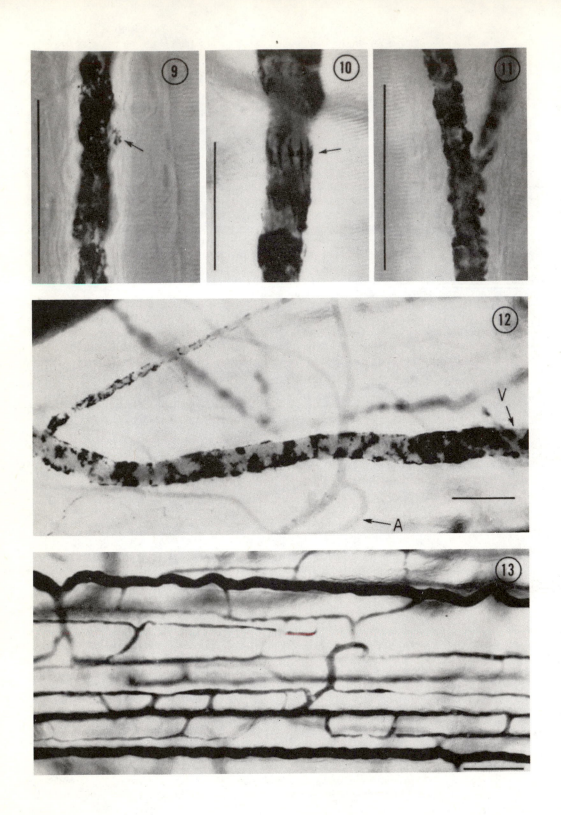

G. Majno, G. E. Palade, and Schoefl, G. I.   *Site of Action of Histamine and Serotonin*   619

Another interpretation which can no longer be held is that which explains the blackening as an expression of *increased phagocytic activity of the endothelium*. This view originated with Jancsó (17–18), who observed that if histamine is painted on the skin of a white mouse, and India ink is injected intravenously, many small vessels in the painted area become black. This effect, later referred to as "Jancsó phenomenon" (19), became the starting point of a series of papers aimed at demonstrating that histamine enhances phagocytosis (20, 21); a summary of this work may be found in a recent monograph on phagocytic stimulation (22).

This is not to say that phagocytosis plays no part in the phenomenon of vascular labeling. It does occur (4, 5), but as a relatively late and probably secondary event, involving the endothelial cells, and more especially the pericytes.

It should be pointed out, of course, that the observations published by the above-named authors remain essentially valid; only the interpretation has changed.

B. LOCALIZATION OF THE VASCULAR DAMAGE IN THE VENULES

If one examines at low magnification a cremaster in which the leaking vessels have been labeled with carbon (Figs. 1, 3) it is not difficult to identify them as branches of the venous tree. The largest venules with traces of deposits have a caliber of 75 to 80 micra. Proceeding upstream, the deposits become heavier, and reach a maximum in venules with a diameter of 20 to 30 micra; then decrease, and finally stop when the caliber has reached about 7 micra: that is, approximately the diameter of a red blood cell. This distribution of carbon

deposits clearly suggests that the venules 20 to 30 micra in diameter are the most sensitive vessels. In fact, when the injury is slight, as at the periphery of the injection site, these are the only vessels to show any blackening at all.

The number of blackened vessels is so great as to suggest, at first sight, that all of the capillary system is affected. However, if the same preparation is compared with another one in which all the blood vessels have been filled with an opaque mass (Figs. 3 and 4) it becomes obvious that there is a vast system of very fine vessels which are almost completely free of carbon deposits. These vessels, to which we will refer, for the time being, as "unlabeled capillaries," are not easily visualized in our ordinary preparations, because they are incompletely filled with blood. Their caliber is the same as—or less than—the diameter of a red blood cell, and ranges approximately from 4 to 7 micra. Their basic pattern is not that of a tree, as is the case for the blackened vessels, but rather that of a three-dimensional network, with oblong meshes running parallel to the muscle fibers and often aligned in a ladder-like arrangement (Figs. 5, 6, 8, 13).

These observations are in complete agreement with our previous electron microscopic study (4), in which a striking feature of the cremaster muscle after injection of histamine or serotonin had been the consistent lack of lesions in the vessels of the smallest caliber. In other words, the vessels which appeared to be the most likely candidates for the term "capillary" did not develop leaks. Their outer diameter (measured on electron micrographs, and taking the basement membrane as a boundary) was 3 to 5 micra. Leaks developed with great regularity in vessels

---

FIGURES 14 TO 16

Aspect of carbon-labeled venules, at varying time intervals after the local injection of histamine. Scale = 100 micra. × 160.

FIGURE 14

Stage of 6 hours. Small clusters of carbon (presumably contained within phagocytic cells) are beginning to appear along the contours of the venules.

FIGURES 15 AND 16

Stages of 1 and 7 days. The carbon is being concentrated in discrete granular masses, presumably intracellular, within and adjacent to the vascular wall. Some carbon also appears in perivascular clusters, probably within phagocytes (*arrows*).

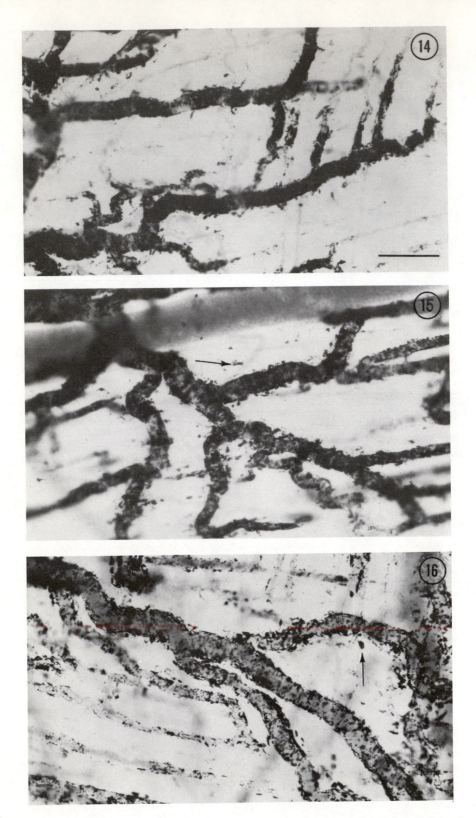

G. Majno, G. E. Palade, and Schoefl, G. I.   *Site of Action of Histamine and Serotonin*   621

about twice this diameter, but whether the vessels represented venules or the finest ramifications of arterioles could not be established by electron microscopy.

Our studies therefore indicate that histamine and serotonin bring out a fundamental difference in response between two types of blood vessels: the finest vessels, 4 to 7 micra in diameter (as measured in the fixed preparations) which remain practically free of demonstrable leaks, and the collecting vessels, from 7 or 8 to 75 or 80 micra in diameter, which develop extensive leaks. It would be tempting to identify these two kinds of vessels with capillaries and venules, respectively. At present, however, there is no general agreement as to the use of the word "capillary," as evidenced by the multiplicity of terms such as protocapillary, precapillary, postcapillary, true capillary, and the like (23). The end-point of the capillary on the venous side is particularly indefinite; it is often extended to include venous vessels (23).

In the past there has been little point in drawing a line between capillaries and venules, because the two types of vessels were generally assumed to be very similar, if not identical, in both structure and function (13). There is, of course, a structural similarity between capillaries and the finest venules: in either case the walls consist of endothelium without a muscular coat; the first smooth muscle cells begin to appear when the caliber reaches 45 to 50 micra (24, 25), and a continuous muscular media is not found until the caliber reaches about 200 micra (24, 25). Therefore, if one were to base the definition of capillary on the absence of smooth musculature, the diameter of the capillaries could reach at least 50 micra. This is a criterion often implied in histopathologic descriptions. Landis called capillaries (in mammals) vessels with a diameter of 5 to 20 micra (26). Among the textbooks of histology, there is a tendency to define the blood capillaries as those vessels which have a diameter "approximately equal to that of the red blood cells which must pass through them" (27). Thus Cowdry (28) states that the capillaries begin when the lumen is reduced to the minimum diameter which will let red blood cells pass freely: "this is considered in man to be about 8 microns. . . . The venous limit of the capillary bed commences where the capillaries run

together to form vessels of larger diameter than 8 microns." For Maximow and Bloom (24) the caliber of the capillaries is closely related to the size of the red blood cells, and "in man it averages about 8 μ." Nonidez and Windle (29) follow the same criterion, and use the figure of 8 to 10 microns. Barrnett (25) states that capillaries "are the blood vessels having generally the smallest lumen and the simplest wall," their diameter varying "between 4 and 12 microns."

It would appear, then, that if we followed the definition of capillary indicated by the above-named textbooks, we could equate with good approximation our unlabeled capillaries with capillaries, and our labeled vessels with venules. In the literature, however, the term "capillary" is used more loosely (23). For the time being, therefore, it is safer to avoid strict reference to given vascular segments, and state that the endothelial leaks induced by histamine and serotonin are found on the venous side of the circulation, with a maximum effect on venules 20 to 30 micra in diameter, decreasing towards the larger veins, as well as towards the finest vessels.

C. COMPARISON OF VASCULAR CHANGES INDUCED BY HISTAMINE AND SEROTONIN

The vascular damage caused by histamine, when tested by the method of carbon labeling, was indistinguishable from that of serotonin. We were unable to convince ourselves that there was any difference either in the topographic distribution of the lesions along the venular tree, or in the actual structure of the carbon deposit.

One cannot avoid some surprise at the observation that two dissimilar agents should bring about—in our experimental system—the same, very specific effect. This leads one, of course, to wonder whether there may not be some common underlying mechanism. According to Woolley, serotonin acts—at the cellular level—by combining with calcium ions and an acceptor substance (30, 31). At present there is little ground for further speculation.

Figures 17 to 19

Further changes in the carbon deposits of the labeled venules; stages of 1, 3, and 10 months, respectively. The structures indicated by arrows represent phagocytic cells. Scale = 100 micra. × 160.

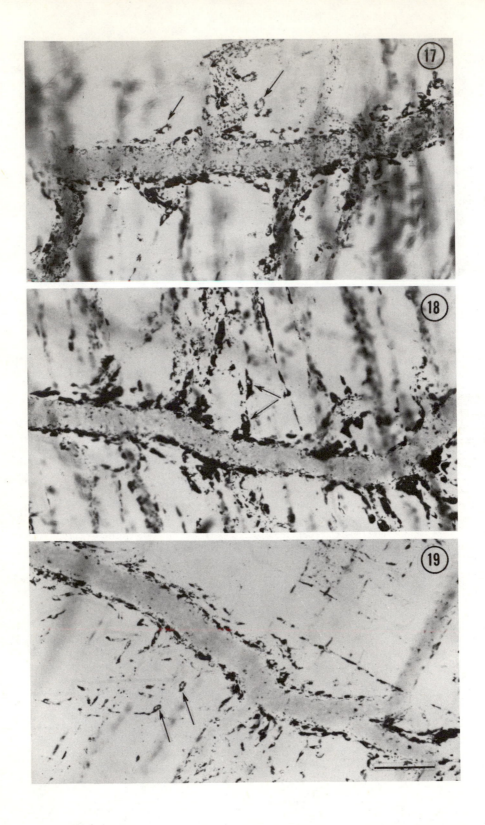

CONCLUDING REMARKS

An objection which could possibly be raised to our experiments is that the doses of histamine and serotonin, however small, could still be high in relation to the amount presumably released as a result of local injury. We have good reason to believe, however, that our results cannot be ascribed to "toxic" levels of the drugs. It is especially instructive to examine the periphery of the injection site, where the drugs are diluted to the minimum dose capable of inducing vascular leakage. Here the elective sensitivity of the venules is particularly obvious.

On the other hand, it should be expected that with very high, toxic concentrations, not only venules but also other vessels might be injured in a non-specific manner. We found evidence of this type of injury particularly after the injection of serotonin. In the very center of some preparations, where the cremaster had been exposed to the highest concentration of the drug, it was occasionally possible to observe very fine black-ened vessels in the typical ladder pattern of the finest capillaries. It seems reasonable to assume that the effect of the drug, at this site, had been of a more drastic, less specific nature; the selective and more "physiological" effect being exerted in the surrounding area. This observation indicates that two types of vascular lesions should be considered; the specific ones, due to pharmacologic effects of mediators, and non-specific ones due to general cell damage. This problem will be dealt with in the next paper of this series.

We have applied the principle of vascular labeling, with carbon, to tissues other than the cremaster (fascia of the abdominal muscles, adipose tissue, mesentery, intestinal wall, testis, eyelid) and in animals other than the rat (mouse, hamster, guinea pig, rabbit, cat, and dog). Histamine was used in all these situations, serotonin in some. The elective sensitivity of the venular tree was confirmed without exception. We therefore have a certain degree of confidence in stating that this is, in all likelihood, a general phenomenon. This conclusion does not necessarily contradict the electron microscopic studies of Alksne (5), who also studied the effect of histamine on vascular permeability, using mouse skin as test tissue. Alksne described endothelial leaks in "capillaries," but did not specify the diameter of the leaking vessels. From three of his illustrations, however (nos. 3, 4, 10), the caliber of the leaking vessel can be estimated, and in each case it falls within the range of a collecting vessel or venule, rather than the terminal capillary network (e.g., about 11 μ in Fig. 3). Alksne noticed, furthermore, that "not all capillaries" were affected, and suggested that this may have depended on a different functional state. It seems more likely that the "unaffected capillaries" may have been the finest. It is worth noting at this point that the vascularization of the skin represents a special case, in that the great majority of the small vessels are venules (32, 33, 13).

If then it is true that two of the major chemical mediators of inflammation, histamine and serotonin, spare the finest vessels (those which are undoubtedly capillaries, whatever definition one may follow) and act selectively on the venular tree, then one may legitimately wonder how these substances could have become almost synonymous with capillary poisons. This is particularly the case with histamine, the oldest and best established of the permeability-increasing factors. In his monograph on histamine, for instance, Rocha e Silva (34) states that histamine increases the permeability of the capillaries, and cites evidence in support. It is quite clear, however, that the arguments advanced do not allow one to distinguish capillaries from other vessels. The local *leakage of dye*, and the increase of *lymph flow*, are, of course, inadequate. The development of *stasis* in the capillaries and venules (stasis is here used in the sense of packing of red blood cells (35)) is often quoted as evidence of a capillary lesion (34). Actually, if stasis appeared first in the venules because of local leaks, it should necessarily develop as a secondary event in the capillaries. As for an *increase in diameter* (the "dilatation of capillaries" so often mentioned by pathologists), careful studies of intact tissues have failed to produce convincing evidence that histamine induces a significant dilatation of the capillary network. Vasodilatation does occur, but in vessels of larger caliber; the terminal capillary network is notable for its more complete injection with blood (36–39). The most logical conclusion seems to be that the dilated capillaries of traditional fame are actually venules filled with stagnant blood. This is quite apparent in some of the published illustrations which are labeled "dilated capillaries": the number of endothelial nuclei or of red blood cells in cross-section clearly betray the vessel as a venule (*e.g.*, Fig. 2 in Menkin (40)).

In closing, it should be mentioned that all topographic studies of the finer vessels are hampered by lack of a rigorous terminology; that is, lack of generally recognized morphologic or functional definitions for each vascular segment. By accumulating more findings such as here presented—the elective sensitivity to chemical agents—it may become possible, in the future, to define more precisely those elusive entities which Lewis (33) felt obliged to group under the noncommittal term of "minute vessels."

It is a pleasure to acknowledge the assistance of Mrs. Monika La Gattuta. For the photographic prints we are indebted to Mrs. Audrey Hadfield.

Dr. Majno's work was performed during the tenure of a Lederle Medical Faculty Award, and subsequently of a Senior Research Fellowship, United States Public Health Service.

Miss Schoefl is now Predoctoral Trainee under a Pathology Training Grant from the United States Public Health Service (2G-113) and held earlier a National Institutes of Health Fellowship (HF-8900). This work was supported by grants from the National Institutes of Health, United States Public Health Service (B-1964, H-5648, and H-5404).

Received for publication, June 7, 1961.

BIBLIOGRAPHY

1. Wright, G. P., An Introduction to Pathology, London, Longmans, Green and Co., Ltd., 3rd edition, 1958.
2. Florey, H. E., General Pathology, Philadelphia, W. B. Saunders Co., 2nd edition, 1958.
3. Cohnheim, J., Neue Untersuchungen über die Entzündung, Berlin, A. Hirschwald, 1873.
4. Majno, G., and Palade, G. E., Studies on inflammation. I. The effect of histamine and serotonin on vascular permeability: An electron microscopic study, *J. Biophysic. and Biochem. Cytol.*, 1961, **11**, 571.
5. Alksne, J. F., The passage of colloidal particles across the dermal capillary wall under the influence of histamine, *Quart. J. Exp. Physiol.*, 1959, **44**, 51.
6. Cohnheim, J., Lectures on General Pathology, London, The New Sydenham Society, 1882, **126**, 242.
7. Feldberg, W., The role of mediators in the inflammatory tissue response, *Internat. Arch. Allergy*, 1956, **8**, 15.
8. Spector, W. G., Substances which affect capillary permeability, *Pharmacol. Rev.*, 1958, **10**, 475.
9. Herzog, F., Endothelien der Froschzunge als Phagocyten und Wanderzellen, *Z. ges. exp. Med.*, 1924, **43**, 79.
10. Stilwell, F., On the phagocytic capacity of the blood vessel endothelium of the frog's tongue and its presumed transformation into wandering cells, *Folia haematol.*, 1926, **33**, 81.
11. Schopper, W., Beobachtungen an der Froschzunge nach Tuscheeinspritzung in die Blutbahn, *Virchows Arch. path. Anat.*, 1929, **272**, 709.
12. Halpern, B. N., Benacerraf, B., and Biozzi, G., Quantitative study of the granulopectic activity of the reticuloendothelial system. I. The effect of the ingredients present in India ink and of substances affecting blood clotting *in vivo* on the fate of carbon particles administered intravenously in rats, mice and rabbits, *Brit. J. Exp. Path.*, 1953, **34**, 426.
13. Krogh, A., Anatomy and Physiology of Capillaries, New Haven, Conn., Yale University Press, 2nd edition, 1929.
14. Volterra, M., Einige neue Befunde über die Structur der Kapillaren und ihre Beziehung zur "sogenannten" Kontraktilität derselben, *Zentr. inn. Med.*, 1925, **46**, 876.
15. Chambers, R., and Zweifach, B. W., Capillary endothelial cement in relation to permeability, *J. Cell and Compar. Physiol.*, 1940, **15**, 255.
16. Chambers, R., and Zweifach, B. W., Intercellular cement and capillary permeability, *Physiol. Rev.*, 1947, **27**, 436.
17. Jancsó, M., Histamine as a physiological activator of the reticulo-endothelial system, *Nature*, 1947, **160**, 227.
18. Jancsó, M., Speicherung. Stoffanreicherung im Retikuloendothel und in der Niere, Budapest, Akadémiai Kiadò, 1955.
19. Mátoltsy, A. G., and Mátoltsy, M., The action of histamine and antihistaminic substances on the endothelial cells of the small capillaries in the skin, *J. Pharmacol. and Exp. Therap.*, 1951, **102**, 237.
20. Biozzi, G., Mené, G., and Ovary, Z., L'histamine et la granulopexie de l'endothélium vasculaire, *Rev. Immunol. et Thérap. Antimicro.*, 1948, **12**, 320.
21. Benacerraf, B., McCluskey, R. T., and Patras, D., Localization of colloidal substances in vascular endothelium. A mechanism of tissue damage. I. Factors causing the pathologic deposition of colloidal carbon, *Am. J. Path.*, 1959, **35**, 75.
22. Gözsy, B., and Kátó, L., Studies on Phagocytic

Stimulation, Canada, University of Montreal, 1957.

23. FULTON, G. P., Microcirculatory terminology, *Angiology*, 1957, **8**, 102.

24. MAXIMOW, A. A., and BLOOM, W., A Textbook of Histology, Philadelphia, W. B. Saunders Co. 6th edition, 1952, **10**, 205.

25. BARRNETT, R., Blood vascular system, *in* Greep, R. O., Histology, New York, Blakiston Co., Inc., 1954, **12**, 273.

26. LANDIS, E. M., The capillary blood pressure in mammalian mesentery as determined by the micro-injection method, *Am. J. Physiol.*, 1930, **93**, 353.

27. COWDRY, E. V., The structure and physiology of blood vessels, *in:* Cowdry, E. V., Arteriosclerosis, New York, The Macmillan Co., 1933, **2**, 53.

28. COWDRY, E. V., A Textbook of Histology, Philadelphia, Lea & Febiger, 2nd edition, 1938, **9**, 110.

29. NONIDEZ, J. F., and WINDLE, W. F., Textbook of Histology, New York, McGraw-Hill Book Co., Inc., 1949, **10**, 134.

30. WOOLLEY, D. W., A probable mechanism of action of serotonin, *Proc. Nat. Acad. Sc.*, 1958, **44**, 197.

31. WOOLLEY, D. W., Serotonin receptors. I. Extraction and assay of a substance which renders

32. SPALTEHOLZ, W., Die Vertheilung der Blutgefässe in der Haut, *Arch. Anat. u. Entwcklngsgesch.*, 1893, 1.

33. LEWIS, T., Blood Vessels of the Human Skin and Their Responses, London, Shaw & Sons, Ltd., 1927.

34. ROCHA E SILVA, M., Histamine: Its Role in Anaphylaxis and Allergy, Springfield, Illinois, Charles C. Thomas, 1955.

35. LANDIS, E. M., Micro-Injection Studies of Capillary Permeability. I. Factors in the production of capillary stasis, Am. J. Physiol., 1927, **81**, 124.

36. DALE, H. H., and LAIDLAW, P. P., Histamine Shock, *J. Physiol.*, 1919, **52**, 355.

37. RICH, A. R., Condition of the capillaries in histamine shock, *J. Exp. Med.*, 1921, **33**, 287.

38. FELDBERG, W., The action of histamine on the blood vessels of the rabbit, *J. Physiol.*, 1927, **63**, 211.

39. FORBES, H. S., WOLFF, H. G., and COBB, S., The cerebral circulation. V. The Action of Histamine, *Am. J. Physiol.*, 1929, **89**, 266.

40. MENKIN, V., Studies on inflammation, XV. Concerning the mechanism of cell migration, *J. Exp. Med.*, 1938, **67**, 145.

serotonin fat-soluble, *Proc. Nat. Acad. Sc.*, 1958, **44**, 1202.

16

Reprinted from *Am. J. Anat.*, **110**(2) 125–153 (1962)

A Quantitative Study of the Hemodynamics in the Living Microvascular System[1]

EDWARD H. BLOCH

Department of Anatomy, Western Reserve University, Cleveland, Ohio

The purpose of this paper is to describe the results of a quantitative study of blood flow in the microvascular system. This study has differed from others, wherein the rheology of blood flow was examined, by employing several methods simultaneously to examine blood flow in living microscopic vessels (Bayliss, '52; Bloch, '56; Harding and Knisely, '58; Jäger, '35; Lutz et al., '50; McDonald, '60; Taylor, '55; Thoma, '27). These procedures have permitted an evaluation of the advantages, limitations, and a statement of what is required, of the methods which may lead to a more complete characterization of the rheology of blood.

These goals were achieved by magnifying the contents of the vessel and recording the blood flow at motion picture framing speeds (fps), up to 8,000 per sec, so that when the film was projected at 16 fps cellular movement was slow enough to trace the pathways of individual cells. Such data were compared with that obtained from vessels by direct visualization with the microscope, television microscopy and cinerecordings taken at 16 to 64 fps.

In spite of numerous studies of cells in flowing blood their behavior had been incompletely analyzed and quantitative data for the peripheral plasma layer and axial stream were sparse (Bayliss, '52; Bloch, '56; Clark and Clark, '35; Jäger, '35; Knisely et al., '44, '47; Krogh, '29; Lutz, Fulton and Akers, '50; Nicoll and Webb, '48; McDonald, '52; Thoma, '27; Vierordt, 1862). The methods in general which had been used were inadequate for discriminating individual cells. Occasionally the recording rates were adequate but data for sequential analyses of cellular movement were not reported (Bayliss, '52; Bloch, '56; Brookes and Monro, '57; Clark and Clark, '35; McDonald and Potter, '49; McDonald, '52a, '60; Monro, '60; Thoma, '27).

The goal of all studies was to obtain data which would assist in understanding the mechanics of the cardiovascular system in regard to: the distribution of blood cells within the vascular system, the influence of cellular movement on the mixing of plasma, the production of murmurs, and the energy required to move blood cells through vascular channels (Bayliss, '52a; Bloch, '53; Fahraeus, '52; Fahraeus and Lindquist, '31; Hale et al., '55; Hamilton, 1884; Hess, '17 Harding and Knisely, '58; Jäger, '35; Knisely et al., '47, '60; Madow and Bloch, '56; McDonald, '52b; Ralston and Taylor, '45; Poiseuille, 1842; Thoma, '27).

METHOD

Animals

Frogs, mice, rats, and rabbits were used.

Anesthesia

Frogs weighing 25–50 grams were anesthetized with 0.6 to 0.7 ml of a 25% solution of ethyl carbamate which was injected subcutaneously and mammals were anesthetized intravenously by injecting 20 mgms of sodium pentobarbitol per kilo body weight.

Surgery

The intestine in frogs was exposed by incising the thoracoabdominal wall with an electrocautery and in mammals by a midline incision using scissors and maintaining hemostasis with clamps and ligatures. To maintain the mesentery flat and maneuverable for microscopic study it was

[1] This work was supported by: The Life Insurance Fund, 1952–1954; The American Heart Association, 1953–1960 and the United States Public Health Service, Grant H-3240, 1957–1960.

125

spread against an optically flat quartz plate by suturing the small intestine to the frame of the plate with 5–0 silk (fig. 10).

The method used to expose the lung of mammals was as follows: a cannula (which was to deliver O_2 to the lung) was inserted into a tracheostomy so that it occupied about three quarters of the opening. (The opening external to the cannula permitted excess gas to escape thereby helping to prevent hyperdistention of the lung.) The right lung was then exposed by making an incision between the fifth and sixth ribs which extended approximately from the parasternal to the mid-axillary line. To achieve hemostasis, ligatures were placed around each rib distal to ends of the anticipated incision.

The liver was exposed by a midline incision of the skin and abdominal muscles extending from the tip of the xiphoid process to the umbilicus.

METHODS OF TRANSILLUMINATION

The quartz-rod method of transillumination was used for studying the circulation of the liver, lung, skeletal muscle and mesentery. Also in the study of the mesentery by transillumination standard microscopy was used.

Due to the intense light required for high speed cinerecording it was necessary to modify the standard quartz-rod method of transillumination. The modifications involved the light source, the temperature control system and the addition of a temperature recording system. A 1,200 watt tungsten filament lamp replaced the 750 watt lamp and was maintained at its optimal light output of 120 volts with an autotransformer. The light was transmitted to the tissue via a modified quartz rod (fig. 8). Information about the maintenance of thermal hemostasis of the intensely transilluminated area was essential. This was achieved by replacing the standard method of temperature control for the irrigating solutions by a servocontrolled proportional feedback system which has been described in detail (Bloch and Haas, '60b). Briefly, in this system of control, the temperature of the irrigating solutions issuing from the tip of the quartz rod and auxiliary irrigating units were maintained at a constant predetermined level through

the use of thermocouples which detected the thermal fluctuations produced by variations in light intensity or flow rate of the irrigating solutions. Such temperature fluctuations acted on the thermocouples to produce small voltages which were amplified and this current activated the heat exchangers of the temperature controlling equipment.

For observing or recording the circulation of the mesentery with monochromatic light the animal was placed on a tray attached to the mechanical stage of a standard microscope. The quality of the images improved not only because it was possible to use a substage condenser, but by placing the microscope on an optical bench, it was possible to obtain critical alignment with the light source (fig. 9). Monochromatic light was obtained with a 250 mm grating monochromator (Bausch and Lomb) which was used to transmit the desired wave length of 407, 414, 435, 550, and 620 mμ. The light source was a 100 watt high pressure mercury lamp (Osram) in conjunction with a power supply which delivered a stable current to the lamp. This light was focussed on the tissue by moving the substage condenser until the edges of the exit slit of the monochromator and the image of the tissue were in focus. The image of the vessel was studied or recorded directly or focussed on the camera of an image orthicon or vidicon television system and the resultant image observed or recorded from a monitor (fig. 9).

Optics

Dry or water immersion lenses were used. For the study of quartz-rod transilluminated tissues both a stereobinocular microscope (4 ×, 6 ×, 8 ×, and 12 × objectives and 12.5 × oculars) and a monocular monoobjective microscope (10 ×, 20 × and 50 × water immersion objectives and 10 × or 12.5 × oculars) were used. On the optical bench a monocular microscope was used. When cinerecording the oculars were either removed or photographic oculars inserted.

Cinerecording

Two high speed cameras were used: and Eastman Kodak Type III and a Wollensak Fastex WF3. The latter camera was similar to the Eastman camera except that the "shutter" was a glass cube and its maximum recording speed was 8,000 fps — twice that of the Eastman camera.

The 16 mm Eastman Kodak High Speed camera was used to record the circulation at framing speeds of 420 to 3,800 per second (figs. 5–7). One hundred feet of film (4,000 frames) were exposed at one time which resulted in the recording of approximately 3,500 sequential images. The film was accelerated slowly by a rheostat mechanically coupled to a 1/5 HP motor which moved the film and the "shutter." Approximately 25 feet of film were needed to reach 80% of the desired framing speed while the remaining 20% was reached gradually. For example, to obtain a framing rate of 3,000 per second, 65 to 70 feet of film were required. In contrast to a standard motion picture camera, in this camera, the film moved continuously. The image which reached the film passed through a "shutter" which consisted of a rotating optically flat glass plate (fig. 1). The ends of the glass plate were capped with metal to act as framers blocking the light to the film until the angle of rotation of the plate to the film plane was such as to reduce the optical distortion to a minimum. Light passed through this "shutter" during approximately 1/5 of the rotation of the plate. (At 3,000 fps the exposure was 1/15,000 second.) The frame frequency was calculated by measuring the length of exposed streaks on the edge of the film. (This exposure was produced by the flashing of an argon lamp mounted in the camera which flashed 120 times per second for a 60 cycle current.)

A 16 mm Kodak Cine Special camera was used to photograph the circulation at 16 or 24 frames per second.

Color and monochromatic film were used in both cameras. Kodachrome Type A, Eastman Ektachrome ER (Kodak SO 270 Type B color reversal film) and Kodak TRI-X negative films were used.

Analysis of the high speed film

The film which was taken at framing rates of 480 to 7,600 per second was projected with a Bell and Howell "Time and Motion" projector either by stopping each frame to study it, using the hand crank for slow motion, or the motor to view them at 16 or 24 frames per second.

The images were projected on graph paper, sketched through sequential frames, counted (by a counter attached to the shaft of the projector) and the magnification of the projected image and rate of movement calculated. Magnification of the projected image was calculated from the initial optical magnification and the projection distance while the rate of cellular movement was calculated from the frame speed which was indicated on the edge of the film and the distance that cells moved between sequential images. These data were inserted into the formula:

$$V = \frac{D}{M} \cdot \frac{T}{C};$$

where V was the velocity in mm/sec; D, the distance in mm that the cell moved when projected; M, the magnification of the projected image; C, the number of frames that the cell had been traced and T, the average frame speed attained during the total number of frames that the cell's pathway was traced.

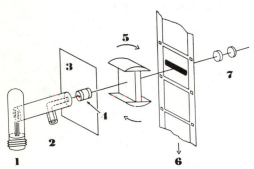

Fig. 1 Diagram of the optical path used for high speed cinerecording. 1. Light source, 2. Light conducting unit (quartz rod with side opening for irrigating solution). 3. Object plane. 4. Microscope optics. 5. "Shutter" of high speed camera. 6. Motion picture film. Vertical bar indicates object in focus which is brought into focus by viewing it through the back of the film with the viewing telescope, 7.

Methods used in determining the peripheral plasma layer and axial stream

These components were analyzed by: direct visualization with the microscope, from motion picture film which had recorded the events at framing rates of 16 to 24 and 480 to 7,600 per second in white light and at wave lengths of 407, 414, 435, 490 mμ; and from images on a monitor produced by an image orthicon or vidicon television system. In selected instances the effect of pressure on these components was determined by direct cannulation of the microscopic vessel (Rappaport et al., '59).

Multiple checks were used to increase the accuracy in measuring the peripheral plasma layer, by measuring it in white light, green light and at 414 mμ where intense absorption of hemoglobin occurred. The image was also displayed on a monitor with a calibrated scale by means of television microscopy which permitted rapid measurement of the layer and simple photorecording. In many instances the measurements were repeated by three different observers. In each instance the elapsed time was recorded between measurements to help in assessing the results.

The microvascular system defined

Before presenting the data, the vessels of the microvascular system are defined: The capillaries, which connect the smallest ramifications of arterioles and venules. Arterioles and venules begin as vessels having a diameter of 3 mm, and decrease in size to connect with the capillaries. The diameter of 3 mm has been selected as the beginning of the microvascular system since this is roughly the limit at which the anatomically unnamed vessels of the arterial and venous systems can be cannulated without optical aid.

RESULTS

To assess the results which were obtained with high speed cinephotomicrography the data will be presented in the following order; from direct visualization with the microscope, from standard cinerecording, from microspectrophotometry and from high speed cinerecording.

The dynamic responses of the circulation can best be appreciated by study of the film. Several films have been made (Bloch, '53, '60, '61).

Direct visualization of the microvascular system

The data which were obtained from direct visualization of the microvascular system were the product of nearly daily observations during the past 25 years in many species; amphibians, common laboratory animals, monkeys and man (Bloch, '56).

The appearance of this system was similar in the unanesthetized and in the average anesthetized animal. The linear velocity of blood flow was so rapid that individual cells in the blood stream were not observed and it was often difficult to determine the direction of flow. In the arterial and venous systems, the blood stream was a homogeneous red column, the axial stream, which sometimes contained a lighter colored central streak and two colorless cell-free peripheral zones, the peripheral plasma layer.

When movement in the blood stream was detected, variations were noted in optical density appearing as interrupted "lines," streamlines, parallel to the wall of the vessel. The streamlines frequently appeared to shift their position from moment to moment, either along the course or across the moving column of blood (figs. 11, 12, 13, 17, 19, 21). This phenomenon was not trustworthy for determining the direction of flow. When longer segments of the vessel were studied which contained a bifurcation, it was often possible to determine the true direction of flow and thereby determine whether the vessel was an arteriole or a venule, by the presence of an additional colorless zone between the confluent streams. Such a zone indicated that the vessel was a venule. Frequently, however, the direction of flow could be identified with certainty only when the vessel was traced to the capillary where cellular discrimination was possible. Other than cellular discrimination and thereby being able to trace the direction of the movement of cells, there were but few criteria which were consistently trustworthy in helping to establish with certainty that the vessel belonged to the arterial or venous system. For example: while it is true that the vessels of the arterial and venous systems were cone shaped, with the smallest dimension or apex directed toward the capillaries, segments of these vessels did not necessarily adhere to this criterion (tables 1 and 2). It was of some value to know that the diameter of arterioles were usually less than the venules which were parallel to them (table 2), but when very short segments of vessel were observed such relationships were not invariably trustworthy. The presence of pulsations of the wall established the vessel as an arteriole. But by direct visualization such pulsations were infrequently observed. And, recognizable color differences between the arterial and venous bloods were not detectable at the microscopic level.

In capillaries the linear velocity of blood flow was slower than in arterioles and generally individual cells could be identified. The flow of the cells was often rapid enough, however, to make it difficult to distinguish their precise orientation when the diameter of the capillary was larger than the red-cell. These cells appeared to be oriented with their smallest dimension in the direction of flow when the diameter of the vessel was less than that of the cells (fig. 26).

The exact site where the capillary began was often impossible to detect. There was little difficulty in determining an arteriole or a venule a little distance from their junction with the capillary. In the arteriole the flow rate was usually much faster and the diameter of the arteriole was *less* than the capillary. A venule was indicated by the confluence of two or more capillaries and with a corresponding increase in the diameter of the vessel.

The above description of the identification of these vessels in life is an over-simplification. In the dynamic responses of living tissue arterio-venous anastomoses can influence the flow patterns. They reverse the normal direction of flow in the peripheral segments of the terminal ramifications of the arteriolar and venous systems. Such pressure response may persist for seconds to perhaps hours, which enhances the difficulty in identifying a particular vessel as an arteriole or venule unless the arterio-venous anastomosis is identified which is not always possible.

The peripheral plasma layer and axial stream

These components were determined in vertical and horizontal mesenteries of the frog and rat. Two thousand seven hundred and fifty measurements were made of which 1,954 were made in the frog (1,146 in arterioles, 808 in venules) and 796 in the rat (338 in arterioles, 458 in venules).

Direct visualization of the peripheral plasma layer and axial stream in white light

The magnitude of the peripheral plasma layer did not change in any segment of vessel unless the linear velocity of flow changed. During tissue movement there was a change in the magnitude of these components which returned to their original dimensions after the movement stopped. In short, for any phase of physiology these components were relatively constant being determined by the type of vessel, its diameter and linear velocity of blood flow.

The peripheral plasma layer was seldom of the same magnitude on both sides of the vessel (tables 3, 4). The difference in magnitude was often considerable. Such differences in magnitude were not due to the gravitational forces of the vessel imposed by the mesentery being vertical or horizontal. Such spatial considerations became important only when the linear velocity of flow decreased sufficiently so that the gravitational forces were greater than the forces which moved the blood forward, a state which did not occur when the flow rate was such that cellular discrimination was not present.

The magnitude of the peripheral plasma layer varied to such an extent in relation to the diameter of the vessel that it was difficult to establish any correlation by simple inspection of these data. The relationship became more apparent when the ratio was calculated between the total peripheral plasma layer, the optically cell free zone on the two opposite sides of the column of blood, and the internal diameter of the vessel and taking the average of these ratios (table 5). When this was done it was found that as the diameter of

TABLE 1

The degree of taper of mesenteric vessels in the frog[1]

Arterioles					Venules			
P	D	L	T		P	D	L	T
65	78	650	− 1° 08′		88	70	1050	+ 0° 59′
107	108	1080	− 0° 93′		88	105	1575	− 0° 37′
105	105	1313	0°		114	105	2450	+ 0° 13′
105	123	1925	− 0° 32′		123	123	2100	0°
117	117	650	0°		140	175	963	− 2° 05′
135	135	1350	0°		140	158	1750	− 0° 35′
135	108	1080	+ 1° 32′		158	175	1313	+ 0° 44′
140	150	3300	− 1° 50′		158	210	1050	− 2° 50′
162	162	2700	0°		189	189	891	0°
193	175	1488	+ 0° 41′		193	175	1488	+ 0° 42′
193	193	1050	0°		193	228	1839	− 1° 05′
216	162	2700	+ 1° 08′		193	175	1050	+ 0° 59′
216	189	2430	+ 0° 38′		193	245	1750	− 1° 42′
245	228	1750	+ 0° 34′		263	210	1138	+ 2° 40′
245	245	2800	0°		263	263	1238	0°
263	263	3500	0°		280	245	1750	+ 1° 09′
265	253	2625	+ 0° 16′		280	263	1750	+ 0° 33′

[1] (P = internal diameter of the vessel in micra toward the heart; D = internal diameter of the vessel in micra toward the capillary system; L = length in micra between P and D; T = degree of taper (sin = P − D/L).)

TABLE 2

A comparison of the internal diameters of mesenteric vessels in the rat which were parallel to each other with their tapers

Vessel	Proximal (P)	Distal (D)	Length between proximal and distal measurement (L)	Angle of taper (sin = P − D/L)
	μ	μ	μ	
Arteriole	210	210	122	0°
Venule	350	350	122	0°
Arteriole	228	210	875	+ 1° 11′
Venule	438	419	875	+ 1° 14′
Arteriole	105	105	875	0°
Venule	175	210	875	− 1° 18′
Arteriole	175	175	1575	0°
Venule	262	227	1575	+ 1° 16′
Arteriole	88	70	1050	+ 0° 59′
Venule	175	123	1050	+ 2° 52′
Arteriole	123	158	1050	− 1° 49′
Venule	263	175	1050	+ 4° 0′
Arteriole	210	210	1050	0°
Venule	385	350	1050	+ 1° 49′
Arteriole	123	140	700	− 1° 23′
Venule	263	263	700°	0°
Arteriole	189	189	2700	0°
Venule	270	297	2700	− 0° 34′
Arteriole	243	216	2700	+ 0° 34′
Venule	378	405	2700	− 0° 34′
Arteriole	140	122	1750	+ 0° 35′
Venule	280	263	1750	+ 0° 33′

TABLE 3

The peripheral plasma layer, axial stream and linear velocity of blood flow in mesenteric arterioles

Internal diameter (ID)	Peripheral plasma layer (PPL)			Linear velocity blood flow[1]	Axial stream	Ratio TPPL:ID
	A	B	Total PPL			
μ	μ	μ	μ		μ	
				FROG		
			(Selected from 1,146 measurements)			
28	2.2	2.2	4.4	4+	23.6	1:6.4
28	4.4	6.5	10.9	3+	17.1	1:2.5
32	4.1	3.5	7.6	1+	24.4	1:4.2
36	2.6	5.2	7.8	4+	28.2	1:4.6
65	6.0	6.0	12.0	4+	53	1:5.4
65	13.0	0	13	1+	52	1:5
74	3.6	3.6	7.2	3+	66.8	1:10
75	3.6	3.6	7.2	3+	67.3	1:10
90	2.7	1.4	4.1	1+	84.9	1:22
90	6.3	4.5	11.5	3+	78.5	1:7.9
90	11.7	9.9	21.6	4+	68.4	1:4.3
102	4.1	9.0	13.1	4+	88.9	1:7.7
105	4.1	9.0	13.1	4+	91.9	1:8
116	3.0	3.5	6.5	4+	109.5	1:18
117	2.7	2.5	5.2	4+	111.8	1:22
137	3.6	0	3.6	4+	133.4	1:38
137	8.1	10.8	18.9	4+	118.1	1:7.3
145	4.5	0	4.5	4+	140.5	1:32
147	7.8	8	15.8	4+	131.2	1:9.3
180	5.4	3.6	9	4+	171	1:20
180	2.7	0	2.7	4+	177.3	1:67
201	9	5.4	14.4	4+	186.6	1:14
202	4.5	2.7	7.2	4+	197.8	1:28
252	4.5	7.2	11.7	4+	240.3	1:21
252	9	8.1	17.1	4+	234.9	1:15
270	5.3	6.3	11.6	4+	258.4	1:23
270	7.2	7.2	14.4	4+	255.6	1:19
				RAT		
			(Selected from 338 measurements)			
5	1.0	1.0	2.0	4+	3	1:2.5
5	1.2	0.8	2.0	4+	3	1:2.5
10	1.5	1.2	2.7	4+	7.3	1:3.7
10	1.5	1.3	2.8	4+	7.2	1:3.6
15	3.1	2.6	5.7	4+	9.3	1:2.6
15	2.5	1.8	4.3	4+	10.7	1:3.5
20	2.3	2.3	4.6	4+	10.7	1:4.4
20	1.3	1.7	3.0	4+	17	1:6.7
23	1.3	1.7	3.0	4+	20	1:7.7
23	2.0	0	2.0	4+	21	1:11.5
33	0	2.0	2.0	4+	31	1:16.5
33	2.6	2.4	5.0	4+	28	1:6.6
35	6.0	6.0	12.0	4+	23	1:3
35	6.3	5.9	12.2	3+	22.8	1:2.8
47	6.9	7.0	13.9	3+	33.1	1:3.4
47	7.0	7.2	14.2	4+	36.8	1:3.3
93	0	2.2	2.2	4+	90.8	1:42
100	2.0	2.5	4.5	1+	95.5	1:22
108	2.5	3.0	5.5	1+	102.5	1:19
130	3.0	3.5	6.5	4+	123.5	1:22
135	3.0	3.0	6.0	4+	129	1:22
135	3.0	3.5	6.5	4+	128.5	1:21

[1] Linear velocity of blood flow. 4+, blood flow so rapid that no cellular discrimination was possible; 3+, cells barely discriminated; 2+, cells readily discriminated; 1+, cells flowing slowly; 0, no flow.

TABLE 4

The peripheral plasma layer, axial stream and linear velocity of blood flow in mesenteric venules

Internal diameter (ID)	Peripheral plasma layer (PPL)			Linear velocity blood flow[1]	Axial stream	Ratio TPPL:ID
	A	B	Total PPL			
μ	μ	μ	μ		μ	
				FROG		
			(Selected from 808 measurements)			
37	8.1	7.2	15.3	4+	21.7	1:2.4
61	5.4	9.0	14.4	3+	46.6	1:4.2
100	12.6	17.1	29.7	4+	70.3	1:3.2
104	1.0	1.7	2.7	1+	101.3	1:38
110	6.3	5.4	11.7	3+	98.3	1:9.4
123	0.5	1.0	1.5	3+	121.5	1:82
134	4.5	3.0	7.5	3+	125.5	1:18
137	6.3	5.4	11.7	3+	125.3	1:12
151	6.3	2.7	9.0	3+	142.0	1:17
180	4.5	0	4.5	3+	175.5	1:40
180	4.5	4.5	9.0	3+	171.0	1:20
230	5.4	9.0	14.4	3+	225.6	1:16
230	8.1	9.0	17.1	3+	212.9	1:14
250	7.2	5.4	12.6	4+	237.4	1:20
273	0	9.0	9.0	4+	264	1:13
275	5.4	7.2	12.6	1+	262.4	1:22
286	9.0	13	22	4+	264.0	1:13
290	11.7	11.7	23.4	4+	265.6	1:13
325	6.0	6.0	12	4+	313	1:28
328	4.5	7.2	11.7	4+	316.3	1:28
360	7.2	5.4	12.6	4+	347.4	1:29
360	5.4	3.6	9.0	4+	351.0	1:40
377	6.0	4.0	10	4+	367.0	1:38
416	13.0	13.0	26	4+	390.0	1:16
				RAT		
			(Selected from 458 measurements)			
8	0.9	1.1	2.0	3+	6.0	1:3.9
8	0.9	1.2	2.1	3+	5.9	1:3.9
10	1.2	1.0	2.2	4+	7.8	1:4.5
10	1.0	1.1	2.1	4+	7.9	1:4.7
13	1.5	1.5	3.0	4+	10.0	1:4.3
13	1.4	1.5	2.9	4+	10.1	1:4.5
14	1.5	1.5	3.0	4+	11.0	1:4.6
14	1.4	2.0	3.4	4+	10.6	1:4.1
16	2.1	1.7	3.8	4+	12.2	1:4.2
16	3.6	4.0	7.6	4+	8.4	1:2.1
18	1.7	2.3	4.0	4+	14.0	1:4.5
18	1.6	2.1	3.7	4+	14.3	1:4.9
20	1.9	1.7	3.6	3+	16.4	1:5.5
20	1.6	2.0	3.6	4+	16.4	1:5.5
23	3.0	4.5	7.5	4+	15.5	1:3
23	1.4	2.0	3.4	4+	19.6	1:6.8
25	3.3	4.0	7.3	4+	17.7	1:3.3
25.1	3.3	3.8	7.1	4+	18.0	1:3.5
30	3.3	3.5	6.0	4+	26.5	1:4.4
30	2.0	3.0	5.0	4+	25.0	1:6
34	3.3	1.6	4.9	4+	29.0	1:7
35	3.2	1.5	4.7	1+	30.3	1:7.5
40	5.3	5.0	10.3	4+	29.7	1:3.9
40	5.7	6.0	11.7	3+	28.3	1:3.4
50	11.0	16.5	27.5	3+	22.5	1:1.8
110	2.7	3.8	6.5	4+	104.5	1:17
110	2.7	4.4	7.1	4+	102.9	1:16

[1] Linear velocity of blood flow. 4+, blood flow so rapid that no cellular discrimination was possible; 3+, cells barely discriminated; 2+, cells readily discriminated; 1+, cells flowing slowly. 0, no flow.

TABLE 5

A comparison of the average ratios of the internal diameter (ID) of mesenteric arterioles and the peripheral plasma layer (PPL)[1]

FROG			RAT		
Internal diameter	PPL:ID		Internal diameter	PPL:ID	
	Arterioles	Venules		Arterioles	Venules
μ			μ		
60–70	1:6	1:7	5–10	1:4	1:4
80–90	1:18	1:15	11–15	1:4	1:5
91–100	1:16	1:18	16–20	1:4	1:5
101–130	1:17	1:19	21–25	1:9	1:4
131–140	1:16	1:19	26–30	1:7	1:6
141–160	1:16	1:24	31–35	1:7	1:6
161–170	1:17	1:24	36–40	—	1:5
171–180	1:24	1:26	41–45	—	1:7
181–190	1:24	1:20	46–50	—	1:7
191–220	1:22	1:24	100–135	1:21	1:13
221–240	1:22	1:26			
241–270	1:21	1:26			
271–300	1:22	1:24			

[1] Total peripheral plasma layer.

the vessel increased the ratio decreased. Or, as the peripheral plasma layer increased the diameter of the vessel decreased. Exceptions occurred.

A study was made of the peripheral plasma layer as it was effected by altering the intravascular pressure locally and by changes in the linear velocity of flow. Linear velocity of flow was influenced by altering the depth of anesthesia or by the local application of epinephrine which increased the local intravascular pressure. A wide variety of responses occurred. The peripheral plasma layer decreased, did not change, or increased as the linear velocity of flow decreased (tables 3, 4). In general as the linear velocity of flow decreased so did the peripheral plasma layer. However, when the linear velocity became sufficiently slow so that the gravitational forces became greater than the propulsive forces engendered by the heart and great vessels sedimentation occurred and the peripheral plasma layer became increasingly larger toward the top of the vessel. When the intravascular pressure increased and the linear velocity of flow decreased due to peripheral constriction occurring after the application of epinephrine locally, (the pressure being measured by an indwelling rigid microcannula connected to a transducer) the peripheral plasma layer decreased. In those instances where the layer increased, cellular sedimentation was occurring.

The axial stream

In the transilluminated blood vessel of the arterial and venous systems the flowing cells appear as a red column, the axial stream, usually surrounded at the periphery by a colorless margin, the peripheral plasma layer. (An axial stream exists essentially only in vessels whose diameters are greater than three to five times the smallest diameter of the species' erythrocyte. Frequently in the center of the stream a more transparent central stream or core is observed.) While the axial stream exists in all vessels but capillaries, difficulties were encountered in detecting and measuring the more transparent core in the microvascular system of the rat. In 796 measurements of the peripheral plasma layer and axial stream in these animals, only 10 measurements of the core were possible. Therefore the results which pertain to this core were data derived from the frog where 208 measurements were made in the arterial and 189 in the venous circulations. The greatest sources of error in measuring this axial core were that it was difficult to establish the peripheral boundary of this core and to determine the velocity of linear flow. These parameters had to be measured almost simultaneously and no entirely satisfactory method was found. The minimum error existed when the linear velocity was rapid and *maximal*. When this occurred maximum contrast existed between this portion of the axial stream and the peripheral portions of the axial stream. But, as "rapid" flow was defined as the lack of visual perception of *any* cellular detail in the stream, there was a rather wide latitude between this and the actual maximal linear rate of flow.

The ratio of the core of the axial stream and the diameter of arterioles was relatively constant for any linear velocity of flow. The ratio was 1:4 for arterioles whose diameters measured 20 to 160 μ and 1:4.4 for those measuring 160 to 300 μ when the linear velocity of flow was rapid. When there was a perceptible, slight, reduction in linear velocity the ratio decreased to 1:2.4 in arterioles measuring 20 to 160 μ but was unchanged for the larger arterioles.

The ratio was 1:1.1 to 1:1.2 for arterioles up to 300 μ for the axial stream (ID:AS) when the linear velocity of flow was so rapid that cellular detail could not be observed or when occasional cellular detail was visible. A similar relationship was found for venules.

In general as the linear velocity of flow increased the diameter of the axial stream decreased. Conversely as the flow rate decreased, the diameter of the axial stream increased, reaching its maximum diameter when flow stopped, but before sedimentation of the cells occurred.

Microspectrophotometric study of the peripheral plasma layer and axial stream

In these studies the mesentery was supported vertically and transilluminated at wave lengths of 355, 407, 414, 435, 519, 625 mμ and in white light. Maximum contrast between the blood and vessel wall was obtained when the tissue was transilluminated at 414 mμ because at this wave length the hemoglobin absorbed intensively turning the column of blood black against a light purple background (figs. 14, 16, 20, 25, 26, 28). When such an image was projected onto the face plate of an image orthicon television camera tube and the image displayed on a monitor there was further control of brightness and contrast of the blood and the vessel wall (fig. 14). These factors helped by

sharply delineating the erythrocytes and the vessel wall, thereby increasing the accuracy in measuring the peripheral plasma layer and axial stream. The more transparent core of the axial stream was not visible at 414 mμ because the blood stream was opaque. Another advantage of studying the blood stream at this wave length was that the leucocytes appeared as colorless globules among the black erythrocytes. They were found to be randomly distributed throughout the blood stream by all methods used in this study. Preponderance of leucocytes at the periphery of the stream occurred only when pathology was present.

The analysis of blood flow with high speed cinephotomicrography

About 800 experiments were made during the past 7 years where the blood flow in the vessels of the microvascular system were recorded with high speed photography. In more than 650 of these experiments blood flow was recorded from the mesentery while about 50 recordings were made from the liver, lung, and skeletal muscle of frogs (*Rana pipiens*). Approximately 75 recordings were made from the mesentery of rats and 25 from the lungs of rabbits. Each recording consisted of 100 feet of film.

In the description of the experiments which follow, the data from the mesenteric circulation were selected as examples, due to the greater number of experiments which were made in this tissue. Similar data were obtained from the circulation in the vessels of the lung and skeletal muscles. No satisfactory data, however, were obtained from the liver.

The peripheral plasma layer

When the film of blood flow in mesenteric arterioles which had been taken at framing speeds of 480 to 7,600 per second was analyzed and compared with film of the *same* vessels which had been taken at 16 or 24 fps, there was considerable difference in the appearance of the peripheral plasma layer. In the control film, 16 or 24 fps, the peripheral plasma layer was a sharply defined clear zone but when the high speed motion picture film was studied the "layer" extended in an irregular manner toward the center of the vessel. Its complex configuration was unstable changing every few msecs. Such spaces or "layers" were interspersed by erythrocytes which slid against the wall and a few msecs thereafter another irregular "peripheral plasma layer" recurred (figs. 18, 20). For example, a peripheral plasma layer in an 80 μ arteriole (frog) extended as much as 30 to 40 μ toward the center of the vessel and was maintained for a distance of approximately 100 μ before changing its configuration. In such instances the cellular components were stable in regard to their position for approximately 100 μ or 5 msecs.

In venules whose diameters ranged between 50 and 500 μ the pattern of the peripheral plasma layer was similar to that of the arterial system (fig. 28). The principal difference was that in venules the rate at which the cells changed their position was slower.

Axial stream

The diameter of the axial stream was not measured *per se* from the high speed motion picture film because of the irregularity in its configuration which has been described in the section on the peripheral plasma layer.

The behavior of erythrocytes in flowing blood

Movement of the amphibian and mammalian erythrocytes was decreased sufficiently in the arterial and venous circulations to trace the pathway of these cells through contiguous frames of the motion picture film when the recording rates were greater than 2,800 frames per second, in frogs under light anesthesia and in rats under deep anesthesia. Under these conditions cellular movement was never stopped entirely, even in terminal arterioles, at framing rates up to 4,000 fps for the amphibian and 7,600 fps in the mammal when the cells were magnified × 200 to × 500. The best cellular discrimination was obtained by using a × 50 water immersion objective with a × 10 ocular. The determining factor in the study of the movement of the cells was the diameter of the vessel. For the frog the limiting internal diameter was approximately 100 to

150 μ and for the rat 30 to 40 μ. The ideal condition was one in which not more than one or two cells were interposed in the optical path, conditions found only at a distance extending 5 to 40 μ from the internal wall of vessels.

The total length that any cell could be followed was a distance of 100 to 150 μ when an initial magnification of 500 × was used. Not infrequently the cell moved out of focus in about half this distance. Both in the rat and frog the forward movement of the erythrocyte was complex in the arterial and venous circulations. In arterioles (*Rana pipiens*) with internal diameters ranging between 150 μ and 35 μ the cells described a helical pathway. The forward movement consisted of an apparent attempt of alignment of the long axis of the cell in the direction of flow. To achieve this a rotational movement of the cell occurred about its short and long axis. During its movement toward the capillary a complex path of motion was described which consisted of a decreasing helical spiral, decreasing as the cell moved toward the center of the moving column of blood. In traversing this pathway the cell produced a "sphere" of disturbance in the plasma and affected other cells by striking them, thereby modifying their flow pattern.

In vessels greater than 150 μ in diameter is was possible to trace cells for short distances, and their pathway, if anything, was more complex than in vessels with smaller diameters. At bifurcations (arterioles) erythrocytes not infrequently first moved 45° to 90° across the width of the tributary vessel before describing the spiral pathway described above.

Adequate analysis of the cellular flow pattern in the arterial system of the rat has been limited to vessels to about 20 μ and then only under deep anesthesia. Most of the analyses have been made from film which recorded the circulation at 3,600 fps. The pilot experiments which were made with the Wollensak Fastex WF3 camera at 7,600–8,000 fps did not stop the movement of cells in arterioles and the quality of the images were inadequate for tracing the pathway of cells; therefore the Eastman Camera was used and the linear velocity of flow reduced approximately to that of the frog's circulation.

The size of the rat's red-cells precluded the analysis of cellular movement in vessels whose internal diameter exceeded 20 to 30 μ due to the overlaying of too many cells in the optical path. (Rat erythrocytes in the circulation measured 3–3.5 μ × 7 μ).

Critical analysis has been possible of the flow of rat erythrocytes in 9 μ to 15 μ mesenteric arterioles when recorded at 3,600 fps. The complexity of the cellular behavior was not appreciated from observing the film at projection rates of 16 fps. At these projection rates the position of erythrocytes was noted to be at various angles in regard to the direction of flow, varying from a right angle to being parallel to the wall (figs. 29, 30). Frequently cells adjacent to each other were oriented differently. In general, the cells had different rates and degrees of orientation from each other. Some red-cells changed their orientation 360° within a distance of 15 μ to 40 μ, equivalent to 2–10 msecs (figs. 2–4). Other cells did not appear to change their position for a distance equal to width of the motion picture frame, approximately 100 μ. It was found that this was not so when the pathway of such cells were traced through sequential frames. Such cells had a "cork screw," helical, pattern of motion similar to that described for the frog.

The distortions of the rat erythrocytes and their alterations in position in the stream are illustrated in figures 2 to 4. Like the amphibian red-cell that of the rat had a helical forward motion turning on its long and short axes but doing so much more frequently. Furthermore considerable cellular distortion occurred, and

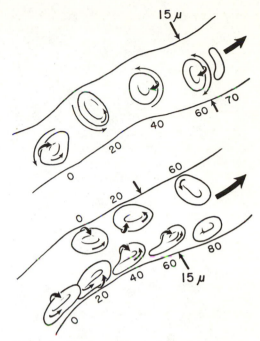

Fig. 3 Cine tracings through sequential frames of the flow pattern of 3 erythrocytes in a mesenteric arteriole of the rat (each exposure 1/15,000 sec or 3,600 fps). The number along the vessel indicates the number of frames between tracings and the arrows (thin) the direction in which the cells were spinning. The broad arrows indicate the direction of blood flow. Note the cellular distortion.

this in vessels which were three to five times wider than the greatest dimension of the cell. Red-cells were compressed, lengthened, folded, or twisted. Undistorted forms existed only a few msecs. In other words the undistorted form occurred no more frequently than the multitude of intermediate forms. Cells were lengthened to 10 or 10.5 μ, being about 50% longer than the normal. Such alterations in shape occurred through distances as short as 15 μ, equivalent to 7 msecs, in straight or curved arterioles, where bifurcations were either proximal or distal.

In venules a similar complexity in the cellular flow pattern existed. Sometimes cells remained in a "lamina" for a long period of time and their rotational changes were slower (figs. 27, 28). The movement of cells in the lamina adjacent to the plasma stream in confluent streams has not been studied.

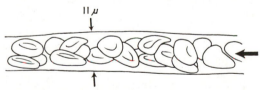

Fig. 2 A cine tracing of a single motion picture frame to illustrate the orientation of erythrocytes in a 11 μ mesenteric arteriole of the rat photographed at 1/15,000 second (3,600 fps). (All cells in the vessel were traced.) Compare with figures 3, 4, 29 and 30.

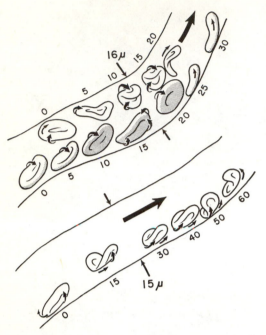

Fig. 4 The same arteriole as in figure 3. Cine tracing of three *other* erythrocytes. Photographic data as in figure 3. Shading denotes the opposite side of the cell. Note lengthening, compression, and folding of cells, occurring within 1/180 to 1/360 sec.

The movement of erythrocytes in vessels whose diameters were approximately that of the cell

The vessels which were of the same magnitude as the cell, or less, were the terminal segments of the arterial system and capillaries.

The orientation of cells in terminal arterioles was also different from what had been expected either from direct visualization or from recordings of this circulation by cinephotomicrography at 16–64 fps. With the standard methods of recording streamlines were seen (fig. 21). Since the vessels were just slightly wider than the longest dimension of the erythrocyte the cells were presumed to be flowing parallel to each other with their shortest diameter oriented in the direction of flow. There was present also a small but constant peripheral plasma layer. When this circulation was analyzed from motion picture film taken at framing speeds of 2,200 to 3,800 per second an entirely different

picture was revealed. The erythrocytes were randomly oriented. Many erythrocytes were oriented with their largest dimension at right angles to the direction of flow (figs. 22 and 23). Other cells had their shortest diameter oriented to the direction of flow or were oriented between these two extremes.

Deformation of the erythrocytes was common (figs. 22–24). Cells which were flowing at right angle to the wall were distorted so that they were either convex or concave.

The number of cells per unit volume of blood varied in terminal arterioles. Per millisecond, the cellular concentration of erythrocytes varied (in 50 μ segments of arterioles) from zero to nearly all cells. In these arterioles plasma skimming had not been observed in the control film nor during direct visualization.

In capillaries whose internal diameters were greater than the largest diameter of the erythrocyte the red cells were oriented similarly to those in arterioles. When the diameter of the vessel was less than that of the erythrocyte the cells were elongated and folded (compare fig. 25 with fig. 26).

A statement of the behavior and distribution of leucocytes as analyzed from high speed cinephotomicrography was not possible because too few of these cells were encountered. When such cells were observed they were randomly distributed in respect to their position in the vessels of the arterial, venous, and capillary systems.

Cellular velocity

The linear velocity was calculated for 51 erythrocytes in arterioles of the frog and 37 in the rat from the high speed film. The velocity of cellular flow in the frog was as follows: in 25 μ arterioles from 3.0 to 19.2 mm/sec with an average of 5.9 mm/sec; in 35 μ arterioles from 2.6 to 9.0 mm/sec with an average velocity of 6.6 mm/sec; and in 150 μ arterioles from 24.0 to 132 mm/sec with an average of 64.4 mm/sec. In the rat the velocity of erythrocytes in 9 μ arterioles averaged 2.23 mm/sec, varying from 1.98 to 2.41 mm/sec; in 13 μ arterioles the average rate was 1.32 mm/sec with a range of 0.74 to 2.16 mm/sec; and in 16 μ arterioles the average rate was 2.13 mm/sec with minimum rate of 1.67 and a maximum of 4.5 mm/sec.

Using the above data, calculations were made to determine how long it would require 100,000 frog erythrocytes to flow through arterioles which were approximately the diameter of the cells. For a flow rate of 2 mm/sec it would require 14 minutes for these cells to flow through a 27 μ arteriole and 7.5 minutes if the rate was 4.5 mm/sec in a 26 μ arteriole.

The dimension of amphibian erythrocytes in the arterial circulation

It was possible to measure the dimensions of frog erythrocytes in arterioles from the high speed film. While many thousands of cells were sketched, 201 were oriented at an angle which permitted measuring one of their three dimensions.

The length of 128 erythrocytes was measured. The average cell's length was 25.1 μ, with a maximum of 34 μ and a minimum of 22 μ.

The width was measurable in 24 cells whose average was 16.1 μ with a minimum of 13 μ and a maximum of 19 μ.

In 49 cells the average thickness was 5.8 μ and it varied between 3 μ and 9 μ.

Film

Adequate exposure for analysis of blood flow was obtained with Kodachrome Type A, Eastman Ektachrome ER and TriX negative films at framing rates to 3,600 per second using white light from the mercury (Osram) or tungsten light sources at microscopic magnification to × 550. Tri-X film has been overexposed at 8,000 fps with the Osram mercury light source at a magnification of × 500. In general, when monochromatic light was used, Tri-X film was most satisfactory. Kodachrome Type A film gave the best definition although normal color balance was not achieved due to the mercury light source and the underexposure which usually occurred at the maximum recording rates.

DISCUSSION

To bring the data of this study into perspective with those of others (Bayliss, '52; Bloch, '56; Brookes and Monro, '57; Harding and Knisely, '58; Jäger, '35; Jeffords and Knisely, '56; Knisely et al., '47, '60; Lutz et al., '50; McDonald and Potter, '49; McDonald, '52b; Ralston and Taylor, '45; Taylor, '55; Thoma, '27) the discussion is divided into: instrumentation, the peripheral plasma layer and axial stream as observed with standard recording methods, and then these data are compared with data derived from high speed cinerecording.

This study has differed from others wherein the rheology of blood was studied by using several methods to examine blood flow in living microscopic vessels. The procedures have permitted an evaluation of the advantages, limitations, and a statement of the requirements of the methods which may lead to a more complete characterization of the rheology of blood *in situ*. To achieve such a goal it is necessary to measure, in the living microvascular system, the volume of blood in a segment of vessel, the rate of flow and the pressure. The present status of the ability to measure these components is as follows:

Blood volume may be calculated in any arbitrarily selected segment of a vessel providing that the vessel is small enough at least to discriminate all of the erythrocytes. Static volume can be determined from the cinephotomicrographic image of the vessel which is projected simultaneously with a calibrated scale whereby the numerical magnitudes are obtained. These values are then inserted into standard formulas for determining the volume of a cone or cylinder. Dynamic cellular (erythrocyte) volumes may be calculated by inserting the values of the dimensions of properly oriented cells in the circulation into formulas which describe the volume of biconcave discs or ellipsoids. (The dimensions of width and length of the frog erythrocytes which were measured in the living circulation, av. 25.1 × 16.1 μ were in agreement with the av. 25.6 × 17.6 μ which were obtained of similar cells *in vitro* suspended in physiological solutions and with the literature (Knisely et al., '60).) Only an average cellular volume can be obtained due to the variation in size of erythrocytes and the probability that platelets or leucocytes may be missed because of superimposed erythrocytes.

While this error will occur, probably its magnitude is small because the number of leucocytes and platelets in such a volume is small and frequently these cells are absent. Thus, the total "cellular" volume is realistically the total red-cell volume.

The linear velocity of cellular flow in the arterial and venous systems can be determined from high speed cinerecording in vessels whose diameters do not exceed 100 μ for the amphibian and 30 μ for the mammalian circulation. In this study the cellular velocities which were calculated were average velocities because the framing rate was determined by measuring the number of frames between the exposed strips of film from the beginning of one strip to the beginning of the next one (25 frames for a frame speed of 3,000 per sec.). It is possible that the rate of film travel may vary during this distance without altering the total length of the strip. While this may be infrequent in occurrence it is a possible source of error which can be eliminated, and was, in a few experiments by photographing a time signal on each motion picture frame. A more serious criticism of the method is that the analysis is sharply limited by the focal depth of the optical system which will only permit the resolution of cells at the periphery of the moving column of blood in vessels whose internal diameters exceed the species' erythrocytes 5 to 10 times.

Historically the linear velocity of blood cells in the microvascular system was first determined by Leeuwenhoek (1798) and since that time many investigators have studied this problem by measuring either cellular flow or whole blood flow in either the gross or microvascular systems (Vierordt, 1862; Tigerstedt, '05; Basler, '27; Brookes and Monro, '57; McDonald, '52a). Of all the methods which have been devised to date, the one that apparently produces the least derangement of vascular physiology and can be used in the unanesthetized and unrestrained animal, is the electromagnetic flow meter (Kolin, '36; Kolin et al., '57; Olmstead, '60). Until a similar method can be developed for the microvascular system the high speed cinephotomicrographic method holds the most promise for measuring cellular flow rates.

The linear velocities of red-cell flow in arterioles obtained in this study represent but special instances of physiology and cannot be considered representative for the species. Considerable more data are needed before representative values can be established.

In this study only one of the many high speed cameras was used to any extent. A variety of high speed cameras were available (Garvin, '51; Industrial Photography, '59). Many of the high speed cameras were not applicable to the study of biological events because of the light intensities required. For example, the light which would be required to expose film at framing rates of 10^6–10^8 per second, would preclude any degree of homeostasis. It would, however, be desirable to utilize cameras with framing rates of 15, to 30,000/sec. Such framing rates will probably be required to study the detail of cellular flow in the microcirculation in small mammals under minimum anesthesia and with adequate magnification. (In the present study, the Eastman camera gave superior images to the Fastex instrument.)

Other methods exist which may be applicable for measuring cellular velocity in the arterial and venous circulations. P. A. G. Monro ('60) and Brookes and Monro ('57) described a method which employed a pulsed cathode ray beam transilluminating the tissue (rabbit ear chamber). The microscopic image of blood flow was transilluminated first at a rate of one msec and the frequency was reduced until there was no apparent movement of the cells; when the frequency was reduced further the apparent direction of cellular motion was reversed. Quantitative data of cellular flow rates were not reported. This method indicates that it is possible to determine the linear velocity of flow in mammals by obtaining cellular discrimination at frequencies below 1,000/sec. In the present study no reversal of flow was seen when the flow was recorded continuously from 480 to 7,600 fps. It would appear that a frequency of 1,000 per sec or less which was used by Monro is an untrustworthy value to use for calculating the linear velocity of cells.

It would be desirable to determine the velocity of plasma flow but at present no methods are available for determining this value in the microvascular system simultaneously with the other parameters.

The other parameter which is required for determining the rheology of blood is the pressure at two points within the microscopic vessel. Since blood flow varies during the cardiac cycle, dynamic pressures must be obtained. Progress is being made to achieve such measurements. Dynamic pressuregrams can be obtained in vessels whose internal diameters are as small as 80 μ (Rappaport et al., '59). At present the smallest useful internal orifice of the cannula is 35 μ whereby an adequate frequency response is obtained.

From this brief review of methods it is suggested that sufficient advances have been made in instrumentation that an approximation of the rheologic characteristics of blood can be made at the microscopic level *in situ* which is anticipated to be more meaningful than determinations made *in vitro*. And these data, when they are inserted into meaningful equations, will characterize the rheology of blood in the living system, the goal since the time of Poiseiulle (1842).

One other method, the image converter system (Wachtel et al., '58), is perhaps worth mentioning for the study of the dynamic morphology of cells in circulating blood. This system has unique advantages for the study of dynamic biologic events because it is a light amplifier, has good resolution, and is relatively simple. With this system it is possible to transilluminate a tissue with light intensities which are equal to or less than those which are used for direct visualization. In this method the image from the microscope is projected on to the face plate of the converter. Within this tube the intensity of the image is amplified and projected on to the distal part of the tube which contains a fluorescent screen. There is a wide range in the frequency at which this image can be displayed. For example an image can be displayed at a frequency of 1×10^{-6} sec (1 μ sec) and be repeated at such a frequency or repeated at msec, sec, or minute intervals. The intensity available on the fluorescent screen however for recording such images on motion picture film is probably of the order of magnitude equivalent to standard recording rates.

No new data were obtained in this study in regard to blood flow in vessels of the microvascular system by standard microscopy using white light. The data were in agreement with other reports (Bloch, '56; Clark and Clark, '35; Knisely, '47; Lutz et al., '50; Nicoll and Webb, '48). Again it was found that the images of cellular blood flow in the microvascular system appear to be so rapid that cellular discrimination is absent in all vessels but capillaries, that visible aggregates are absent, and that the peripheral plasma layer is cell free.

Detailed reports do not exist of blood flow analyzed with television microscopy although investigators have used the vidicon and image orthicon systems in monochrome and color, have indicated some of the advantages gained from the use of television, and have made cinerecordings to illustrate these points (Bloch et al., '56; Warner and Brown, '60). Detailed analysis was not attempted in this study. When white light was used with the monochrome television system, the only gain was the ability to have some control of contrast, most of which resided at the vessel wall and in the tissue. (This discussion is limited to those factors pertaining to information of structure and reaction, not to other factors inherent in these systems such as light and size amplification, which do not necessarily increase resolution and thereby information.)

This study is also in essential agreement with those who state that arteries and veins, of all sizes, are cone shaped with the taper of the cone in the direction of the capillary system. (Capillaries are considered to be cylinders.) The only quantitative data to support this concept is the report of Jeffers and Knisely ('56), although the photographs of many investigators support the concept qualitatively. In this study considerable variation was found in the degree and direction of the taper. Some of the data were in agreement with Jeffers and Knisely and others were not. The discrepancy in the data was not due to animals or tissue since they were similar in both studies and in both the mesentery had to be spread to visualize the vessels. In this study as many as 6 different observers reported similar results with regard to the variation in the direction of the "normal" taper although there was some difference in the magnitude of the measurements made by these observers. Perhaps the data reported by Jeffers and Knisely were selected deliberately to illustrate the general principle of taper, with which this report concurs. The important point is that in the characterization of blood flow, its rheology, the direction of the taper of the vessel cannot be taken for granted but must be determined.

It is surprising that published quantitative data were absent on the magnitude of the peripheral plasma layer and axial stream in the living-microvascular system although every time the system is observed these parameters are seen. The relation of peripheral plasma layer and axial stream to the internal diameter of vessel are important factors in the study of the rheology of blood because the ratio of cells to plasma would affect the viscosity of the fluid. It has been repeatedly demonstrated *in vitro* that the viscosity of blood decreases as the diameter of the tubes decrease especially in those which are comparable in size to those in the living microvascular system (Bayliss, '52, '59; Fahraeus and Lindquist, '31; Hagenbach, 1860; Haynes, '60; Poiseuille, 1842; Taylor, '55). Such a decrease in viscosity is presumably due to a decrease in the number of cells per unit volume of blood. This was indicated by the change in ratio of the peripheral plasma layer and the diameter of the vessel. The ratio of the peripheral plasma layer was found to decrease as the vessel decreased in size, with a ratio of 1:4 in the smaller vessels to a ratio of 1:20 or more for the larger vessels of the microvascular system.

The question of the ability to measure the peripheral plasma layer accurately, has been questioned recently (Bayliss, '59). In the past this layer has been noted with such ease that at one time it was suggested that a membrane existed between the peripheral plasma layer and the axial stream because they were so sharply demarcated (Thoma, '27). Recently Taylor ('55) and Bayliss ('59) have applied absorption microscopy to the study of blood (human, dog) flow through narrow glass tubes. Bayliss ('59) has found that in no experiment was the transmittance of a magnitude which would indicate that all of the erythrocytes had left the peripheral plasma layer. Furthermore, the increase in transmittance was not correlated with the reduction in apparent viscosity, nor was it possible to determine to what degree the erythrocytes were oriented in the direction of flow. Corroborative evidence of the presence of erythrocytes in the peripheral plasma layer was also obtained in the present study when blood flow was examined with monochromatic light at a wave length at which intense absorption of hemoglobin occurred and the stream observed with either standard or television microscopy. And like Bayliss found, it was not possible to state to what extent the cells were oriented in the direction of flow as the flow rates increased except when the flow became pulsatile, at which time the erythrocytes were randomly oriented during the time of zero flow. (Zero flow, however, has never been demonstrated during the normal cardiac cycle in the arterial vessels of the mesentery, the lung or in skeletal muscles. Pulsatile flow, with a zero flow component, was produced artificially by the local application of epinephrine.) Also, when dynamic pressures were determined in the vessel, simultaneously, with flow and the peripheral plasma layer, wide variations occurred in flow and pressure, without a significant alteration in the peripheral plasma layer. One consistent finding was that as the diameter of vessels decreased, the peripheral plasma layer increased; the smaller the vessel the larger the peripheral plasma layer, capillaries excepted.

What was learned of blood flow that had not been known when the data of blood flow, determined by standard methods, were compared with data derived from the high speed cinerecording method?

Perhaps one of the most unexpected results of the analysis was the finding that streamlines were no indicator of either cellular orientation or position. This fact was most significantly demonstrated in the smaller branches of the arterial system. When the flow of blood was observed either with the microscope directly, or from film which recorded this flow at normal framing speeds, obvious streamlines were present suggesting that the cells were flowing parallel to each other. This was emphatically not the case when this flow was studied from the high speed film. There was found to be a random orientation of the cells. Then why did the flow appear streamlined? Probably because the edges of groups of randomly oriented cells were fused in the visual integrating system of the observer as well as by the film (standard recording frequencies) to give the appearance of streamlines. Therefore neither the eye nor the standard photographic procedures were capable of resolving the true position or orientation of the cells.

The rate of reorientation of the cells especially in the mammalian (rat) arterial circulation was surprisingly rapid. Such changes could occur within a few msecs. This fact was not determined even from study of the high speed film at normal projection speeds but only by tracing single cells through sequential fields. There does not appear to be any indirect evidence that this could occur.

The concept and fact is common knowledge that capillaries can contain primarily plasma when ingress to the vessel has been partially occluded (Krogh, '29). This phenomenon of plasma skimming, however, had not been observed in the arterial or venous system when the diameter of the vessel was greater than the largest dimension of the erythrocyte. In this study it was demonstrated by analysis of the high speed film, that the cellular concentration per unit volume could vary and therefore "plasma skimming" could occur in these vessels. This was found in both the amphibian and mammalian circulations and is suggestive that it may be a common pattern of cellular flow.

The question has been raised by the *in vitro* studies of Bayliss ('59) that the peripheral plasma layer is not free of erythrocytes and by the present study where standard methods of visualization were combined with monochromatic light whereby occasional erythrocytes were found in this layer. The presence of cells in this layer was elucidated further from the analysis of blood flow with high speed cinerecording. Erythrocytes were found frequently in very close proximity to the wall, apparently touching the wall or 1–2 μ from it, sometimes in nearly every frame of the film. Also in nearly every frame the "peripheral" plasma layer extended varying distances from the wall to the center of the vessel (in arterioles measuring 10 to 100 μ often to the center of the vessel or 1/3 to 1/4 of this distance). So far the largest volume of data has been obtained from the amphibian circulation and the results have been corroborated in the mammalian (rat) circulation. An explanation must exist to account for the apparent discrepancy between the appearance of the peripheral plasma layer as observed by direct microscopic observation in contrast to the appearance of this layer in the high speed film. It is suggested that this discrepancy is due to a lack of contrast of the erythrocytes adjacent to the wall of the vessel, a decrease in their number because of volume and shallowness of the optical path at the sides of the vessel, coupled with bands of plasma which extend for various distances toward the center of the vessel. The summation of these factors produces the classical peripheral plasma layer. While the absorption studies and television microscopy indicate the presence of erythrocytes in the peripheral plasma layer the true state of affairs could not be appreciated until this zone was analyzed with a method which produced cellular discrimination.

It has been frequently demonstrated that erythrocytes deform readily, but this has been seen invariably only in vessels whose diameter were less than the erythrocyte (Krogh, '29; Nicoll and Webb, '48). That considerable deformation could occur of the erythrocyte, especially the mammalian erythrocyte, in vessels which were *larger* than such cells has not been reported. High speed recording has shown that not only are the cells deformed as they flow through vessels which are considerably larger than they are, but they can alter their spatial position in the vessel at rates which can be of the order of msecs. Because of these activities there must be considerable agitation of the plasma and therefore it is questionable that a "still" layer of plasma exists of any appreciable magnitude adjacent to the wall of the vessel (Bayliss, '52).

The *in vitro* studies of Vejlens ('38), Müller ('48) and Taylor ('55) and in *in vivo* studies of McDonald ('52, '60) and Prec et al. ('49) have indicated that the parabolic velocity profile of blood flow was not consonant with the classical concept of lamellar flow, but more akin to that of turbulent flow (Bateman, '56; Reiner, '49; Reynolds, 1883). This study extends these concepts to the living microvascular system by the presentation of data of the behavior of erythrocytes in the arterial and venous systems.

Finally, one may well ask what name should be given to describe normal blood flow in the arterial and venous systems — laminar, mixed or turbulent flow. According to the majority of students of blood flow it is laminar in the peripheral circulation while it may be turbulent in short segments of the central circulation (Bayliss, '52; Burton, '60; Hale et al., '55; Hess, '17; Potter and McDonald, '52; McDonald, '52a; Prec et al., '49; Ralston and Taylor, '45; Thoma, '27). They have derived their opinion from the study of blood flow in the vessels of the macrovascular system by a variety of methods (in a few instances from high speed cinerecording, up to 1,500 fps) and from the study of blood flow in narrow glass tubes. Recently, Taylor ('55) has questioned this concept of laminar flow and has presented evidence that it is neither laminar nor turbulent and he suggests that it be called "mixed." In this study the flow was found to consist of a complex pattern where erythrocytes spin about their long and short axes, deform readily, and travel across the "lamina" in an irregular helical spiral. So far no length of vessel has been found in which a stable pattern was established, although an attempt is made to orient the cell with its smallest dimension in the direction of flow. Such a pattern does not conform to the classical description of laminar flow. Therefore the least accurate name to describe the normal flow of blood in the microvascular system is "laminar." Perhaps before applying an-

other name to replace the well established name of "laminar" to normal blood flow, it would be more useful to continue, repeat and extend the study of blood flow with high speed cinephotomicrography and other methods which can produce cellular discrimination so that a thorough description of normal flow can be made, and then consider replacing the current name with a more appropriate one.

SUMMARY

Quantitative aspects of the rheology of blood, its dynamic morphology, were determined in the living microvascular system of the mesentery, lung and skeletal muscles.

Blood was analyzed with the following methods: direct visualization with the microscope, television microscopy, absorption microspectroscopy, dynamic pressuregrams, standard and high speed cinephotomicrography, where recording rates to 7,600 fps were used.

Quantitative data were presented for the peripheral plasma layer and axial stream as determined by standard methods.

The current status of the methodology was examined for obtaining data from the living microvascular system which could be inserted into formulas to characterize the rheology of blood in the living rather than to withdraw the blood, as is done now, and then determine its flow characteristics.

Blood flow was described as determined by direct microscopic visualization, television microscopy, absorption spectroscopy and standard cinephotomicroscopy and then contrasted with data obtained from high speed cinephotomicrography.

High speed cinephotomicrography of cellular blood flow revealed that the standard methods gave an imperfect understanding of cellular flow. Cellular flow was found to be complex and could not be designated as laminar.

The major features of cellular blood flow elucidated in this study from high speed cinephotomicrography were as follows: The forward motion of erythrocytes was a complex pattern which could be roughly described as an irregular helical path which decreased in diameter in the direction of flow. Erythrocytes spun around their short and long axes. Erythrocytes deformed, compressed, elongated, twisted and folded rapidly, within msecs, in all vessels of the microvascular system. Streamlines were no indication of cellular orientation.

The data were discussed in relation to current concepts of blood flow.

LITERATURE CITED

Bateman, H. 1956 Turbulent flow. In: Hydrodynamics. H. L. Dryden, F. D. Murnaghan and H. Bateman. Dover Publications, Inc., pp. 335–492.

Bayliss, L. E. 1952 Rheology of blood and lymph. In: Deformation and flow in biological systems. Ed. by A. Frey-Wyssling. Interscience Publishers Inc., New York, pp. 355–418.

———— 1959 The axial drift of the red cell when blood flows in a narrow tube. J. Physiol., 149: 593–613.

Basler, A. 1927 Eine Methode zur Untersuchung der Strömungsgeschwindigkeit in den Blutcapillaren. Handbuch der Biologischen Arbeitsmethoden, Abt. V, Teil 4, 2 Hälfte. Ed. by E. Abderhalden. Urban und Schwarzenberg, Berlin.

Bloch, E. H. 1953 In vivo high speed cinephotomicrography: technic and application (motion picture). Anat. Rec., 115: 383.

———— 1956 Microscopic observation of the circulating blood in the bulbar conjunctiva in man in health and disease. Ergebnisse d. Anatomie u. Entwicklungsgeschichte, 35: 1–98.

———— 1960 High speed cinephotomicrography of hemodynamics (motion picture). Fed. Proc., 19: 89.

———— 1961 Principles of hemodynamics in the microvascular system (motion picture). Anat. Rec., 139: 340.

Bloch, E. H., and A. Nordstrom 1953 A camera stand for cinephotomicrography. Photographic Science and Technique, 19B: 47–49.

Bloch, E. H., L. Warner, M. C. Brown and J. W. Christensen 1956 Color television of microcirculation (motion picture). Anat. Rec., 124: 476.

Bloch, E. H., and R. H. Hass 1960 The thermal control of tissue used in quartz rod transillumination. Ibid., 138: 261–280.

Brookes, A. M. P., and P. A. G. Monro 1957 Application of a flash cathode ray tube to the study of the circulation in live tissue. In: Proceedings of the Third International Congress on High-Speed Photography. Ed. by R. B. Collins. London, Butterworth Scientific Publications, pp. 142–143.

Burton, A. C. 1960 Hemodynamics and the physics of the circulation. In: Medical physiology and biophysics. Ed. by T. S. Ruch and J. F. Fulton. W. B. Saunders Company, Philadelphia, Chapt. 29, pp. 643–666.

Clark, E. R., and E. L. Clark 1935 Observations on changes in blood vascular endothelium in the living animal. Amer. J. Anat., 57: 385–438.

Fahraeus, R. 1952 The viscosity of normal and pathological blood. In: Deformation and flow in biological systems. Ed. by A. Frey-Wyssling. Interscience Publishers, New York, pp. 489–499.

Fahraeus, R., and T. Lindquist 1931 Viscosity of blood in narrow capillary tubes. Am. J. Physiol., 96: 562–568.

Garvin, E. L. 1951 Bibliography on high-speed photography. SMPTE, 56: 93–111.

Hagenbach 1860 Ueber die Bestimmung der Zähigkeit einer Flüssigkeit durch den Ausfluss aus Röhren. Ann. Phys. (Lpzg), 19: 385–426.

Hale, J. F., D. A. McDonald and J. R. Womersley 1955 Velocity profiles of oscillating arterial flow with calculations of viscous drag and the Reynold's number. J. Physiol., 128: 626–640.

Hamilton, M. B. 1884 On the circulation of the blood-corpuscles considered from a physical basis. Ibid., 5: 66–90.

Harding, F., M. H. Knisely 1958 Settling of Sludge in human patients. Angiology, 9: 317–341.

Haynes, R. H. 1960 Physical basis of the dependence of blood viscosity on tube radius. Am. J. Physiol., 198: 1193–1200.

Hess, W. R. 1917 Über periphere Regulierung des Blutzirkulation. Pflügers Arch., 168: 439–490.

Industrial photography 1959 A directory of high speed cine cameras. Industrial Photography, 8: 35–38.

Jäger, A. 1935 Die Anordnung und Stellung der roten Blutkörperchen im strömenden Blut. Pflügers Arch., 235: 705–722.

Jeffords, J. V., and M. H. Knisely 1956 Concerning the geometric shapes of arteries and arterioles. Angiology, 7: 105–136.

Knisely, M. H., W. K. Stratman-Thomas, T. S. Eliot and E. H. Bloch 1944 Microscopic pathological circulatory physiology of rhesus monkeys during acute Plasmodium knowlesi malaria (motion picture). M. H. Knisely, The Medical College of the State of South Carolina, Charleston, South Carolina.

Knisely, M. H., E. H. Bloch, T. S. Eliot and L. Warner 1947 Sludged blood. Science, 106: 431–440.

Knisely, M. H., L. Warner and F. Harding 1960 Ante Mortem settling. Angiology, 11: 535–588.

Kolin, A. 1936 An electromagnetic flow meter. Proc. Soc. Exper. Biol. and Med., 35: 53–56.

Kolin, A., N. Assali, G. Herrold and R. Jensen 1957 Electromagnetic determination of regional blood flow in unanesthetized animals. Proc. Natl. Acad. Sci., 43: 527–540.

Krogh, A. 1929 The anatomy and physiology of capillaries. Yale University Press, New Haven, pp. 5, 7–12.

Leeuwenhoek, A. van 1798 Certain positions laid down by the author respecting the circulation of the blood in an Human body, with his opinion respecting the manner of exhibiting the circulation by the injection of quicksilver. In: The selected works of Anthony van Leeuwenhoek. Samuel Hoole. Henry Frey, London. Part the first, 231–330.

Lutz, B. R., G. P. Fulton and R. P. Akers 1950 The neuromotor mechanism of the small blood vessels in membranes of the frog (*Rana pipiens*) and the hamster (*Mesocricetus auratus*) with reference to the normal and pathological conditions of blood flow. Exper. Med. and Surg., 8: 258–287.

Lutz, B. R., and G. P. Fulton 1954 Living microscopic blood vessels: Normal and pathological conditions (motion picture). G. P. Fulton, Boston University, Department of Biology, Boston, Mass.

Madow, B., and E. H. Bloch 1956 The effect of erythrocyte aggregation on the rheology of blood. Angiology, 7: 1–15.

McDonald, D. A. 1952a The velocity of blood flow in the rabbit aorta studied with high speed cinematography. J. Physiol., 118: 328–339.

——— 1952b The occurrence of turbulent flow in the rabbit aorta. Ibid., 118: 340–347.

——— 1960 Blood flow in arteries. Williams and Wilkins, Baltimore.

McDonald, D. A., J. M. Potter 1949 Blood streams in the basilar artery (motion picture). American Medical Association, 535 N. Dearborn Street, Chicago, Illinois.

Monro, P. A. G. 1960 Measurement of corpuscular velocity in small blood vessels. Anat. Rec., 136: 357–358.

Müller, A. 1948 Über das Druckgefälle im Blutgefäszen, insbesondere in den kapillaren. Helv. Physiol. Acta., 6: 181–195.

Nicoll, P. A., and R. L. Webb 1948 Subcutaneous blood flow in the bat's wing (motion picture). Audio-Visual Center, Indiana University, Bloomington, Indiana.

Olmstead, F. 1960 Measurement of cardiac output in unrestrained dogs by an implanted electromagnetic meter. In: Medical Electronics. Ed. by C. N. Smyth, Iliffe and Sons Ltd., London, pp. 327–334.

Poiseuille, J. L. M. 1842 See Regnault.

Prec, O., L. N. Katz, L. Sennett, R. H. Rosenman, A. P. Fishman and W. Hwang 1949 Determination of kinetic energy of the heart in man. Am. J. Physiol., 159: 483–491.

Ralston, H. J., and A. N. Taylor 1945 Streamline flow in the arteries of the dog and cat. Ibid., 144: 706–710.

Rappaport, M. B., E. H. Bloch and J. W. Irwin 1959 A manometer for measuring dynamic pressures in the microvascular system. J. Appl. Physiol., 14: 651–655.

Regnault 1842 Rapport sur la memoire de M. le docteur Poiseuille ayant pour titre: Recherches experimentales sur le mouvements des liquids dans les tubes de tres-petits diameters. C. R. Acad. Sci., Paris, 15: 1167–1186.

Reiner, M. 1949 Deformation and flow. H. K. Lewis and Co. Ltd., London.

Reynolds, O. 1883 An experimental investigation of the circumstances which determine whether the motion of water shall be direct or sinuous, and of the law of resistance in parallel channels. Phil. Trans., 174: 935–982.

Taylor, M. 1955 The flow of blood in narrow tubes. Austr. J. Exp. Biol. Med. Sci., 33: 1–14.

Thoma, R. 1927 Die experimentell-mathematische Behandlung des Blutkreislaufes. In: E. Abderhalden's Handbuch der biologischen Arbeitsmethoden. Abt. V., Teil 4/ii, 1103–1260. Urban und Schwarzenberg, Berlin.

Tigerstedt, R. 1905 Die Geschwindigkeit des Blutes in den Arterien. Ergebn. d. Physiol., 4: 481–516.

Vejlens, G. 1938 The distribution of leucocytes in the vascular system. Acta path. et microbiol. Scandinav., suppl., 33, pp. 1–241.

Vierordt, K. 1862 Die Erscheinungen und Gesetze des Stromgeschwindigkeit des Blutes. Max Hirsch, Berlin, 212 pp.

Wachtel, M. N., D. D. Doughty and A. E. Anderson 1958 The transmission of secondary emission image intesifier. In: Image intensifier symposium, October 6–7, U. S. Department of Commerce, O.T.S., 151813.

Warner, L., and M. C. Brown 1960 Techniques for studying the microcirculation in the eye. Anat. Rec., 138: 399–408.

PLATE 1

5   The Eastman Kodak High Speed Camera positioned over the microscope to record blood
    flow in the lung of the rabbit simultaneously with additional time mark pulses (3 on
    each motion picture frame) from an oscilloscope which is focussed on the film by the
    side lens of the camera. (Enlarged from a 16 mm motion picture frame.) For a de-
    scription of the camera stand see Bloch and Nordstrom, '53.

6   The Eastman Kodak High Speed Camera. (D) Film supply spool; (A) Argon timing
    lamp; (S) Shutter Mechanism; (M) dichroic mirror for positioning image from the side
    lens onto the film; (V) viewing telescope; (T) film take up spool.

7   Simplified photograph illustrating the arrangement of the high speed camera (C) with
    a monoobjective microscope (M) and the light conduction quartz-rod system (R) when
    used to record the circulation in vertically mounted tissue. (Enlarged from a 16 mm
    motion picture frame.)

8   The modified quartz rod. (S) Delivery tube for the irrigating solution and (T) thermo-
    couple.

9   Arrangement for transilluminating tissue with monochromatic light. (G) Grating
    monochromator and light source; (M) monocular monoobjective microscope mounted on
    a modified milling machine head; (C) camera (Image Orthicon); (O) optical bench.

10 Vertically supported mesentery in position for being transilluminated (T) Irrigating tip
    which contains a thermocouple. (Enlarged from a 16 mm motion picture frame.)

146

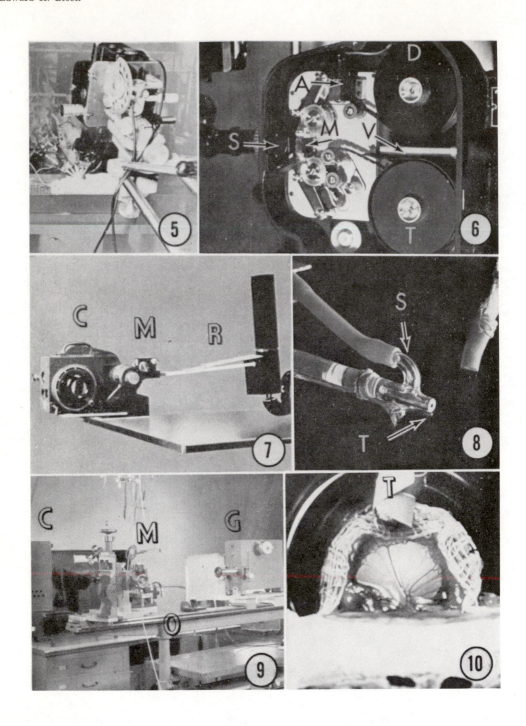

11 Arterial blood flow (frog) photographed with white light at 24 fps in a horizontal mesentery. Note streamlines (S), lack of cellular detail in the axial stream and the apparent absence of a peripheral plasma layer. (Enlarged from a 16 mm motion picture frame.)

12 Arterial and venous blood (rat) transilluminated a wave length of 510 mμ and photographed at 24 fps in a vertical mesentery. (A) Arteriole. (B) Venule. Compare with figure 11. Note streamlines lack of cellular detail in blood stream and indistinct peripheral plasma layers. (C) Indicates confluence of peripheral plasma layers in the major stream. Arrows indicate direction of flow. (Enlarged from 16 mm motion picture frame.)

13 Blood flow in a terminal arteriole and capillary (frog). Photographed with a wave length of 490 mμ at 16 fps in a vertical mesentery. (A) Arteriole. (C) Capillary. (S) Streamlines. Compare with figures 11, and 12. (Enlarged from a 16 mm motion picture frame.)

14 Photograph of a monitor (Image Orthicon Camera chain) depicting an image of a 30 μ mesenteric arteriole (frog) which was being transilluminated at a wave length of 414 mμ. Contrast has been accentuated to demonstrate the edge of the vessel wall. Absorption of the hemoglobin in the erythrocytes has turned the flowing column of blood black (note that the column of blood extends nearly everywhere to the luminal surface of the arteriole. (Photographed at 1/10 sec.)

15 Mesenteric arteriole of the rat transilluminated with white light and photographed at 1/1,000 sec on 35 mm film. Note indistinctness of the peripheral plasma layer. Compare with figure 16.

16 The same mesenteric arteriole as illustrated in figure 15 transilluminated at a wave length of 414 mu and photographed 35 secs later.

148

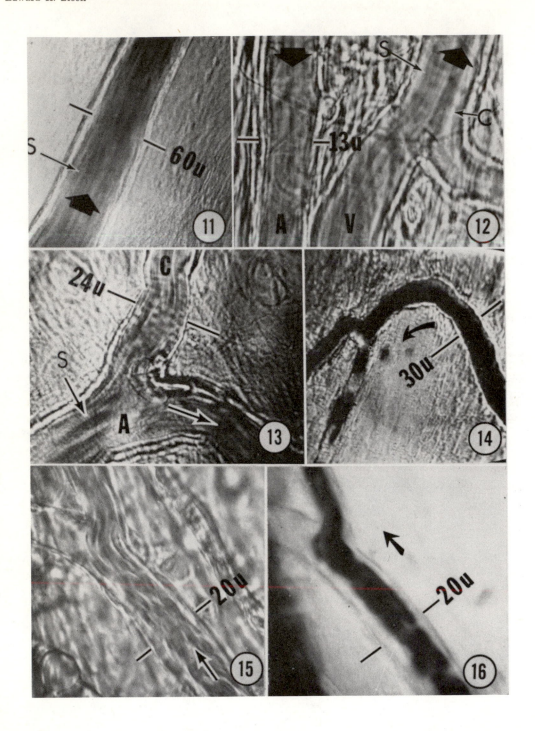

PLATE 3

17 Arterial blood flow photographed in a horizontal mesentery (frog) in white light at 24 fps. Note streamlines and lack of cellular detail. This was the control for the circulation illustrated in figure 18. (Enlarged from a 16 mm motion picture frame.)

18 The same vessel as in figure 17 except the circulation was photographed at 2,600 fps. Note the orientation of the cells and the peripheral plasma layer. Elapsed time between the two recordings approximately three minutes. (Enlarged from a 16 mm motion picture frame.)

19 Arterial and capillary flow in a vertically suspended mesentery (frog) transilluminated with light of 490 mμ. (A) Arteriole. (C) Capillary. Note streamline flow, lack of cellular detail, thick wall and indistinct peripheral plasma layer.

20 The same blood flow and vessels as in figure 19 except they were transilluminated with light at a wave length of 414 mμ and recorded at 3,000 fps. In the arteriole note plasma spaces and irregular peripheral plasma layer. Some erythrocytes are oriented parallel to the wall and in the direction of flow, others at various angles. Note the position of the erythrocytes in the capillary. (Enlarged from a 16 mm motion picture frame.)

21 Blood flow in an arteriole with a capillary branch in a vertical mesentery (frog) transilluminated with white light and recorded at 24 fps. Note streamline flow in arteriole and erythrocytes (temporarily) impinged upon the fork of the vessel. Note streamlines in the capillary. (Enlarged from a 16 mm motion picture frame.)

22 The same vessels as in figure 21 except that the flow was recorded at 3,700 fps. (Enlarged from a 16 mm motion picture frame.

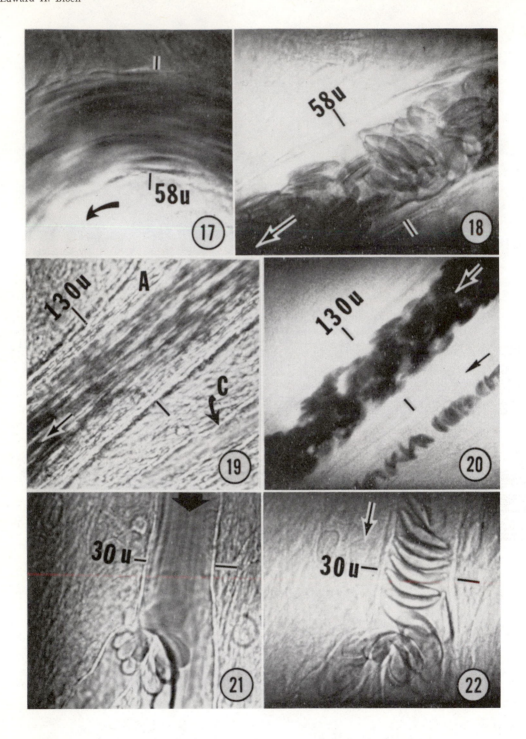

23 The same vessel as illustrated in figure 22 photographed a few msecs later than the image depicted in figure 22. (Enlarged from a 16 mm motion picture frame.)

24 Blood flow in a terminal arteriole of a vertical mesentery (frog) transilluminated with light at a wave length of 435 mμ and at 3,000 fps. Note the shape of the erythrocytes, the plasma spaces between cells, and the peripheral plasma layer. (Enlarged from a 16 mm motion picture frame.)

25 Blood flow in a "dilated" capillary of a vertical mesentery (frog) transilluminated at a wave length of 414 mμ. (Still photograph, 1/1,000 sec.) Compare orientation of cells with figure 26.

26 Blood flow in a partially constricted capillary (other data similar to figure 25. Compare orientation of cells with figure 25. (Still photograph, 1/1,000 sec.)

27 Blood flow in venules of a vertical mesentery (frog) transilluminated with light at a wave length of 510 mμ and photographed at 24 fps. (Enlarged from a 16 mm motion picture frame.)

28 The same vessels as in figure 27 but flow was recorded at 2, 600 fps and the tissue transilluminated with light at a wave length of 414 mμ. Note orientation and distribution of erythrocytes. (Enlarged from a 16 mm motion picture frame.)

29 Blood flow in an arteriole of a vertical mesentery of the rat transilluminated with white light and recorded at 3,600 fps. Note unequal cellular distribution and cellular orientation. Compare with figure 2. (Enlarged from a 16 mm motion picture frame.)

30 Arterial blood flow in the vertical mesentery of the rat transilluminated with white light and recorded at 3,600 fps. The orientation of the cells is illustrated more clearly in figures 3 and 4. (Enlarged from a 16 mm motion picture frame.)

152

349

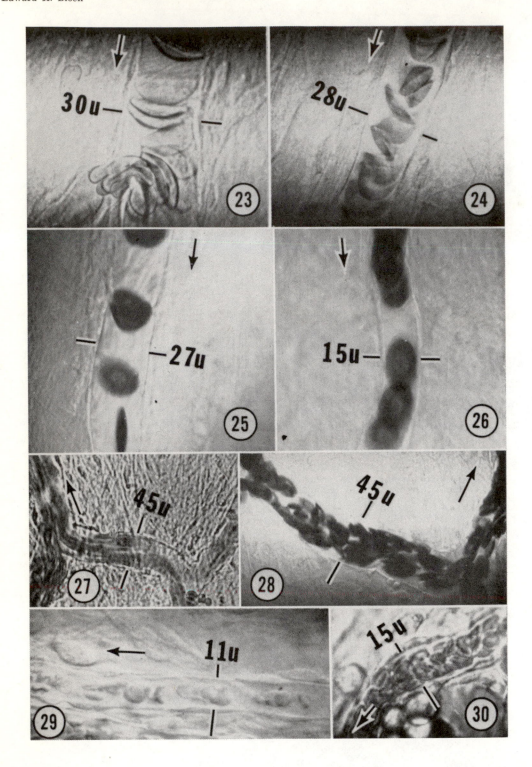

17

Reprinted from *Arch. Int. Pharmacodyn. Ther.*, **139**(3–4), 455–469 (1962)

TRANSMURAL PRESSURE AND VASCULAR TONE — SOME ASPECTS OF AN OLD CONTROVERSY [1]

BY

Björn FOLKOW

(Received for publication 1-2-1962).

INTRODUCTION

In 1902 BAYLISS (1) put forward the interesting hypothesis that the distension, offered by the blood pressure, might serve as an adequate stimulus for the vascular smooth muscles and contribute to the maintenance of their tonic activity. The hypothesis was based on a series of carefully performed experiments, which, however, were not entirely unequivocal, and on analogies to the responses of other types of smooth muscles when exposed to stretch.

Since then the Bayliss hypothesis has been much debated, starting with a critical study by ANREP (2) in which he concluded that BAYLISS's experimental results could be explained by other mechanisms. BAYLISS was not convinced that his hypothesis was invalid and left the question open in his monograph "The vasomotor system" (3) by stating that "... on the whole I fear that we must regard the question as undecided."

During recent years much interest has been devoted to the validity of this hypothesis and opinions are still divided, to say the least. Since the present author has been concerned with this problem for several years, it was thought to be of interest to try to evaluate the Bayliss hypothesis in the light of more recent studies.

---

[1] This paper is dedicated to Professor C. HEYMANS on the occasion of his 70th birthday.

I. *Basal vascular tone and its background.*

It might be suitable to start with the important question of whether the vascular bed, or some of its haemodynamically more important sections, exhibits any smooth muscle tone after acute elimination of all central nervous and bloodborne excitatory influences. Should no such "basal vascular tone" be demonstrable, it would automatically rule out the significance of strictly *local* vasomotor activity including that suggested by Bayliss. This would then point to neurohormonal mechanisms as the only relevant sources of vascular tone.

In earlier years it was often taken for granted that vascular tone was due solely to neurohormonal influences. Surprisingly few studies examined more directly whether any truly basal tone exists, and if so, the extent and location within the vascular bed. On the other hand, a great number of scattered data can be extracted from the wealth of studies dealing with other aspects of the circulation, which, when put together, help to shed light on this problem.

It is fairly easy to demonstrate that at least the resistance vessels of several haemodynamically important vascular circuits do exhibit a considerable basal tone, and that its extent varies from one tissue to the other. In order to demonstrate basal tone it is necessary to compare the flow resistance after acute vascular denervation with the resistance remaining at maximal vasodilatation. To be comparable both resistance measurements must be performed at the same pressure level because of the distensibility of the vessels.

Such comparisons reveal that, in the resting and otherwise normal organism, the acutely denervated vessels of e.g. skeletal muscle, myocardium, brain and intestine maintain a considerable tone. Other vessels, such as the cutaneous arteriovenous anastomoses, are almost maximally dilated after symapathectomy. The possibility exists that the residual tone exhibited by the vessels is due to bloodborne vasoconstrictor agents, and that the observed regional differences in tone are due to differences in sensitivity to such agents. However, the cutaneous arteriovenous anastomoses, which exhibit almost no tone after denervation, have the greatest sensitivity to such agents of all the vessels studied. This suggests that, in the 'resting' intact organism, the blood contains only insignificant amounts of vasoconstrictor agents, and that the vascular tone remaining after denervation is truly 'basal', in the sense that it is of strictly local origin (4, 5). A wealth of scattered data in the literature can, as mentioned, be taken to support such a view.

The question then arises as to whether the tone of the vascular smooth muscles is due to some locally originating, but extrinsic factor, or is truly intrinsic, that is, inherent in the muscle itself. In this sense, an independent nerve cell plexus or secretory cells situated in the vascular walls could be looked upon as extrinsic factors. Intrinsic myogenic activity, or automaticity, is a well known phenomenon in many other types of smooth muscles, with the exception of the 'multi-unit' variants which, for performing their special functions, must be completely dominated by their nervous supply (5, 6, 7). It is obvious that a rhythmic, more or less unsynchronized myogenic activity of the vascular contractile elements will create a basal tone, which, if present in the resistance vessels, would express itself as an enhanced resistance to flow. The characteristics of the 'vasomotion phenomenon' of e.g. precapillary sphincters strongly suggest the existence of myogenic activity in the vascular bed, at least in some of its sections.

Most histologists at present appear to deny the existence of local independent nerve plexuses in the vascular walls (8) which at one time or another have been implicated in most local vascular events. Even if such plexuses could be demonstrated to exist, it would certainly have to be shown that they were the true origin of the basal vascular tone and not merely an integrating, local communication network. Further, it would only mean that automaticity would be ascribed to nervous instead of smooth muscle elements. This would solve no problems, but, rather, add new ones. In fact, not even the propagation of responses, known to occur along the vascular walls under certain circumstances, requires independent local nerve plexuses. Such a spread seems to take place along the muscle elements themselves (9, 10). Other local sources of extrinsic influences may exist. Scattered chromaffine cells, which could presumably release catechol amines or closely related substances, have been identified in some tissues along small vessels, especially veins (11). However, there is nothing to indicate that such cells are responsible for any 'spontaneous' secretion of vasoconstrictor agents that could be the origin of the basal vascular tone. Presumably these cells are controlled by the sympathetic nervous system rather than being a link in a strictly local control system. Furthermore, they are not concentrated in that vascular section where the basal tone is most pronounced, the precapillary resistance vessels. All the agents known to be locally produced by the metabolism of the tissues have, if anything, a vasodilator influence and, therefore, would tend to depress basal tone.

Moreover, recent experiments show that the basal vascular tone is not reduced when all sources of vasoconstrictor agents, whether centrally or locally controlled, are depleted by intense reserpine treatment (7). This finding also excludes the remote possibility that some sort of axon reflex mechanism, operating along the ramifications of the centrally controlled vasoconstrictor fibres, could be responsible for the basal tone.

It is then reasonable to conclude that basal vascular tone is an expression of a truly myogenic activity. From all points of view, this seems the simplest and most attractive explanation available. Basal tone is probably a consequence of the rhythmic, 'spontaneous' variations of membrane potential, typical for the 'visceral' smooth muscles. When these rhythmic variations are pronounced enough they result in a complete membrane depolarization and contraction.

It has also been shown that the basal tone is essentially confined to the precapillary resistance vessels (7). Presumably it is most pronounced within the sections closest to the capillary level. It is evident that there must exist a considerable difference in the extent of myogenic activity of various smooth muscle effectors. This appears to be related to the particular series-coupled vascular section to which the smooth muscle belongs. In this regard, the smooth muscles of the precapillary vessels behave more like 'visceral' smooth muscles, while those of the venous capacitance compartment behave more like 'multi-unit' smooth muscles, to use Bozler's terminology (12), in that they almost lack basal tone and their control is entirely dependent upon neurohormonal mechanisms. No doubt such vascular smooth muscle differentiation is, however, more a matter of quantity than quality. This is illustrated by the fact that in some tissues the smallest veins, which are a part both of the post-capillary resistance vessels and the capacitance vessels, can show considerable myogenic activity (13, 14, 15). Isolated arteries or veins sometimes exhibit a slight or moderate 'spontaneous activity' (10, 16). However, it appears that the precapillary vessels form the only consecutive compartment of the vascular bed, which exhibits a haemodynamically important basal tone. This basal tone is important in that it markedly affects such functional aspects of a vascular circuit as total flow resistance, capacitance function and the ratio of precapillary to postcapillary resistance, which is one of the main determinants of transcapillary filtration exchange (7).

In summary the following conclusions may be drawn:

1) The *basal vascular tone*, varying in extent from one vascular circuit to the other, appears to be a consequence of a truly myogenic activity and is confined mainly to the precapillary resistance vessels. These vascular smooth muscle cells therefore have much in common with the 'visceral' type of smooth muscle. This basal tone is especially pro-

nounced in tissues characterized by marked variations in metabolic needs, (e.g. myocardium and skeletal muscle) and/or by a high priority for blood supply, where extrinsic restrictions of the supply cannot be tolerated (myocardium and brain). In such tissues a considerable, locally controlled 'blood flow reserve' is created by the tone inherent in the precapillary myogenic activity. This 'reserve' is promptly mobilized as needed by the inhibitory influence of locally produced metabolites on basal tone. Broadly speaking it may be stated that for the different 'parallel-coupled' resistance vessels a roughly inverse relationship exists between the extent of basal tone and the superimposed constrictor fibre control.

2) The basal tone appears to be small or even negligible in vascular compartments which serve the system as a whole rather than local needs. The performance of these compartments calls for a dominating central control with little allowance for interfering local mechanisms. As examples of this the capacitane vessels, acting as filling regulators for the pump, and the cutaneous shunt vessels, subserving temperature regulation, can be mentioned. Accordingly, such vascular compartments are almost entirely dominated by their vasoconstrictor fibres and may, therefore, be said to belong to the 'multi-unit' type of smooth muscle.

3) If the distension offered by the transmural pressure significantly affects the vascular tone as BAYLISS suggested, then previously mentioned results make it clear that such a mechanism may only be expected to affect the precapillary resistance vessels, since these are the vessels, which under normal conditions, exhibit a haemodynamically significant basal tone.

II. *The influence of the transmural pressure on basal vascular tone.*

In dealing with the possible influence of transmural pressure on basal vascular tone it may be advisable first to discuss briefly some considerations of interest for the experimental analysis. If other factors remain constant, a raised transmural pressure can be expected to distend a vascular circuit, including its resistance vessels. Though their distensibility is small in terms of bore change, it is nevertheless of considerable haemodynamic significance due to Poiseuille's relationship between internal radius and flow resistance. It follows that if other factors are considered to be constant, then: a) an increase in arterial pressure alone will increase flow *more* than the pressure head, as the concomitantly elevated transmural pressure will distend the vessels. The pressure-flow curve will therefore be convex to the pressure axis. Further, b) equal increases of arterial and venous pressures will increase flow in spite of the unchanged pressure head, because of the vascular distension. Lastly, c) an increase in venous pressure alone will decrease flow but this decrease will be *less* than that expected from the decreased pressure head, because again, the raised transmural pressure will cause a vascular distension. These results, which have been found experimentally (17, 18, 19), are the results that one would predict if the vascular bed were considered to be passively distensible, and in which such variable as viscosity and smooth muscle activity were kept constant. Some special exceptions do exist. Presumably, at some point vascular distension is cheched by the rigid fibrous jacket around the vessels. Also if a vascular circuit is enclosed within a rigid capsule, secondarily raised tissue pressure may curtail the effects of a raised arterial pressure (20, 21, 22, 23).

Consider now the circumstance in which counteracting smooth muscle adjustments occur within the precapillary resistance vessels in the situations a), b), and c) above. If such 'active' adjustments exactly balance the distensibility, they will make the resistance vessels behave as if they were truly rigid. Only very rapid pressure shifts would then be able to reveal the fact that there were two opposing forces influencing the flow resistance, since the relative slowness of the smooth muscle adjustments would cause them to lag behind the effects caused by the physical distensibility (19, 24).

In the circumstance in which the counteracting smooth muscle adjustments were so extensive as to more than overcome the physical consequence of the distensibility, then the following effects would be expected in the three alternatives; a) flow would increase *less* than the pressure head, creating 'flow autoregulation' with the pressure-flow curve concave to the pressure axis; b) flow resistance would tend to increase and hence flow decrease; c) flow would tend to decrease *more* than the pressure head because of the concomitant 'active' resistance increase.

By proper variations of the arterial and venous pressures, performed during exact flow and resistance measurements results such as those just described have been found. In this way it is possible to reveal counteracting smooth muscle adjustments. If pressure shifts are made rapidly enough or if the smooth muscle adjustments are eliminated then the usually masked effects of vascular distensibility may be observed.

Several technical precautions have to be taken. It would, for instance, appear to be of little relevance to draw conclusions concerning possible pressure-induced smooth muscle adjustments of the precapillary resistance vessels by performing model studies on isolated larger arteries and veins. The smooth muscles of these sections of the vascular bed normally exhibit little or no basal tone, behaving more like 'multi-unit' smooth muscles. Therefore they can be expected to exhibit little or no 'active' response to a continuous transmural stretch stimulus (10, 16, 25). This does not deny that blunt mechanical stimuli may depolarize these smooth muscle cells causing a contraction or, if some automaticity is awakened, a contraction may even be induced by a moderate stretch (10, 16). However, to reveal what happens in the 'visceral' type of smooth muscle of the precapillary resistance vessels, which is the haemodynamically relevant problem, these vessels must be studied under circumstances in which their environment is as normal as possible. Too often experiments have been devised which markedly derange the chemical environment of these vessels and expose them to vasodilator and/or vasoconstrictor factors which are not normal constituents of the blood or the tissue fluid. Myogenic activity is a subtle cell phenomenon, which is easily interfered with. Technical artefacts may eliminate what was intended to be studied. It is obvious that artificial perfusions with plasma substitutes must markedly change the local smooth muscle environment with respect to its oxygen and carbon dioxide tension, pH, etc. Such changes will certainly affect the activity of the precapillary resistance vessels markedly, since they normally respond promptly to any changes in these factors. At best a feeble trace of myogenic activity and 'active' reactions to pressure-flow changes may be expected under such circumstances. Further, blood perfusion with artificial pump systems, often used with the intention of keeping the system under complete control, will also markedly derange the smooth muscle environment. The slightest handling of the blood cells, in cats and dogs, leads to cell damage. Large amounts of vasodilator agents can be released from the erythrocytes (26). The results of a recent study (27) can be shown to be due to such artefacts. Also vasoconstrictor agents, such as 5-hydroxytryptamine are known to be released from other blood cell elements, under certain circumstances. As these substances, which are not present in the blood of the intact circulations, tend to accumulate in the artificial circuit, they will soon completely dominate the behaviour of the vascular smooth muscles. Such conditions may mask such subtle mechanisms as myogenic activity and autoregulatory flow adjustments. The same vascular circuit can, in fact, be shifted from almost perfect flow autoregulation to a passively distensible tube system, simply by letting the arterial inflow pass through an artificial pump (26). To draw a parallel, it would be meaningless to estimate the myogenic activity of intestinal strips and the effects of a distension stimulus, if the strips were kept in an organ bath flooded with smooth muscle-depressing drugs. It is true that several precautions can be taken to minimize the damage inflicted on the blood cells, but the use of the normal heart and arterial system for supplying the blood, with the flow measurement devices inserted on the venous outflow side, appears to be by far the best way of maintaining normal vascular reactivity.

With these considerations as a general background, the principal results, obtained in pressure-flow studies in the abovementioned alternatives a), b), and c) will be discussed. Pressure-flow studies in alternative a), in which the changes in the transmural pressure are in the same direction as the changes in pressure head, can only rarely provide unequivocal information concerning a mechanism such as that proposed by BAYLISS for the following reason. Increasing arterial pressure alone will increase both the transmural pressure and the pressure head. According to the Bayliss hypothesis, the increased transmural pressure would cause a constriction of the resistance vessels. However, the increased pressure head will increase the flow, which would then reduce the level of locally produced vasodilator metabolites, and this would tend to cause a constriction of these same vessels. Decreasing arterial pressure, obviously would cause a dilatation by either mechanism, and in either case it would be very difficult to say which mechanism was responsible. However, if such an experiment failed to reveal any autoregulatory adjustments of vascular tone then this would strongly contradict Bayliss's hypothesis.

A great many studies have revealed the existence of a more or less pronounced flow autoregulation in the brain, skeletal muscle, myocardium, intestines, and kidney (for lit. see e.g. 24, 28, 29, 30). These are the tissues where some basal vascular tone can be demonstrated. The fact that no significant flow autoregulation occurs in skin areas, dominated by the specialized A-V shunt vessels which practically lack basal tone, suggests that the autoregulation phenomenon may result from a modulation of the myogenic activity (24).

One of the very first series of studies, which lent strong support to Bayliss's hypothesis, was performed on the cerebral vessels by FOG (31, 32, 33). Arterioles on the surface of the brain were observed directly during arterial pressure changes under circumstances in which it was unlikely that flow-dependent local chemical changes could be made responsible for the vascular responses. In most other studies of flow autoregulation carried out by changing arterial pressure, vascular adjustments due to flow-dependent changes in local chemical environment can hardly be excluded.

In this respect the kidney, to some extent, is an exception. An increase in renal blood flow and ultrafiltration will automatically tend to increase renal metabolism by the increased tubular reabsorption activity. Such a factor will tend to minimize the flow-induced changes in chemical environment of the vascular smooth muscles within this organ. But the kidney exhibits perhaps the most pronounced flow autoregulation of all tissues. Kidney autoregulation has attracted great interest for several decades but opinions are still much divided concerning its genesis. MILES et al. (34) presented results which suggested an 'active' smooth muscle mechanism, a view further strengthened by the experiments of THURAU and KRAMER (35, 36) and WAUGH et al. (30, 37, 38). When taken together these results appear to be most convincing, but there is also strong experimental support for a purely physical mechanism. On close study of these apparently contradictory results it is tempting to assume that both mechanisms exist. WAUGH has been able to show that on deliberate elimination of a smooth muscle-dependent autoregulatory component a less effective though sometimes quite powerful 'physical' component is revealed. This latter mechanism, originally suggested by WINTON (20) has recently been carefully explored by HINSHAW et al. (21, 22, 23). When arterial inflow pressure is raised, the rigid renal capsule causes the tissue pressure to rise markedly, making the effective intrarenal rise of pressure head far smaller than predicted. The quite peculiar characteristics of renal structure and function are a prerequisite for such a mechanism. As several studies of renal flow autoregulation have been performed with the aid of arterial perfusion circuits, it is difficult to judge when, and to what extent the suggested 'active' and 'passive' components have dominated the haemodynamic events. As mentioned, it is quite possible that both mechanisms do exist, in which case it may be reasonable to assume that the 'active' component normally dominates renal haemodynamics. Whatever the case it seems advisable to be cautious about making definite statements, since the renal circulation is such a complex haemodynamic problem.

In experiments using alternatives b) and c) it is easier to evaluate whether the transmural pressure *per se* constitutes an adequate stimulus for the maintenance of vascular smooth muscle tone. In alternative b) the pressure head is kept unchanged while only the transmural pressure is varied. In alternative c) the pressure head is reduced when transmural pressure is raised and *vice versa*. This latter alternative has the drawback that the Bayliss mechanism is counteracted, not only by the vascular distensibility, as in b), but also by flow-dependent chemical environment changes, which may well mask it more or less completely. This suggests that alternative b) offers the most unequivocal way to prove or disprove Bayliss's hypothesis, if nervous and similar extrinsic influences can be excluded.

Experiments performed by the author in 1949 (39) on acutely and chronically denervated vascular circuits, while not exactly reproducing the situation outlined in alternative b), are nevertheless similar enough to see the operation of the Bayliss mechanism. Equal reductions in blood flow to the hind part of the cat were produced either by partial arterial obstruction or partial venous obstruction, and observations made on the extent of the reactive hyperaemia following release of the obstruction. In both cases during the period of reduced flow one expects relaxation of the precapillary resistance vessels due to the relative accumulation of metabolites. With reduction in arterial pressure the decreased transmural pressure, according to the Bayliss hypothesis, would also relax these same vessels, while the increased transmural pressure from venous obstructions would constrict these vessels. Since there would be an appreciable lag in the smooth muscle adjustments of the precapillary resistance vessels following sudden release of the obstruction, it would be expected, then, that the extent of the reactive hyperaemia would be greater in the former case than in the latter. This is the observed result and is in strong support of the Bayliss hypothesis. A parallel was drawn to the then recent experiments by BOZLER (40) on the myogenically active ureter, in which a continuous distension was found to cause a lasting increase in the 'spontaneous' discharge of the smooth muscle elements. It was, however, also obvious that the pressure-induced 'facilitation' of the myogenic vascular tone was fairly moderate, as compared with such dominating mechanisms as the superimposed constrictor fibre control and locally produced 'vasodilator metabolites'. Nevertheless, the Bayliss mechanism evidently is of great interest for the appreciation of how vascular tone is established and normally controlled.

When the Bayliss mechanism works in synergism with the flow-dependent local chemical changes, the locally induced reactions of the precapillary vessels can be powerful enough to keep mean capillary pressure rather constant even if arterial pressure is changed from 200 down to 40 mm Hg. These local mechanisms must be considered to be of great importance for keeping mean capillary pressure and hence the filtration exchange as constant as possible (7). The local mechanisms must be of especial importance in vascular circuits, where normally the extrinsic nervous influence is weak or absent. It is likely that wherever basal vascular tone constitutes the important basis for the vascular control, the transmural pressure acts as a continuous modulator of this basal tonic activity, sometimes in synergism with, sometimes in antagonism with extrinsic control mechanisms. Furthermore, the quantitative balance between these essentially local control mechanisms and the extrinsic ones certainly varies between the different circuits in the control of the pre-capillary resistance vessels. All these aspects must be considered whenever vascular control is discussed.

The operation of the Bayliss mechanism has been confirmed and extended in several different studies (e.g. 29, 41), and has also been demonstrated in man (41, 42, 43, 44, 45). It has been debated, as to exactly how the reactions are brought about. GASKELL and BURTON (46) have pointed out that Bayliss's hypothesis appears to contain a paradox insofar as the transmural pressure distension must be imagined to cause a lasting shortening of the smooth muscles beyond their initial length. Then, however, the stimulus would have eliminated itself. For such reasons GASKELL and BURTON suggested that the regional resistance increase, seen when venous pressure was raised (as in alternative c), might be a consequence of a 'veni-vasomotor reflex'. It was suggested that there was some sort of local reflex arch with its 'receptor' end within the highly distensible venous compartment and its 'effector' end within the arteriolar section. It has previously been discussed that no independent local nerve plexuses appear to exist. Furthermore responses of this character are seen also in chronically denervated vascular beds. They are present also when local anesthetic agents are locally administered (29). Moreover, it has recently been shown (7) that vascular reactions of this type are, if anything, more vivid in animals totally depleted of vasoconstrictor agents that might serve as transmittors for central or local nervous or neuro-hormonal mechanisms. As has been mentioned earlier, our experiments suggest that the Bayliss mechanism is for all practical purposes confined to the precapillary resistance vessels, where myogenic basal tone is present.

Also, the fact that the Bayliss mechanism implies a positive feed-back mechanism raises another theoretically important objection. It follows that if the pressure-induced vasoconstriction raises the pressure head, this will in turn accentuate the vasoconstriction, and so on.

A clue to the solution of these two apparently serious objections can be derived from some studies on other types of myogenically active smooth muscles. BOZLER (40) observed in the ureter and BÜLBRING (47) in the isolated intestinal strip that distension increased the *rate* of the 'spontaneous' discharge. It thus appears as if distension facilitates the inherent rhythmic activity so that the rate of the contraction cycles increases. It is then easy to understand why the Bayliss mechanism is not demonstrable in vessels, which normally do not exhibit any significant myogenic activity, (the cutaneous A-V shunts or the capacitance venous compartment) or when a normally present myogenic activity is depressed by vasodilator agents (26). It is not a contradiction that blunt-mechanical stimuli, such as pinching, can produce powerful contractions in vessels that usually exhibit no myogenic activity. Any stimulus, even mechanical ones, if intense enough, can produce membrane depolarization in resting muscle cells and induce a contraction.

It is reasonable to assume that the interrelationship between myogenic activity and distension would be valid wherever myogenic activity is exhibited. It has also been reported that the 'spontaneous' vasomotion of the venules in the bat's wing increases its rate when these vessels are distended (14, 15). When this interpretation is applied to the smallest precapillary resistance vessels, which exhibit the haemodynamically most significant myogenic activity, it would mean that the time fraction, occupied by the constriction phase, tends to increase at the expense of relaxation phase. Such a phenomenon is seen in any rhythmically activated muscle, when driven at increasing rates, whether the myocardium or skeletal muscle. The integrated *haemodynamic* result of a distension, inducing an unsynchronized increase of myogenic activity of the thousands of precapillary smooth muscles, would be an increase in vascular tone (49). If the rate of the unsynchronized spontaneous activity of the muscle cells is increased enough, it will express itself haemodynamically as an *increase* in resistance to blood flow. Such a view implies a paradox only if the rate of the contraction cycles is increased to the point at which a true summation of the contractions occurs. The consequent fusion of the contractions here implies a lasting shortening of the individual smooth muscle with no relaxation-elongation. Presumably the facilatory influence of moderate, continuous stretch on the myogenic activity cannot be further enhanced when fusion of the contractions begins. In addition to this there will be a limit set by the relative refractory period. If so, this may create the natural and effective 'brake' on the positive feed-back mechanism. It would automatically tend to keep the pressure-induced resistance increase within moderate limits, with the critical point set where the contraction cycles appear so frequently that summation occurs. No doubt, intense *extrinsic* excitatory influences can produce a truly 'tetanic' contraction, resulting in maximal vasoconstriction. Such a view is in harmony with the fact that flow autoregulation usually vanishes when the arterial pressure rise becomes too high. It would further explain why there is no trace of flow autoregulation if the blood vessels are continually exposed to high concentrations of vasoconstrictor agents, such as barium ions (19), which in all probability induce a tetanic contraction of the smooth muscle cells.

Concluding remarks: An interpretation of the Bayliss mechanism in terms of recent, well-documented findings dealing with the functional characteristics of myogenically active smooth muscles has been presented. No paradoxes or hypothetical nervous mechanisms are involved. The principle applied is that simple distension causes a continuous facilitation of the *rate* of the inherently evoked contraction cycles. Though this is a positive feed-back mechanism, it can be expected to be selflimiting when the rate of contraction becomes high enough to cause summation. At this point the distension stimulus will automatically eliminate itself.

In a way, the myogenically active vascular smooth muscles of the pre-capillary resistance vessels, like those of the intestine (48), appears to act as a sort of spontaneously active mechano-receptor. Because of their built-in contraction system they will function as a single cell 'receptor-effector unit', serving a purpose similar to the more complexly organized excitatory proprioceptor reflex of the skeletal muscles. Superimposed on this locally controlled, primitive mechanism are the specific cardio-vascular proprioceptor reflex arcs which constitute a neurogenically mediated integration and balancing system that often completely overrule the local single-cell mechanism and give priority to the needs of the cardiovascular system as a whole. Their centralized reflex control has, in its turn, many analogies to the vestibular and neck receptor influences on the supraspinal control of the somatomotor system.

Part of the studies discussed was supported by a grant from the School of Aviation Medicine AF 61 (052)-286, USA.

REFERENCES

1. — BAYLISS, W. M. *J. Physiol.*, 1902, *28*, 220.
2. — ANREP, G. v. *J. Physiol.*, 1912, *45*, 307.
3. — BAYLISS, W. M. 'The vasomotor system'. London, 1923.
4. — LÖFVING, B. and MELLANDER, S. *Acta Physiol. Scand.*, 1956, *37*, 134.
5. — FOLKOW, B. 'Hypotensive drugs', p. 163. Pergamon Press, London and New York, 1956.
6. — FOLKOW, B. *Physiol. Rev.*, 1955, *35*, 629.
7. — FOLKOW, B. and ÖBERG, B. *Acta Physiol. Scand.*, 1961, *53*, 105.
8. — HILLARP, N. Å. Handbook of Physiology, Neurophysiology II, 1960, 979.

9. — HILTON, S. M.   *J. Physiol.*, 1959, *149*, 93.

10. — FURCHGOTT, R. F.   *Pharm. Rev.*, 1955, 7, 183.

11. — ADAMS-RAY, J., NORDENSTAM, H. and RHODIN, J.   *Acta Neuro-veg.*, 1958, *18*, 304.

12. — BOZLER, E.   *Experientia*, 1948, *4*, 213.

13. — NICOLL, P. A. and WEBB, R. L.   *Ann. N. Y. Acad. Sci.*, 1945, *46*, 697.

14. — WIEDEMAN, M. P.   *Circ. Res.*, 1957, *V*, 641.

15. — WIEDEMAN, M. P.   *Circ. Res.*, 1959, *VII*, 238.

16. — WACHHOLDER, K.   *Pflüg. Arch.*, 1921, *190*, 222.

17. — WEZLER, K. and SINN, W.   'Das Strömungsgesetz des Blutkreislaufes'. Ed. Cantor KG/Aulendorf, Würstl. 1953.

18. — PHILLIPS, F. A. Jr, BRIND, S. H. and LEVY, M. N.   *Circ. Res.*, 1955, *III*, 357.

19. — FOLKOW, B. and LÖFVING, B.   *Acta Physiol. Scand.*, 1956, *38*, 37.

20. — WINTON, R. R.   Harvey Lect. 1951-52, ser. 47, p. 21. Acad. Press Inc. New York.

21. — HINSHAW, L. B., DAY, S. B. and CARLSSON, C. H.   *Amer. J. Physiol.*, 1959, *197*, 309.

22. — HINSHAW, L. B., BALLIN, H. M., DAY, S. B. and CARLSSON, C. H.   *Amer. J. Physiol.*, 1959, *197*, 853.

23. — HINSHAW, L. B. and WORTHEN, D. M.   *Circ. Res.*, 1961, *IX*, 1156.

24. — FOLKOW, B.   *Acta Physiol. Scand.*, 1952, *27*, 99.

25. — BURNSTOCK, G. and PROSSER, C. L.   *Amer. J. Physiol.*, 1960, *198*, 921.

26. — FOLKOW, B.   *Acta Physiol. Scand.*, 1952, *27*, 10.

27. — ZSOTEŘ, T.   *Canad. J. Biochem. Physiol.*, 1961, *39*, 653.

28. — KETY, S.   'The control of the circulation of the blood', Suppl. Vol., p. 176. W. M. Dawson & Sons Ltd., London, 1956.

29. — JOHNSON, P. C.   *Amer. J. Physiol.*, 1960, *199*, 311.

30. — WAUGH, W. H. and SHANKS, R. G.   *Circ. Res.*, 1960, *VIII*, 871.

31. — FOG, M.   "Om pialarteriernes vasomotoriske reaktioner", Copenhagen, 1934.

32. — FOG, M.   *Arch. Neurol. Psychiat.*, 1937, *37*, 351.

33. — FOG, M.   *J. Neurol. Psychopath.*, N. S., 1938, *1*, 187.

34. — MILES, B. E., VENTOM, M. G. and DE WARDENER, H. E.   *J. Physiol.*, 1954, *123*, 143.

35. — THURAU, K. and KRAMER, K.   *Pflüg. Arch.*, 1959, *268*, 188.

36. — THURAU, K. and KRAMER, K.   *Pflüg, Arch.*, 1959, *269*, 77.

37. — WAUGH, W. H. and HAMILTON, W. F.   *Circ. Res.*, 1958, *VI*, 116.

38. — Waugh, W. H.   *Circ. Res.*, 1958, *VI*, 363.

39. — Folkow, B.   *Acta Physiol. Scand.*, 1949, *17*, 289.

40. — Bozler, E.   *Amer. J. Physiol.*, 1947, *149*, 209.

41. — Hilton, S. M.   *J. Physiol.*, 1953, *120*, 230.

42. — Wood, J. E., Litter, J. and Wilkins, E. W.   *Circ. Res.*, 1955, *III*, 581.

43. — Greenfield, A. D. M. and Patterson, G. C.   *J. Physiol.*, 1954, *125*, 508.

44. — Coles, D. R., Kidd, B. S. L. and Patterson, G. C.   *J. Physiol.*, 1956, *134*, 665.

45. — Coles, D. R. and Greenfield, A. D. M.   *J. Physiol.*, 1956, *131*, 277.

46. — Gaskell, P. and Burton, A. C.   *Circ. Res.*, 1953, *I*, 27.

47. — Bülbring, E.   *J. Physiol.*, 1955, *128*, 200.

48. — Bülbring, E.   Lectures on the Scientific Basis of Medicine, Vol. VII, 1957-58, p. 374. Western Print. Serv. Ltd, Bristol.

49. — Folkow, B.   *Circ.*, 1960, *XXI*, 760.

Reprinted from *Circ. Res.*, **12**, 375–378 (Apr. 1963)

Dimensions of Blood Vessels from Distributing Artery to Collecting Vein

By Mary P. Wiedeman, Ph.D.

■ In a recent study, measurements of lengths, diameters, and numbers of vessels contained in a peripheral vascular bed from distributing artery to arterial capillaries were made in the living animal.[1] From the data, total cross-sectional areas of the various portions of the arterial tree were calculated and compared with values from similar measurements of vessels in fixed tissue. In the living animal, a linear increment in total cross-sectional area was found from artery to arterial capillary, differing markedly from the long accepted concept of small increases in total area from artery to arteriole followed by a tremendous increase in area at the level of the capillaries. It was suggested at that time that the wide variance in results of the two studies was due mainly to inaccurate estimates in fixed tissue of the numbers of the various types of vessels, especially the capillaries. Further consideration reveals that vessel diameters may be a more important factor in accounting for the variance.

In this paper, lengths, diameters, and numbers of the collecting vessels are presented, thus completing measurements of a total vascular bed from a major distributing artery to its accompanying vein in the living animal. Comparisons are made with similar measurements and computations from fixed tissue.[2]

Methods

The site used for measurements of the collecting vessels was the wing of the common brown bat (Myotis). The vessels in this subcutaneous area were observed in the intact, unanesthetized animal. An eyepiece micrometer was used to measure the length and inside diameter of the vessels

From the Department of Physiology, Temple University School of Medicine, Philadelphia, Pennsylvania.

Supported in part by Research Grant H-2880 (C5) from the National Heart Institute, U. S. Public Health Service.

Received for publication October 15, 1962.

at magnifications of 400 × and 1200 × depending on the size of the vessel being measured.

In general, the beginning and end of a venous vessel were determined in the same manner as had been used for measuring the arterial vessels in the same category. For example, the major artery was said to end at its first bifurcation while the major vein was considered to begin at the point where two large veins form a junction. An arterial bifurcation or a venous junction were easily differentiated from the branches or tributaries of these vessels.

Small veins are defined here as vessels which empty into the major vein. Their origin was found to be in general parallel to an arterial arcade, except that in the case of venous vessels the two paths of blood flow diverge rather than converge.

Venules are defined as the vessels which empty into small veins. Venules receive blood from smaller vessels, called here post-capillary venules, which in turn originate from the capillary network. In the report on arterial vessels from this laboratory,[1] a capillary was defined as a distributing vessel which arose as a side branch of an arteriole and it ended at the point where an inflowing tributary joined it, the newly formed vessel now becoming a post-capillary venule.

Results

Table 1 shows that the average length of a major vein was essentially the same as its accompanying artery while the diameter of the vein was greater than that of the artery by one-half. The major vein had twice as many inflowing tributaries as the major artery had branches. The cross-sectional area of each of the vessels was calculated and the average of these values revealed that the cross-sectional area of the major vein was more than twice that of the artery.

The average length of a small vein was the same as the average length of the small artery that ran adjacent to it, but the diameter of the small vein was twice the diameter of the small artery. Small veins had one-half again as many vessels flowing into them as small arteries had distributing branches, and the

TABLE 1
Dimensions of Blood Vessels in the Bat's Wing

Vessel	Average length mm	Average diameter μ	Average number of branches	Number of vessels	Total cross-sec area μ²	Capacity mm³ × 10⁻³	Per cent of capacity
Artery	17.0	52.6	12.3	1	2,263*	38.4	10.1
Small artery	3.5	19.0	9.7	12.3	4,144	14.4	3.8
Arteriole	0.95	7.0	4.6	119.3	5,101	4.7	1.2
Capillary	0.23	3.7	3.1†	548.7	6,548	1.5	0.39
Post-capillary venule	0.21	7.3		1,727.0	78,233	16.4	4.3
Venule	1.0	21.0	5.0	345.4	127,995	127.9	33.7
Small vein	3.4	37.0	14.1	24.5	27,885	94.7	25.0
Vein	16.6	76.2	24.5	1	4,882	81.0	21.4

*Average of individual cross-sectional areas.
†Calculated.

total cross-sectional area (average of areas of individual vessels times number of vessels) of the small veins was almost seven times as large as the total cross-sectional area of the small arteries.

Arterioles and venules had the same length, but the average diameter of the venules was three times greater than the average diameter of the arterioles. There were about the same number of post-capillary venules emptying into the venules as there were capillaries leaving the arterioles. The total cross-sectional area formed by the venules was the largest in the entire vascular bed, exceeding by 25 times the total cross-sectional area formed by the arterioles.

Post-capillary venules were about the same length as the capillaries although they had a diameter twice as large. Post-capillary venules were three times more numerous than arterial capillaries. By calculation, each arterial capillary must give rise to three post-capillary venules on the average. Although there were equal numbers of post-capillary venules emptying into venules and arterial capillaries originating from arterioles, there were almost twice as many venules to receive these small vessels as there were arterioles to supply the capillaries. A diagrammatic representation of the vascular bed in figure 1 shows a possible arrangement to account for the large numbers of venous vessels. The results of the measurements are summarized in table 1.

Figure 2 indicates that the total cross-sectional areas produced by division of arterial vessels and confluence of venous vessels show a linear increment from artery to capillary, a marked rise at the post-capillary venules, and a still further increase at the level of the venules. At the small veins, the area decreases sharply and this is followed by a small decrease to the major vein. A comparison of these values obtained from measurements in the living animal with those computed by Green[2] using Mall's[3] data on fixed material is reasonably similar with the exception of the total cross-sectional area of the capillaries. Green[2] states that his data are very rough since many assumptions are necessary. One assumption frequently made relates to the diameter of a capillary vessel which is estimated to be about eight microns, based on the diameter of the mammalian red blood cell. The two curves presented in figure 2 for total cross-sectional area can be made to agree more closely if one accepts the view that the diameter of a capillary is approximately four microns as measured in the living animal, rather than the estimated value of eight microns (see dashed line in figure 2). In defense of accepting such a diameter for the capillary, a survey of the literature reveals that in instances where the diameter was actually measured rather than estimated, the majority of the values fall well below eight microns as shown in table 2. More specifically, according to a recent compilation[4] in which 36 capillary diameters from different mammals are given, only four are based on actual measurements and these four values are 3, 3.8, 4.6, and 5 microns. The remaining normal values, in gen-

Circulation Research, Volume XII, April 1963

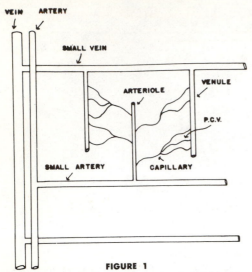

FIGURE 1

Diagrammatic representation of relationships between arterial and venous vessels in a terminal vascular bed.

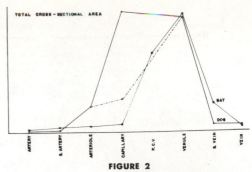

FIGURE 2

Comparison of total cross-sectional areas from the living bat by Wiedeman and from the dog by Green[2] who used measurements from fixed mesenteric vessels.

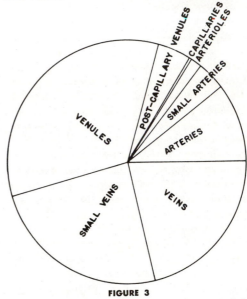

FIGURE 3

Percentage of total volume of blood contained in various portions of the vascular bed.

eral around seven microns, are estimates based on red blood cell diameters.

Calculations of the capacity of each of the various portions of the vascular bed and the per cent of the total volume of blood each portion contains, shows that the venous vessels can contain 80% of the total blood in the peripheral vascular bed (fig. 3).

Discussion

The importance of having measurements of the lengths, diameters, and numbers of vessels formed by the ramifications of a distributing artery and the convergence of the collecting venous system lies in their defining the proper relationships between the various portions of the vascular bed. Actual values for lengths, diameters, and numbers of vessels have no real significance except perhaps at the capillary level where one would expect some uniformity of vessel diameter in all mammals with red blood cells of comparable size. It is meaningless to define an artery or arteriole on the basis of its diameter, or to define a capillary in this manner. The assignment of a name to a specific vessel should be determined by its position and function in the vascular system.

The most outstanding difference between

previously accepted values and those reported here is the determination of that portion of the vascular bed with the greatest total cross-sectional area. If the vascular bed considered in this living animal is acceptable as being representative of peripheral vascular beds, excluding those which serve specific organs, then the greatest total cross-sectional area is formed by the venules rather than by the capillary network.

It is recognized that the number of capillary vessels reported here may be somewhat

Circulation Research, Volume XII, April 1963

TABLE 2

*Measured Capillary Diameters in Various Mammals**

Animal	Site	Condition	Capillary diameter
Dog[3]	Villus, small intestine	Injected and fixed	8.0
			5.0
Guinea Pig[5]	Abdominal wall	Injected India ink	3.5
	Diaphragm		5.0
Rabbit[6]	Skeletal muscle	Injected and	5.2
		fixed	2.5
	Heart		5.0
Mouse[7]	Mesentery	In vivo	3.0 -10.0
Rabbit[8]	Ear	In vivo	5.5
Mouse[9]	Skeletal muscle	In vivo	5.6
Guinea Pig[4]	Abdominal wall	?	3.0
			3.8
			4.6
	Diaphragm	?	5.0
Human[10]	Nail bed and	In vivo	5.0 -12.0
	conjunctiva		5.0 - 3.5
			3.5 - 2.0
Dog[11]	Heart	In vivo	4.0

*Arranged by dates of publication from Mall[3] in 1888 to Reynolds et al.[11] in 1958.

smaller than is actually the case, and perhaps the vessels referred to as post-capillary venules should be included with the arterial capillaries in calculations of area and capacity of the network. The fact remains, however, that these are two different types of vessels. The capillary as seen in this preparation is a non-muscular distributing vessel marking the termination of arterial outflow, while the post-capillary venule, with its larger diameter, is truly a collecting vessel returning blood to the venous system.

Summary

Measurements of lengths, diameters, and numbers of post-capillary vessels were made in the bat's wing. The cross-sectional area and capacity in the various portions of the vascular bed were calculated.

The greatest total cross-sectional area in the entire vascular bed was found in the venules, a result not in agreement with similar reports made by others using measurements from vessels in fixed preparations. This discrepancy probably results from disagreement regarding the diameter of capillary vessels.

Calculations to determine the per cent of total volume in each portion of the vascular bed showed that the venous system accounts for as much as 80% of the total vascular volume.

References

1. WIEDEMAN, M. P.: Lengths and diameters of peripheral arterial vessels in the living animal. Circulation Research 10: 686, 1962.

2. GREEN, H. D.: Circulation; physical principles. *In* Medical Physics, edited by O. Glasser. Chicago, Year Book Publishers, 1944.

3. MALL, F.: Die Blut- und Lymphwege im Dünndarm des Hundes. Ber. Sachs. Ges. (Akad.) Wiss. 14: 151, 1888.

4. Handbook of Biological Data, edited by W. S. Spector. Philadelphia, W. B. Saunders Co., 1956, p. 284.

5. KROGH, A.: The Anatomy and Physiology of Capillaries. New Haven, Yale University Press, 1929, p. 65.

6. STOEL, G.: Ueber die Blutversorgung v. weissen u. roten Kaninchenmuskeln. Zeitsch. f. Zellforsch. u. mikr. Anat. 3: 91, 1925.

7. ZWEIFACH, B. W., AND KOSSMAN, C. E.: Micromanipulation of small blood vessels in the mouse. Am. J. Physiol. 120: 23, 1937.

8. CLARK, E. R., AND CLARK, E. L.: Caliber changes in minute blood vessels observed in the living mammal. Am. J. Anat. 73: 215, 1943.

9. ALGIRE, G. H.: Determination of peripheral blood pressure in unanesthetized mice during microscopic observation of blood vessels. J. Nat. Cancer Inst. 14: 865, 1954.

10. LANDAU, J., AND DAVIS, E.: Capillary thinning and high capillary blood pressure in hypertension. Lancet 1: 1327, 1957.

11. REYNOLDS, S. R. M., KIRSCH, M., AND BING, R. J.: Functional capillary beds in the beating, KCl-arrested and KCl-arrested-perfused myocardium of the dog. Circulation Research 6: 600, 1958.

Circulation Research, Volume XII, April 1963

19

Reprinted from *Microcirculation as Related to Shock*, D. Shepro and G. P. Fulton, eds., Academic Press, Inc., New York, 1968, pp. 161–180

RHEOLOGICAL ASPECTS OF LOW FLOW STATES

P-I. BRÅNEMARK

I. INTRODUCTION

According to definition, shock is characterized as a volumetric discrepancy between available circulating blood and the vascular system of the body. Shock results in impairment of tissue structure and function due to the fact that the peripheral parts of the circulatory system—the microcirculation—cannot provide the tissue cells with their environmental requirements. The resulting homeostatic disturbances call for restoration of circulatory function.

II. PATHOPHYSIOLOGICAL MECHANISMS AND RHEOLOGY

A. FACTORS INFLUENCING FLOW

In attempts to clarify the pathophysiological mechanisms in shock much interest has been devoted to the flow properties of blood. These are influenced by many different physical factors, e.g., radius of vascular

161

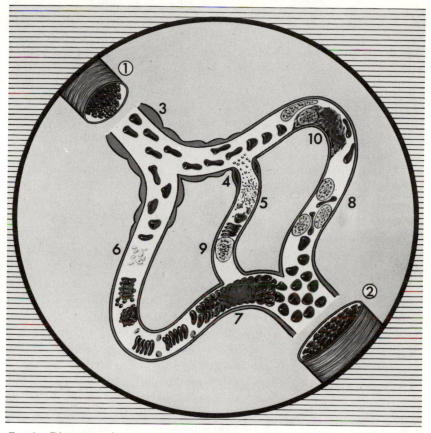

Fig. 1. Diagrammatic representation of factors influencing distribution and flow of blood in a microvascular compartment.

(1) and (2) Volume of blood per unit time reaching and leaving the area via major vessels.

(3) The distribution and flow of blood in the microcirculation is controlled by sphincters located in the arteriolar vessels. These constrictor-dilator mechanisms are controlled via the nervous system, but are also influenced by local tissue metabolites, etc.

(4) In the true capillaries there are no muscle cells, changing the radius of the vascular tube. However, the endothelium, or endothelium-periendothelium by changes in cellular form, can participate in directing the flow of blood to different parts of the microvascular system, according to nutritional demands. The architectural arrangement of the microvessels is also a determining factor in microcirculatory distribution of blood.

(5) Normal plasma constituents may in low flow states and stasis interfere with the structure of blood cells. Thus, the presence of chylomicra may induce changes in granulocytes, leading to cellular disruption and liberation of injury-provoking factors.

(6) In low flow states, and especially in stasis, platelets may form loose aggregates,

tube, form of endothelial surface, character of marginal plasma zone, form and shape of blood cells, and flow velocity. Viscosity as measured *in vitro* varies with hematocrit flow velocity, size of vessel, and temperature. [Bayliss (1962); Copley (1963); Frasher (1965); Somer (1966); Wayland (1965a, b).]

B. LIMITATIONS OF THE INDIRECT METHOD

Due to the character of the problem indirect methods were used in previous studies of investigation, which limited the possibilities for interpretation of rheological events within the body. Although important contributions have been made concerning the physical properties of blood, especially with respect to viscosity, the problem still persists: Do these figures obtained *in vitro* give an accurate picture of what goes on in the circulation? Furthermore, it should be emphasized that the viscosity data so far obtained concern major vessels but not the microvascular system, where the pathological mechanism is located in shock and where treatment should be instituted.

In order to delineate qualitatively the problem of microcirculatory disturbances in shock, detailed information about microvascular architecture and flow as well as interrelation between blood cells, plasma, and endothelium is required. In addition, flow controlling and distributing factors of constrictor or dilator type must be considered (Fig. 1). The literature in this field contains a large number of reports concerning microcirculatory studies of shock in animals and man, but so far very little has been done with respect to what happens in a microvascular

---

which are readily broken up and which do not seem to cause circulatory impairment. If, however, the tissue is locally injured by direct trauma or hypoxemia platelets may also form dense aggregates, in which the platelets stick together. This results in formation of a microthrombus, which often moves freely in the plasma and therefore leaves the area as a microembolus, when flow again starts.

(7) When flow velocities are reduced, erythrocytes appear in rouleaux formations. These are broken up again into their cellular components, when flow is reestablished. In prolonged stasis, the cellular outlines may lose their definition, and the red cells then form a mass of tightly packed cells. Even then, however, single, normally plastic erythrocytes leave the vessel, when flow is released. Only a minor pressure and flow velocity increase is required to achieve this transformation from cell mass to separate, freely circulating erythrocytes.

(8) Intravascular granulocytosis, which accompanies tissue injury, interferes with flow of blood. The degree of circulatory hindrance depends on how firmly the granulocytes adhere to the endothelium.

(9) Sometimes the granulocytes appear as rigid cells, which may block flow temporarily or permanently.

(10) Wall-adhering thrombi, consisting of fibrin, platelets, erythrocytes, and granulocytes occur in low flow states in tissue injury.

area in man at low flow states, as judged by direct microscopic analysis at high resolution.

C. Experimental Procedures

We have approached the problem of rheology of blood in low flow states in man by studying a microvascular region in the light microscope by a chamber technique, which enables structural analysis at a resolution level of 1 micron, includes dynamic evaluation, and permits control of blood flowing through the area so that different degrees of impairment of circulation can be produced. It is important to emphasize that this

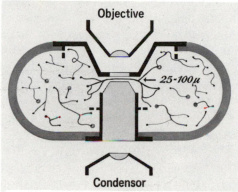

FIG. 2. Principle of chamber technique used for vital microscopic analysis of low flow states in man. The diagram shows a transverse section of the skin tube with installed chamber.

investigation is not a study of shock in man, but instead an attempt to perform rheological analyses in the microcirculation of man under controlled conditions. This type of approach thus provides another source for data without removing the blood from the body.

The observations were performed in healthy volunteers 20–25 years of age. On the inside of the left upper arm a twin pedicled skin tube was prepared, in which after a healing period a titanium chamber (Fig. 2) was installed. The space in different chambers varies between 25 and 100 microns. The chamber space is filled with ingrowing tissue and is vascularized. These vessels and their constituents were studied in a modified light microscope. The vital microphotograms illustrated in this paper were recorded with an objective 55 × N.A.O.85 on Gevaert Scientia film 39 C56 and 45 C62 at an exposure time of 1/10,000 second (Brånemark, 1966; Brånemark and Jonsson, 1963a, b).

In order to obtain variations in flow of blood in the tissue studied, the pedicles of the skin tube were compressed to varying degrees resulting in reduced flow or complete blockage of flow. The microvascular system in the chamber was studied with respect to analysis of low flow states 2–3 months after installment of the chamber. At this time there was normal vasomotion in the area and the tissue had a mature appearance.

III. RHEOLOGICAL ANALYSIS OF MICROCIRCULATION IN MAN

A. PLASMA SKIMMING PHENOMENA

Reduction in the amount of blood per time unit passing the chamber tissue resulted in plasma skimming phenomena in several capillaries and venules. These vessels without corpuscular flow were, in fact, difficult to discern optically (Fig. 3) unless platelets occasionally passed together with the plasma in them or chylomicra disclosed their presence after a fatty meal. The platelets and chylomicra thus acted as plasma "visualizers" and in most cases these particles were seen moving, indicating plasma circulation. Thus, even if no corpuscles are seen circulating— which is the only way of identifying simultaneous plasma circulation at low or medium microscopic resolution—flow might nevertheless occur in the plasma compartment.

This implies that, although only minor parts of a microvascular system are perfused by blood cells in low flow states and in shock, plasma movements may still be capable of furnishing the nutritive requirements of the tissue, especially if the tissue is in a state of hypothermia.

B. CORPUSCULAR DISTRIBUTION

The distribution of corpuscles in a microvascular compartment is influenced by many factors: the architecture of the capillary bed, (including the angle at which a capillary vessel leaves the stem branch), corpuscular flow velocities, and sphincter activities (Fig. 4a,b). Even minor changes in intravascular pressure conditions appear to exert an influence on the flow and distribution of blood. Thus, blockage of one venule, for instance, often changes the circulatory patterns in a large area, sometimes 100–150 microns from the structural origin of blockage.

C. PULSATIONS OF CORPUSCULAR FLOW

The connective tissue vessels studied in this chamber normally exhibit pulsations in corpuscular flow, often at a rate of eight to ten per minute. These rhythmic flow alterations do not seem to be directly related to the pulse rate, but could be influenced by changes in sympathetic tone during the respiratory cycle. They could also be influenced by local metabolites and other factors affecting arteriolar sphincters. Even in low flow states pulsating movements are seen (Fig. 5a–d).

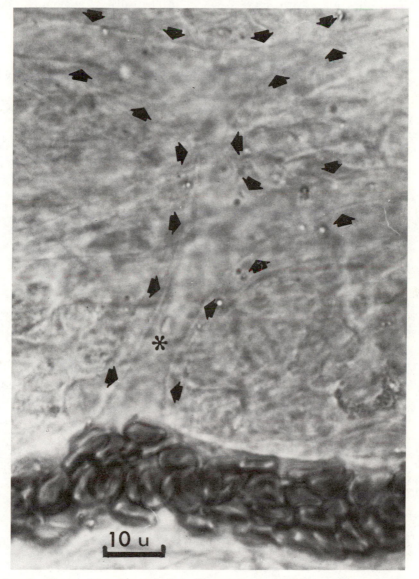

FIG. 3. Plasma skimming with flow illustrated by a platelet at the asterisk. The capillary-venular vessels are indicated by arrows. Red cells are only passing in the venule at bottom of picture.

D. CELL ADHESION AND AGGREGATION DURING HYPOVOLEMIA

Under normal flow conditions erythrocytes, granulocytes, and platelets do not show any tendency to adhere to each other or to the endothelium. Plasma constituents of particulate type, such as chylomicra, do not form aggregates or adhere to the endothelium (Fig. 6). Under normal conditions the red cells are very plastic, granulocytes are moderately plastic and deformable, and platelets behave like rigid discs.

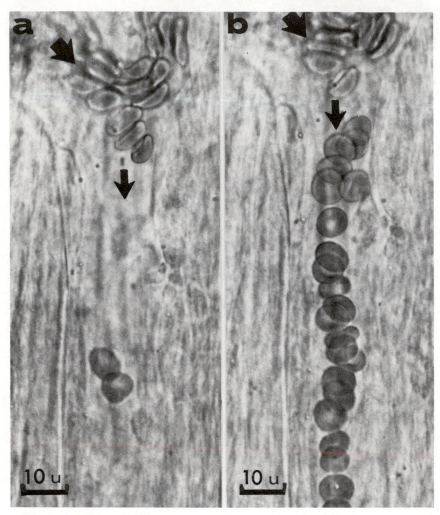

FIG. 4. Example of plasma skimming in venule, with two red cells, indicating flow in (a) and a row of erythrocytes in the same vessel in (b). Arrows indicate direction of flow.

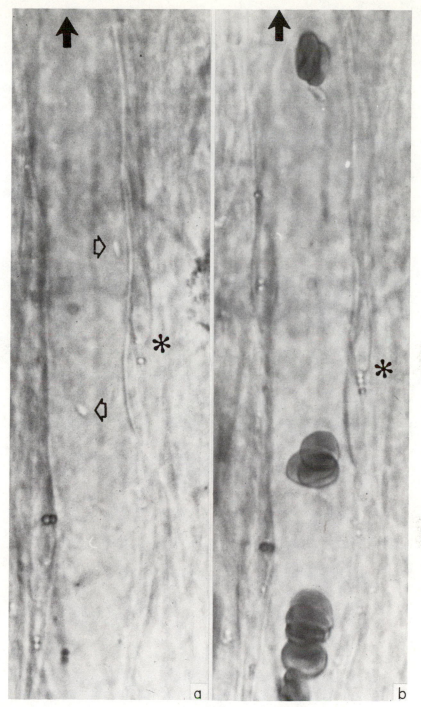

Fig. 5a–d. Variation of corpuscular flow in a venule in a series of vital micro-photograms recorded with a few seconds' interval. Arrows indicate direction of flow.

168

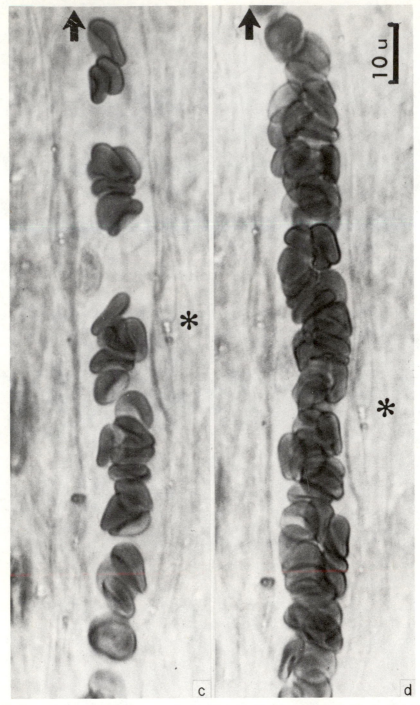

Observe platelets at open arrows in (a). Asterisk denotes endothelial-periendothelial structural complex.

169

When flow velocities in the microcirculation are reduced to 0.2–0.1 mm per second (normal 0.5–0.8 mm/second) erythrocytes form characteristic rouleauxs (Fig. 7a–c). These may be composed of a long, continuous row or chain of red cells consisting of 20–30 cells. Often, however, the erythrocytes appear in short rouleauxs, composed of four or five cells,

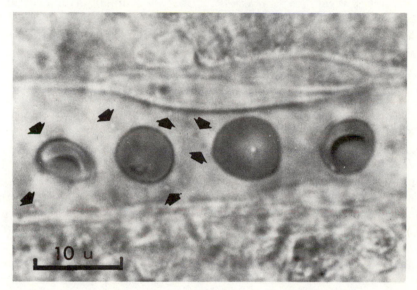

FIG. 6. Capillary at endothelial nucleus and periendothelial cell. Flow velocity in this case was only 0.2, but the red cells move as separate bodies. Observe the chylomicra, indicated by arrows. Two chylomicra are overlying the two red cells at the right-hand side of the figure and appear with increased contrast and definition at this site. The fat particles do not adhere to form aggregates to each other, the red cells, or the endothelium in this noninjured vessel.

which move with slight ryhthmic pulsations (Fig. 8) in the center of the vessel.

In blocked venular segments, rouleauxs consisting of five to ten erythrocytes are often seen moving slowly in the center of the vessel. Granulocytes as separate cells move in the space between the red cells, as do separate erythrocytes also. Even in complete standstill of the blood some erythrocytes appear as separate cells in close proximity to rouleauxs and these cells do not join the rouleauxs, although they often are very close to or moving and sliding along these red cell formations. Platelets are also found in the same plasma zone, but more often they move slowly alongside the endothelium without, however, sticking to the vessel wall. These patterns are found even when the circulation is completely blocked but the corpuscles are moving in the plasma "pockets."

The rouleauxs do not exhibit any tendency to adhere to the endothelium or the endothelial plasma layer, even in long-standing stasis for 2 hours. When flow is released the rouleaux formations immediately break up again. The erythrocytes do not seem to adhere to each other to any appreciable degree and they exhibit normal deformability; this is the case even when flow has been occluded for 1 or 2 hours.

In cases where the ratio erythrocytes/plasma is high (which means high hematocrit), especially occurring in venules in low flow states or stasis, the red cells are often compressed by transmitted pulsations to a brownish-red mass of cells, with hardly discernible cellular outlines. In overall views of such a microvascular region it may look as though these venules and capillaries were blocked by a plug of red cells (Figs. 9, 10). When the circulation starts again, however, this mass of cells is readily—even at slow flow rates—broken up again into its cellular constituents. Single red cells of normal shape, behavior, and deformability leave the area and again join the circulation. It thus appears as if only a slight force were required to transfer the cells to normal circulating conditions.

Direct microscopic observation at high resolution of this condition in man reveals that there is no identifiable adhesion between the resting cells and the endothelium. The red cells leave the resting cell mass without any appreciable sticking tendency to each other.

The studies so far performed in man have disclosed that flow can be reestablished and structurally and functionally normal erythrocytes "regained" after complete, controlled stasis for up to 3 hours.

The endothelium did not show any significant swelling under these circumstances, and its integrity was further elucidated by the fact that when flow was reestablished, blood cells were not sticking to the endothelium.

E. STRUCTURAL STABILITY OF HEMOCYTES AND ENDOTHELIUM DURING LOW FLOW STATES OR STASIS

It is a significant finding that in the human microcirculation erythrocytes, granulocytes, and platelets, as well as the vascular endothelium, do not change their structure or function at the light microscopic level of recognition when the circulation is slowed down or blocked for as long as 3 hours. This statement is valid for connective tissue microvessels under the prevailing experimental conditions. Observations on animal tissues such as skeletal muscle and peripheral nerve have shown similar patterns; in fact, it has been possible to regain as much as 70% of microvascular function after complete and controlled local circulatory standstill for 12 hours in a peripheral nerve.

In this connection it should be mentioned that the more-or-less highly differentiated tissue cells and their resistance to circulatory impairment is a factor that is probably more important for the long-term prognosis of the tissue than is microvascular resistance.

F. PLATELET AND GRANULOCYTE INTEGRITY IN LOW FLOW STATES OR STASIS

In low flow states, or in complete stasis, granulocytes and platelets remain as separate cells and do not tend to adhere to each other or to

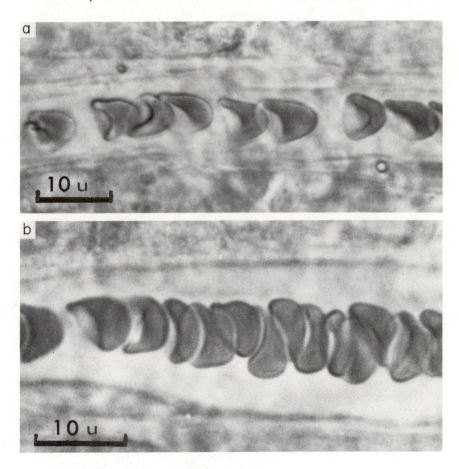

form clusters of cells, as do the erythrocyte rouleauxs. This is a particularly important phenomenon to emphasize. Thus, the assumption (presented in theoretical calculations of cellular behavior in low flow states) that cells join and adhere to each other in resting conditions is not correct for granulocytes and platelets and only partly correct for erythrocytes.

That platelets even in 2–3 hours' blockage of the circulation still preserve their cellular integrity is a fundamental phenomenon in interpretation of intravascular clotting mechanisms. Only if tissue injury is added does intravascular thrombosis occur. This may be in the form of loose platelet aggregates, firm platelet aggregates, forming microemboli, or—if the endothelium is damaged—in form of mixed microthrombi consisting of fibrin, platelets, erythrocytes, and granulocytes (Figs. 11–13). The wall-adhering thrombi may form a partial or complete obstruction

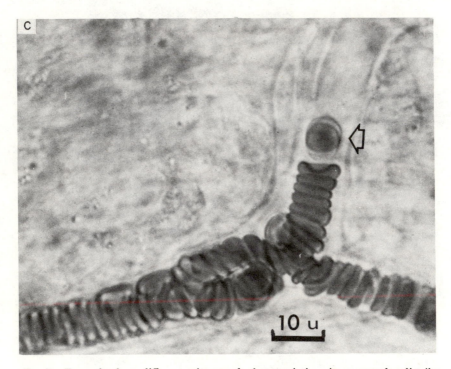

FIG. 7. Examples from different microvessels show variations in corpuscular distribution and shape at varying flow velocities. In (a) the red cells are moving separately at a velocity of 0.8 mm per second. In (b) the erythrocytes are lying close together at a velocity of 0.3 mm per second, but have not formed rouleauxs. In (c), at almost stagnant flow at a rate of 0.05 mm per second, a typical rouleaux formation has occurred. Observe the two free erythrocytes at arrow.

to flow, but often a part of the thrombus, or the whole clot, leaves the site of formation and is then transformed into an embolus.

G. TISSUE DAMAGE AND RHEOLOGICAL EFFECTS

When, in addition to reduced flow rates, the tissue is damaged, blood cells may adhere to the vessel wall, singly or in clusters. A prominent feature is the occurrence of wall-adhering granulocytes. These may form a hindrance to the circulation, but even when many white cells are

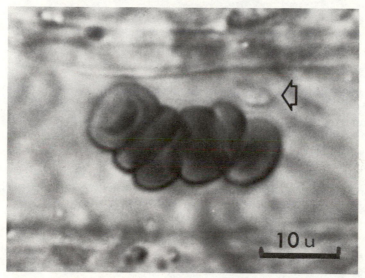

FIG. 8. Venule with stasis for 30 minutes. The red cells have formed a rouleaux, but there is also a platelet (see arrow) moving freely in the plasma without adhering to the red cells or the endothelium.

sticking to the endothelium (forming a pavement on the vessel wall) erythrocytes, granulocytes, and platelets are still capable of passing between the adhering white cells due to their plasticity or to the labyrinthian lumen still present. Considerations of circulatory conditions in a damaged tissue have direct bearing on the problem of shock in those cases where large tissue areas are injured, as in severe burns. Not only the vitality of the damaged tissue but also the survival of the patient are dependent on the reversibility of microcirculatory impairment.

Sometimes rigid granulocytes occur that may completely block a capillary or venule. This, in turn, may change flow patterns in retrograde direction far away from the site of sticking (Fig. 14a,b). The blockage may be permanent, leading to infarction and tissue necrosis.

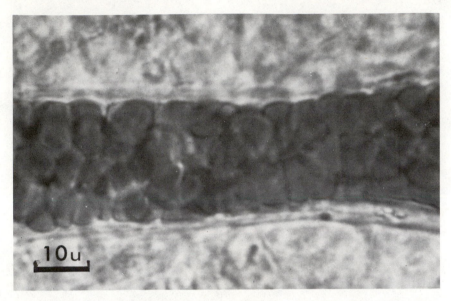

FIG. 9. Venule densely packed with red cells but still with discernible cellular margins.

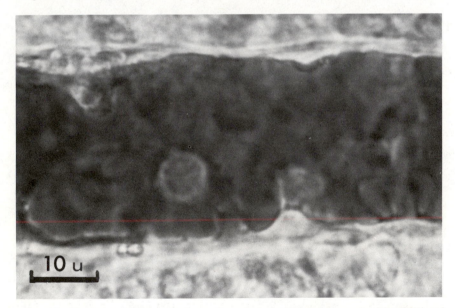

FIG. 10. Appearance of venule in prolonged stasis (1½ hours) and with additional tissue injury (ultraviolet radiation). The erythrocytes seem to have merged into a mass of cells; separate cellular details cannot be identified. There are also signs of endothelial damage.

When chylomicra are present in a blocked microvascular segment it has been observed in some cases that granulocytes have changed over a period of 30–60 minutes. Signs of disruption of the granulocytes have occurred, possibly resulting in release of enzymes promoting the development of a vicious circle of microcirculatory pathology, including blood cells, plasma, endothelium, and periendothelium.

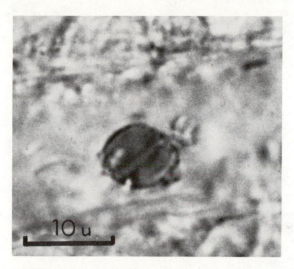

Fig. 11. Structurally abnormal platelets adhering to erythrocytes in a stagnant venule: an early step in intravascular clotting after tissue injury.

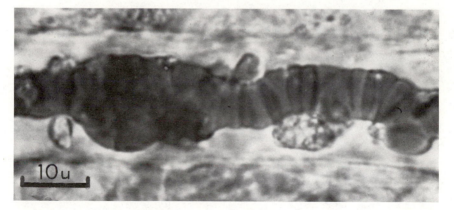

Fig. 12. Firm platelet emboli moving freely in plasma pockets in slow flow venule; red cells in rouleaux formation.

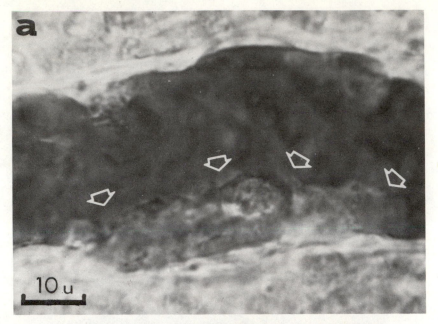

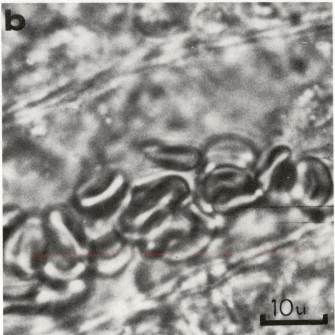

FIG. 13. (a) Wall-adhering mixed thrombus (indicated by arrows) in a stagnant
venule after tissue injury. (b) The same region of the microvascular system when flow
is again released after 3 hours complete microcirculatory standstill (an enlargement
of a 16 mm cinerecording of the dynamic events involved in restitution of flow).

177

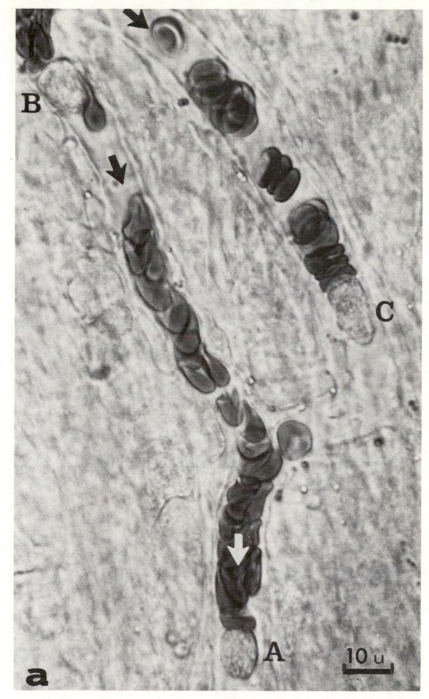

Fig. 14. (a) Capillary system showing granulocytes that are: deformable, circulating (A); deformable, wall-adhering, partly blocking (B); and rigid, completely blocking (C).

178

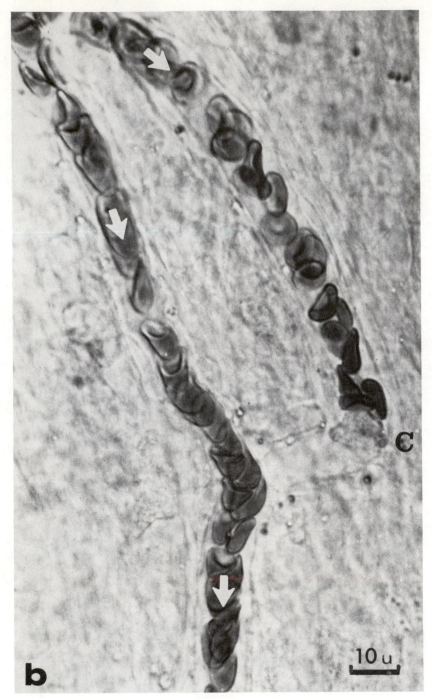

In (b) the rigid cell (C) has been pushed slightly forward and the two other cells (A) and (B) have left the area.

179

IV. CONCLUSIONS

Thus, vital microscopic analysis at high resolution of low flow states in the microcirculation of man discloses that even in the presence of long-standing reduced or blocked flow, erythrocytes, granulocytes, and platelets behave like single cells and maintain their shape and functional characteristics. If erythrocytes appear in rouleaux formations, these immediately break up again as soon as flow is reestablished. Even if the red cells have merged into a mass of cells, with loss of optical definition of cellular outlines, cellular integrity is still preserved; only a slight increase in flow is required to break up the cell accumulation into separate cells. Stasis alone is not sufficient to induce intravascular clotting or adhesion of erythrocytes or granulocytes to the endothelium; additional injury is required to initiate these mechanisms.

Furthermore, these studies in low flow states in man have revealed that some of the assumptions, hitherto accepted, concerning the shape and behavior of blood cells and plasma (defined as rheology of blood and based on *in vitro* tests, theoretical deductions, and investigations at low microscopic resolution levels) are not in agreement with the actual pathophysiological mechanisms in the living human tissue. The most important finding in this study is, however, that the microvascular system of man can sustain several hours of reduced or blocked flow, yet return to almost normal nutritive circulatory functional levels.

ACKNOWLEDGMENTS

The author's investigations reported in this paper were supported by grants from National Institutes of Health, HE-5724 USPHS, the Swedish Medical Research Council, and the Swedish Cancer Society.

The vital microscopic observations in man were performed in cooperation with U. Breine. Research assistance by Miss M. Dunér, Miss Y. Winsnes, and Mr. V. Kuikka is gratefully acknowledged.

REFERENCES

Bayliss, L. E. (1962). *In* "Handbook of Physiology," Circulation, Vol. 1., p. 137. Williams & Wilkins, Baltimore, Maryland.
Brånemark, P-I. (1966). *Med. Biol. Illus.* **XVI:2**, 100-108.
Brånemark, P-I., and Jonsson, I. (1963a). *Biorheology* 1, 143-146.
Brånemark, P-I., and Jonsson, I. (1963b). *J. Roy. Microscop. Soc.* 82, 245-249.
Copley, A. L. (1963). *Proc. 4th Intern. Congr. Rheology* (Part 4). Wiley, New York.
Frasher, W. G. (1965). *Bibliotheca Anat.* 5, 23-32.
Somer, T. (1966). *Acta Med. Scand. Suppl.* 456.
Wayland, H. (1965a). *Bibliotheca Anat.* 5, 2-22.
Wayland, H. (1965b). *Bibliotheca Anat.* 5, 33-46.

Reprinted from *J. Gen. Physiol.*, **52**, 29s–61s (1968)

Dynamics of Transcapillary Fluid Exchange

CURT A. WIEDERHIELM

From the Microcirculation Laboratory, Department of Physiology and Biophysics, University of Washington School of Medicine, Seattle, Washington, 98105

ABSTRACT   Fluid balance at the capillary level has been simulated with an analogue computer program, based on experimental data on regional differences in capillary permeability, surface areas, and hydrostatic pressures. The program takes into account fluid and protein fluxes into and out of the interstitial space. Solutions are obtained for tissue hydrostatic pressure, tissue fluid osmotic pressure, interstitial space volume, and lymph flow. Simulation of a variety of physiological experiments and clinical disease states has yielded reasonable agreement between experimental data and data obtained by computer analysis. Dilution of the interstitial plasma protein pool with a consequent reduction of its oncotic pressure appears to be a major factor, which prevents edema unless plasma oncotic pressures are reduced by 10–15 mm Hg or, alternatively, venous pressures are elevated by a similar amount. The computer analysis in all instances yields positive values for tissue pressure, in agreement with experimental data obtained by needle puncture. The negative tissue pressures observed in subcutaneous capsules can be reproduced in the computer program, if the interface between the capsule and the surrounding interstitial space is assumed to have the properties of a semipermeable membrane.

Partition of body fluids between the circulation, on the one hand, and the interstitial and intracellular spaces, on the other, is normally maintained within narrow limits. The mechanism maintaining this precise partition is still not well understood, but a balance of capillary hydrostatic and colloid osmotic pressures is generally acknowledged to play an important role, as originally pointed out by Starling (1). Current views on capillary water balance are summarized in Fig. 1, which is based on experimental data of Starling (1) and Landis (2). The graphs illustrate the relationship between hydrostatic pressures along the length of a capillary and the colloid osmotic pressure of plasma proteins.

The oncotic pressure of plasma (π_{PL}) averages 25 mm Hg (3), corresponding to a plasma protein concentration of 7%. The hdyrostatic capillary pressures are averages based on extensive series of pressure recordings in skin capillaries of man by Landis (2). In arterial capillaries (Fig. 1 *A*, left), the pressures averaged 32 mm Hg (P_A). The hydrostatic pressures in the venous capillaries (Fig. 1 *A*, right) averaged 15 mm Hg (P_v). The transcapillary flux of fluid is governed by the difference in the hydrostatic and colloid osmotic pressure of the plasma; thus fluid is filtered from the capillary into the tissues in the arterial end of the capillary, and it is reabsorbed from the tissues into the capillary at the venous end. The hydrostatic pressures in the arterial and venous ends of the capillary bracket the colloid osmotic pressure, and the amount of fluid filtered at the arterial end is similar to the volume reabsorbed at the venous end.

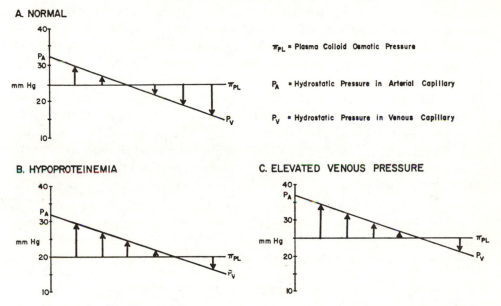

FIGURE 1.   Diagram of hydrostatic and colloid osmotic pressures along a capillary. *A*, normal values; *B*, hypoproteinemia; *C*, elevated venous and arterial capillary pressure.

This equilibrium of filtration and reabsorption has been considered an essential feature of the mechanism which prevents excessive shifts of fluid between the blood and the interstitial space. Such an equilibrium would be unstable, however. If the colloid omsotic pressure of the plasma is reduced in hypoproteinemia, the equilibrium would be disturbed, as shown in Fig. 1 *B*. If the plasma osmotic pressure is reduced to 20 mm Hg, filtration occurs along almost the entire length of the capillary, and excessive fluid accumulation should occur in the interstitial space. This finding is contrary to clinical experience, however; edema does not occur until the plasma protein concentration has fallen to almost half its normal value (4–6). A similar disturbance of equilibrium would result if venous and arterial capillary pressures were elevated, as in heart failure or venous obstruction (Fig. 1 *C*). Increasing hydrostatic pressures in the arterial and venous ends of the capillary by 5 mm Hg produces filtration along virtually the whole length of the capillary. Experimental data indicate, however, that edema does not develop until venous pressures are elevated by at least 10–15 mm Hg (7–9). Thus protective mechanisms appear to exist which limit the shift of fluids over a range of ± 10 mm Hg around the normal hydrostatic and colloid osmotic pressures found in capillaries. The traditional capillary model fails to explain this feature of fluid balance at the capillary level.

Since the formulation of this model, much quantitative information relating to capillary function and structure has accumulated. This information indicates that the mechanism maintaining the partition of fluid between the circulation and the interstitial space is considerably more complex than indicated by the traditional capillary model. An equilibrium of fluid exchange in the traditional model implies three unstated assumptions: (*a*) the permeability to water and solutes is uniform throughout the capillary; (*b*) the surface areas of the arterial and venous ends of the capillary networks are identical; and (*c*) the hydrostatic and colloid osmotic pressures of tissue fluid are negligible compared to the corresponding blood values. The objectives of this report are, first, to examine the validity of these assumptions, and, second, to expand the traditional model of the capillary to include experimental data on regional differences in permeability, capillary surface area, permeability to protein, and lymph flow. Finally, these factors will be incorporated into equations describing fluid exchange at the capillary level; these equations will be subjected to computer analysis. Data obtained from the computer analysis will be compared with experimental data.

REGIONAL DIFFERENCES IN CAPILLARY PERMEABILITY

Substantial experimental evidence indicates that different regions of the capillary network in many different peripheral vascular beds are not uniformly permeable to solutes of intermediate molecular weight. The classical studies of Rous et al. (10) indicated that water-soluble dyes generally escaped more rapidly from venous capillaries and venules than from arterial capillaries in the mammalian skin. Similar studies by Mori et al. (11) demonstrated similar differences in permeability in the capillary networks of frog and rabbit mesenteries, and also in rabbit ear chambers.[1] Landis also showed that plasma albumin tagged with Evans blue dye escaped eventually through spotty leaks in venous capillaries and venules (12). Regional differences in permeability to a large dye molecule do not necessarily imply similar differences in permeability to water.

For this reason, a series of experimental studies were undertaken which were

---

[1] K. Mori. Personal communication.

designed to yield a quantitative measurement of the permeability to water in arterial and venous capillaries in the frog mesentery. The filtration rates in capillary segments in the frog mesentery were measured with an indirect densitometric technique, which has been described elsewhere (13). The experimental data indicated that permeability to water was approximately similar in arterial capillaries, midcapillaries, and venules. Venous capillaries, however, were approximately twice as permeable to water as the arterial capillaries. A similar set of data was also gathered in an independent study by Intaglietta (14), in which capillary filtration rates were measured by the Landis micro-occlusion technique. His data indicated that the permeability of venous capillaries in the frog mesentery averages 60% higher than that of the arterial capillaries. The assumption of uniform permeability of the capillary network thus is not justified in all cases. The elevated permeability to water at the venous end of the capillary tends to favor reabsorption, and thus leads to a relative dehydration of the tissues.

REGIONAL DIFFERENCES IN CAPILLARY SURFACE AREA

The second assumption in the traditional capillary model, that the surface areas available for filtration and reabsorption are similar, may also be challenged. That the subpapillary capillary loops in human skin are asymmetrical is well known. Characteristically, the arterial limb of the capillary is considerably smaller than the venous limb. Davis and Lawler measured the diameter of many skin capillaries, finding on the average that the venous limb is 50% larger than the arterial limb (15). The apex of the loop has generally the same dimension as the descending venous limb. Landis' measurements in the capillaries also indicated that the hydrostatic pressure at the apex of the capillary loop was lower than the plasma colloid osmotic pressure, and thus is presumably the site of reabsorption (2). The apex of the capillary loop should thus be included as a part of the venous limb for functional as well as morphological reasons. However, the surface area of the two capillary segments is difficult to estimate, as their lengths were not measured separately. The subpapillary venular plexus in man possesses a considerably larger surface than the capillaries. Wetzel and Zotterman (16) measured the surface area of the subpapillary venular plexus and of the skin capillaries. The objective of their studies was to evaluate the relative contribution of venules and capillaries to skin color, and their surface area values refer to a projection of these vessels on the skin surface. The capillary loops run perpendicular to the skin, in contrast with the venular plexus, which lies parallel to the skin. The total capillary surface area, however, can be calculated by assigning 200 μ (15) as an average value for the length of the capillary loops. The surface area values recalculated in this manner have been listed in a previous publication (13). The ratio of the surface areas of the venular plexus and of capillaries ranged from a low of 0.82 in the skin of the knuckle to a high of 5.7 in the skin of the cheek. The average ratio for skin in six different regions was 2.0. The surface area of the venules is thus about twice that of the capillaries. The estimate of capillary surface area, however, includes both arterial and venous capillary segments. The area available for reabsorption in venous capillaries and venules, then, is at least 6 times as large as that available for filtration at the arterial end of the capillary. In a recent study, Wiedeman (17) measured dimensions and counted the vessels in the different categories of the microvascular bed in the bat wing. Recalculation of her data indicated that the surface area of venous capillaries was about 6 times larger than that of the arterial capillary (13). The relatively larger surface area of the venous capillaries tends to favor the reabsorption process, and thus lead to a relative dehydration of the tissues.

PLASMA PROTEIN CONCENTRATION IN INTERSTITIAL FLUID AND TISSUE PRESSURE

With few exceptions, the capillaries in peripheral vascular beds are somewhat permeable to plasma protein. It is generally conceded that the plasma protein passes through the capillaries through a system of large pores with sizes ranging from 250 to 350 A. Microscopic evidence indicates that these leaks or large pores are most frequent in the walls of venous capillaries and venules (12). Landis perfused capillaries in the frog mesentery with albumin solution tagged with Evans blue dye. About 10–12 sec after this perfusion was begun, the dye escaped in spotty leaks predominantly around venules and venous capillaries.

The relative order of magnitude of the plasma leakage through the large-pore system may be estimated from data in studies by Grotte (18). Grotte injected solutions of dextran of varying molecular radius into the circulation of dogs and subsequently measured plasma and lymph concentration of dextran. He found, as would be expected, that the concentration of dextran in the lymph decreased with increasing molecular radius. Even the largest dextran molecules, however, were found in lymph, in a concentration about 10% of the plasma concentration. Grotte estimated that for 34,000 small pores of 35 A radius only one of the large leaks with an estimated radius of 250 A was present. This value may represent an overestimate, however, since his derivation was based on the net filtration in the capillary bed, and the concentrating effect of reabsorption was not included.

In some of Grotte's experiments, however, the lymph concentration of dextran was found to be 5% of the plasma concentration under conditions of venous congestion (venous pressure = 50 mm Hg). Under these circumstances, filtration occurs along the whole length of the capillary. Recalculation of his data, with this value for dextran concentration and with the revised figure for the radius of the small-pore system (42 A) obtained by Landis and

Pappenheimer (3), yields a value of one large leak for every 24,000 small pores. It may be deduced from Grotte's data that, for every milliliter of plasma filtered through the large-pore system, 19 ml of fluid is filtered through the small-pore system during venous congestion.

Our best estimates of interstitial fluid protein concentration are based on tracer techniques, in which tagged plasma proteins were injected into the circulation. When the tagged proteins had equilibrated with the extravascular protein pool, partition of the proteins between the circulation and the extravascular compartment could be estimated. Several studies on the distribution of various plasma protein fractions have been reported from different laboratories (19–22). These studies indicate that 24–50% of the total plasma protein pool is found in the interstitial space. Three of the four studies indicate that 50% of the plasma proteins were located extravascularly. Since the interstitial space occupies approximately 3.3 times the plasma volume in mammals, the corresponding protein concentration in tissue fluid would amount to 2.1%. This is in the same general range as the protein concentration in lymph from extremities, which has been reported by several authors to range from 1.1 to 2.4% (23–25). A protein concentration of 2.1% is equivalent to an osmotic pressure of approximately 5 mm Hg, which would be sufficient to disturb seriously the equilibrium of filtration and reabsorption.

The magnitude of hydrostatic pressures in tissue fluid, i.e. the tissue pressure, has been subject to controversy. McMaster and other investigators inserted small hypodermic needles (25–30 gauge) into the tissue (26). A small volume of fluid was then injected into the tissues, and the equilibrium pressure was measured. This technique has yielded values of 1–5 mm Hg for tissue pressure. The method has been criticized, however, on the grounds that fluid injected into the tissue distorts tissue elements, and pressure recorded in this manner may simply represent elastic rebound phenomena. Furthermore, insertion of the needle might be associated with injury to capillaries and lymphatics along the needle track, possibly leading to increased local transudation of fluid and artificially elevated pressures. Recently, tissue pressures have been measured in the Microcirculation Laboratory with a pressure-recording technique which utilizes ultramicroscopic glass micropipettes as pressure transducers. Details of the technique have been described elsewhere (27). Pressures recorded in the subcutaneous tissues of the bat wing range from 0 to 4 mm Hg in virtually all locations of the wing web.[2] The tips of the micropipettes are less than 1 μ in diameter, and minimal interference with normal tissue structure is thus ensured.

An alternative method for recording tissue pressure was suggested by Guyton (28), who implanted perforated spherical capsules subcutaneously in

[2] C. A. Wiederhielm. Unpublished observations.

a large group of animals and 4 wk later recorded the hydrostatic pressures in the free fluid space within the capsule. Hydrostatic pressures in the capsules were always negative, averaging −6.3 mm Hg. Guyton felt that the intra-capsular pressure was representative of tissue pressure, since, when Evans blue dye was injected into the capsule under positive pressure, the dye could be traced into the tissues surrounding the capsule. The formation of edema, either by infusion of large volumes of physiological saline or by venous compression, was associated with an elevation of the pressure within the capsule into the positive range. A good correlation was then obtained with tissue pressures recorded by insertion of needles into the connective tissue. The presence of negative pressures in the tissue space creates additional problems, however. A direct consequence would be increased capillary filtration, which would add to the effect of the high colloid osmotic pressure of tissue fluid. Furthermore, the transport of tissue fluid into lymphatics against a hydro-static pressure gradient is difficult to visualize, particularly since electron micrographs of lymphatic capillaries indicate large spaces between endothelial cells, similar to those seen in liver sinusoids (29). The following general conclusions may be drawn from the studies quoted in the first section of the paper. (*a*) Capillary permeability to water is not uniform along the length of the capillary, but may be 50–100% larger in the venous capillary than in the arterial capillary. (*b*) The surface area of the arterial capillaries is not identical with that of the venous capillaries in all tissues, but may be only one-sixth to one-fourth of the surface area of the venous capillary. (*c*) The average protein concentration in interstitial fluid is not negligible, but may be as high as 2–3%, with corresponding colloid osmotic pressures of 5–8 mm Hg. (*d*) Measurements of hydrostatic tissue pressure have yielded contradictory results. Measurements obtained by direct puncture, either with hypodermic needles or with ultramicroscopic glass micropipettes, yield tissue pressures ranging from 0 to +5 mm Hg, whereas pressures recorded in subcutaneous capsules are negative and average −6 mm Hg.

In the following section of this report, these deviations from the traditional model have been incorporated into a revised model.

COMPUTER ANALYSIS OF CAPILLARY WATER BALANCE

The basic considerations on which the computer analysis is based are illustrated in Fig. 2 *A* and *B*. In the simulation program, fluid and protein fluxes into and out of the interstitial space and the compliance of the interstitial space were considered. The volume of the interstitial space is dependent on four separate fluid fluxes into and out of the space (Fig. 2 *A*). Filtration occurs from the capillary at the arterial end of the network; also plasma leaks into the interstitium through the large-pore system in the venous capillaries. At equilibrium these two inward fluxes are balanced by reabsorption of fluid into the venous capillaries and smallest venules, and also by removal of tissue fluid through lymphatics. The equations describing the magnitude of these fluid fluxes are as follows.

$$\text{Filtration: } F = K_A A_A (P_A - P_T - \pi_{PL} + \pi_T) \tag{1}$$

where K_A represents the permeability of the arterial capillary to water, A_A the surface area of the capillary, P_A the hydrostatic pressure in the capillary,

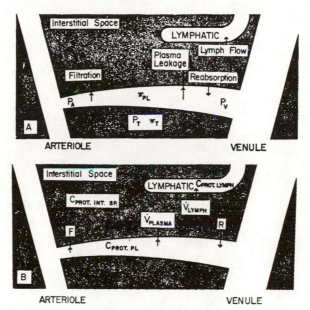

FIGURE 2.   Fluid and protein fluxes in interstitial space. A, Fluid fluxes: P_A = arterial capillary pressure; P_V = venous capillary pressure; π_{PL} = plasma oncotic pressure; P_T = tissue pressure; π_T = tissue fluid oncotic pressure. B, Protein fluxes in interstitial space: $\dot{V}_{plasma}$ = plasma leak through large-pore system; $\dot{V}_{lymph}$ = lymph flow; $C_{prot.\ pl}$ = protein concentration of plasma; $C_{prot.\ lymph}$ = protein concentration in lymph.

P_T the hydrostatic pressure in the tissue of the interstitial space, π_{PL} the colloid osmotic pressure of plasma, and π_T the colloid osmotic pressure of tissue fluid. A similar equation describes reabsorption.

$$R = K_V A_V (P_V - P_T - \pi_{PL} + \pi_T) \tag{2}$$

where K_V and A_V represent the permeability and surface area of the venous capillaries, respectively, and P_V is the hydrostatic pressure in the venous capillary. The plasma leakage through the large-pore system is a bulk flow, and is mainly determined by the hydrostatic pressure gradient across the venous capillary wall. Thus

$$\text{Plasma leakage: } \dot{V}_{plasma} = K_1(P_V - P_T) \qquad (3)$$

When the tissue pressure exceeds the venous capillary pressure, plasma leakage is assumed to be zero. The lymph flow is assumed to be a linear function of the tissue pressure. Thus

$$\text{Lymph flow: } \dot{V}_{lymph} = K_2 P_T \qquad (4)$$

Lymph flow is also assumed to be zero for negative tissue pressures. In equilibrium, the algebraic sum of the fluxes into and out of the interstitial space must be zero. If an input variable, e.g. venous capillary pressure or colloid osmotic pressure of plasma, is changed, net flux changes transiently, leading to a change in interstitial space volume before a new equilibrium is established. The change in interstitial space volume is

$$\Delta V = \int_0^t (F + \dot{V}_{plasma} + R - \dot{V}_{lymph})\, dt \qquad (5)$$

As a first approximation, the hydrostatic pressure of tissue fluid was assumed to be a linear function of the change in tissue volume.

$$\text{Tissue pressure: } P_T = K_4 \Delta V \qquad (6)$$

where K_4 represents the compliance of the interstitial space. At a given volume of the interstitial space, which might be considered a reference volume (V_0), tissue pressure is zero. The total interstitial space volume under varying input conditions, then, is

$$V = V_0 + \Delta V \qquad (7)$$

A similar set of expressions may also be derived for protein fluxes into and out of the interstitial space (Fig. 2 *B*). The protein flux into the interstitial space through the large-pore system is

$$\dot{Q}_{prot.\ leak} = \dot{V}_{plasma}\, C_{prot.\ pl}, \qquad (8)$$

where $C_{prot.\ pl.}$ is the concentration of protein in the plasma. Similarly, the protein flux removed from the interstitial space by the lymphatics is

$$\dot{Q}_{prot.\ lymph} = \dot{V}_{lymph}\, C_{prot.\ lymph} \qquad (9)$$

where $C_{prot.\ lymph}$ is the concentration of protein in the lymph. The protein content of lymph and tissue fluid is assumed to be identical. Thus

$$C_{prot.\ lymph} = C_{prot.\ int.\ sp.} \qquad (10)$$

The quantity of protein in the interstitial space may be represented by a time integral of the differences of these two protein fluxes. Thus

$$Q_{\text{prot.}} = \int_0^t (\dot{Q}_{\text{prot. leak}} - \dot{Q}_{\text{prot. lymph}}) \, dt \qquad (11)$$

The concentration of protein in the tissue fluid may then be determined.

$$C_{\text{prot. int. sp.}} = \frac{Q_{\text{prot.}}}{V} \qquad (12)$$

Colloid osmotic pressure in the tissue fluid was assumed as a first approximation to be a linear function of the protein concentration. Thus

$$\pi_T = K_3 C_{\text{prot. int. sp.}} \qquad (13)$$

TABLE I

ASSUMED NORMAL VALUES FOR PARAMETERS
USED IN COMPUTER ANALYSIS

Parameter	Value
Arterial capillary pressure (P_A)	35 mm Hg
Venous capillary pressure (P_V)	15 mm Hg
Plasma oncotic pressure (π_{PL})	25 mm Hg
K_A/K_V	0.6
A_A/A_V	0.25
$K_A A_A/K_V A_V$	0.16
Plasma leakage	5% of total exchange
Interstitial space compliance	60%/mm Hg

It should be emphasized that the equilibrium is established by osmotic pressures, and any errors introduced by the assumption that the plasma proteins obey Van't Hoff's law will be reflected in values for the protein concentration rather than in the osmotic pressures.

The majority of the terms in the preceding equations represent experimentally determined input variables as listed in Table 1. Solutions are sought for steady-state values of the tissue fluid osmotic pressure (π_T) and hydrostatic tissue pressure (P_T). The solution for these two parameters in turn determines changes of interstitial volume (ΔV) and lymph flow ($\dot{Q}_{\text{lymph}}$).

A schematic of the analogue computer program is shown in Fig. 3. The two operational amplifiers in the upper left-hand corner are connected in an adder-subtracter configuration, and yield values for the net pressures for filtration and reabsorption. After multiplication by the coefficients $K_A A_A$ and $K_V A_V$, a measure of filtration and reabsorption is obtained. The additional two operational amplifiers on the left side of the figure, with their coefficient potentiometers, generate the remaining two fluxes, the plasma leak and lymph flow. The diodes in the output circuits impose unidirectional flow through the large-pore system and through the lymphatics. The coefficient potentiometer K_5 establishes the relationship between plasma and protein leakage. The four fluid fluxes are added algebraically, yielding a measure of net flux, which after integration yields a measure of changes in the interstitial volume (ΔV). The coefficient potentiometer K_4 represents interstitial compliance, and relates tissue pressure to the change in interstitial volume. The net flux

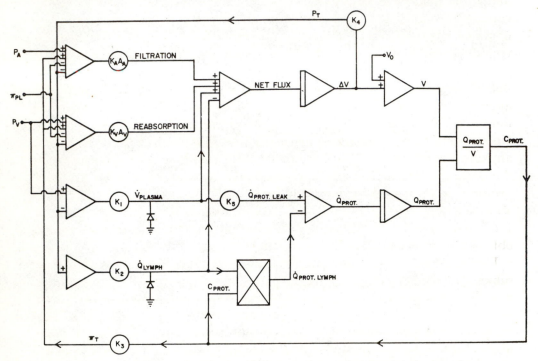

FIGURE 3. Diagram of analogue computer program. For a description, see the text.

of protein into the interstitial space is also derived from the output of the two operational amplifiers (Fig. 3, lower left). The net flux of protein ($\dot{Q}_{prot.}$) represents the difference of the protein flux through the large pore system and the lymph. By integrating the net flux, the quantity of protein ($Q_{prot.}$) in the interstitial space is derived. Dividing this quantity by the interstitial volume (V) yields a value for the protein concentration in the interstitial fluid. The coefficient K_3 relates this concentration to the colloid osmotic pressure of the tissue fluid.

Time scaling was not attempted in this first generation of the simulation program; only steady-state solutions were sought. A rigorous solution for transient events would require inclusion of nonlinearities in the relationship between protein concentration and colloid osmotic pressure of plasma proteins, and also the interstitial compliance. These were not included at this time because of analogue computer limitations.

RESULTS

Normal Values and Simulation of Lymphedema and Inflammation

Ten input and output variables were recorded on an eight-channel strip-chart recorder, as shown in Fig. 4. Recordings of colloid osmotic pressure for plasma and tissue fluid were multiplexed on one channel, and arterial and venous capillary pressures were multiplexed on another. Fig. 4 *A* shows a recording obtained in experimental simulation of lymphedema. The first 5 mm of the recording represent the normal state. Interstitial volume in the normal state was considered to be 100%, and changes in interstitial volume were subsequently shown as percentages of the initial volume. The tissue pressure was approximately +1 mm Hg. Colloid osmotic pressures of plasma and tissue fluid were 24 and 10 mm Hg, respectively. Filtration under these conditions amounted to 15 AU, and reabsorption, to 9 AU. Plasma leakage, as expected, amounted to only a small fraction of the sum of filtration and reabsorption, on the order of 0.4 AU. Lymph flow was 5 AU; arterial and venous capillary pressures were 35 and 14 mm Hg, respectively. Lymph flow amounted to approximately 30% of the filtration. The computed tissue pressure value of 1 mm Hg agrees with McMaster's observations (26) and also with results obtained in this laboratory.

Lymphedema was simulated by reducing lymph flow to zero and recording subsequent changes in the different parameters. The most striking feature is a dramatic increase in interstitial volume, amounting to over 900%. If the interstitial space is assumed to represent 20% of the tissue volume, this increase in interstitial space would correspond approximately to a doubling of the tissue volume, which is not uncommonly observed in severe lymphedema. Associated with the drastic increase of interstitial volume, tissue pressure is elevated to about 13 mm Hg, which approximates the pressure in the venous capillary. The oncotic pressure of tissue fluid rises to levels approaching the plasma colloid osmotic pressure. Relatively small changes were observed in both filtration and reabsorption, mainly because of the parallel increases in tissue hydrostatic and oncotic pressures, which cancel each other. Plasma leakage decreases toward zero as the hydrostatic pressure gradient across the venous capillary is progressively reduced with increasing tissue pressure. Many clinical features of lymphedema thus can be simulated by the computer program.

Increased capillary permeability to protein, associated with an inflammatory reaction, may also be conveniently simulated with the computer (Fig. 4 *B*). In this computer run, inflammation was simulated by increasing the

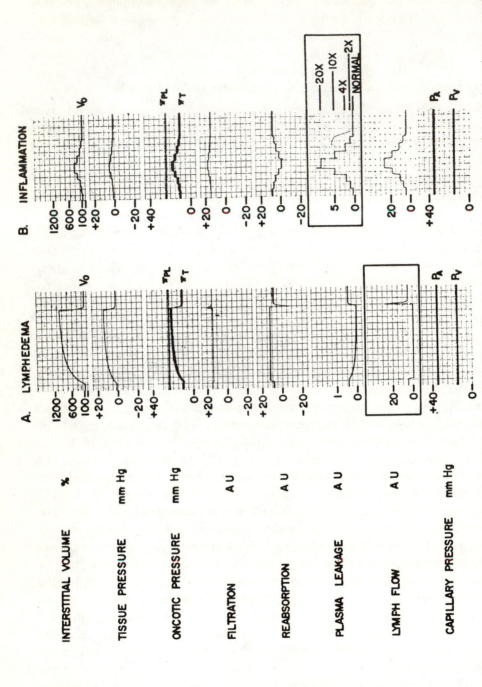

FIGURE 4. Simulation of lymphedema and inflammation. The eight recorder channels show recordings of 10 input and output variables. Oncotic pressures of plasma and tissue fluid are multiplexed on the third recorder channel. Arterial and venous capillary pressures are multiplexed on the eighth recorder channel. The altered input parameter is indicated by a frame.

plasma leakage from normal to 2, 4, 10, and 20 times normal. Edema, re-flected in the increased interstitial volume, was less pronounced than in the case of lymphedema. With a 20-fold increase in permeability to protein, interstitial volume increased only 3-fold. Tissue pressure showed a moderate elevation to +5 mm Hg. Colloid osmotic pressure of tissue fluid increased from a normal of 10 mm Hg to a peak of approximately 16 mm Hg. There was a slight increase in filtration, and a marked depression of reabsorption, presumably because of the elevated tissue fluid protein concentration. Lymph flow increased dramatically from a normal of 5 AU to a maximum of 26 AU. The higher removal rate of tissue fluid by means of lymphatics probably accounts for the relatively small accumulation of fluid in the interstitial space.

Even though it is reassuring that pathological processes may be reproduced in some detail by means of a computer program, its greatest value rests in the ability to elucidate basic physiological mechanisms, as described in the next section.

Effects of Changing Plasma Oncotic Pressure and Venous Pressure

As pointed out in the first section of this report, a protective factor appears to exist which limits major shifts of fluid from the circulation into the inter-stitial space, unless changes in either plasma oncotic pressure or venous pressure are larger than 10–15 mm Hg. In order to elucidate the nature of this protective mechanism, the plasma oncotic pressure or, alternatively, the venous pressure was changed in separate computer runs (Figs. 5 and 6). Fig. 5 illustrates an experiment in which the plasma oncotic pressure was changed from 40 to 0 mm Hg and then returned. With hypertonic pressures, the interstitial volume was reduced about 30%. Changing the colloid osmotic pressure from 40 to 20 mm Hg produces relatively slight changes in the interstitial volume. As the plasma osmotic pressure is reduced to less than 15 mm Hg, however, each stepwise change in oncotic pressure leads to progres-sively larger changes in interstitial volume. When the plasma oncotic pressure is reduced to zero, the interstitial volume increases by 500%. The change in interstitial volume is associated with a moderate increase in tissue pressure, from a low of less than +1 mm Hg in the hypertonic range to a peak of +8 mm Hg when the plasma oncotic pressure is zero. It is particularly noteworthy that each incremental change in plasma oncotic pressure is followed by an almost identical change in oncotic pressure of tissue fluid, as shown in the third recorder channel. As the plasma oncotic pressure is reduced below 20 mm Hg, however, the changes in tissue oncotic pressure become progressively smaller. Filtration increases moderately as the plasma oncotic pressure is decreased; reabsorption is markedly reduced, however. In fact, when the plasma oncotic pressure is reduced to 10 mm Hg, reabsorption in the venous capillary is supplanted by filtration. Plasma leakage shows a gradual decrease

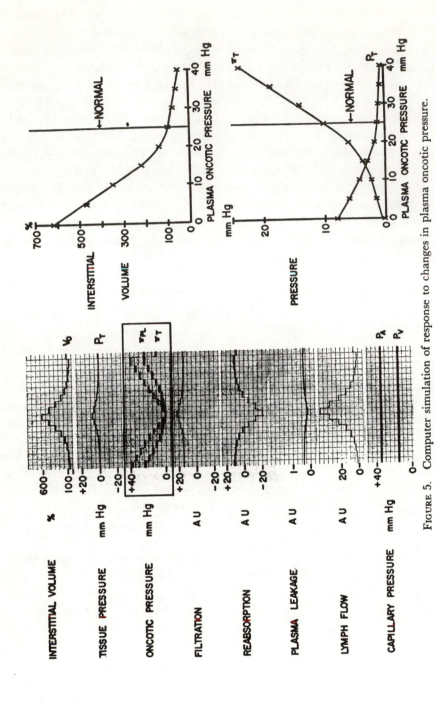

FIGURE 5. Computer simulation of response to changes in plasma oncotic pressure.

associated with progressively increasing tissue pressure. Lymph flow increases dramatically, and reaches a peak of 43 AU as compared with a control value of 5 AU.

The maintenance of a relatively constant interstitial volume can be demonstrated by plotting interstitial volume against plasma oncotic pressure (Fig. 5, top right). Over a range of plasma oncotic pressure from 40 to 20 mm Hg, the change in the interstitial volume is relatively insignificant. When the plasma oncotic pressure is reduced below 15 mm Hg, interstitial volume increases dramatically. At a plasma oncotic pressure of 15 mm Hg, the interstitial volume has approximately doubled, equivalent to 1+ edema. The compensatory changes which maintain the interstitial volume relatively constant are illustrated in the graph in Fig. 5, bottom right. This graph shows a composite plot of tissue pressure and tissue fluid oncotic pressure against plasma oncotic pressure. At hypertonic plasma oncotic pressures, the oncotic pressure of tissue fluid is high. Each decremental decrease of plasma oncotic pressure is reflected in an almost identical decrease in the tissue fluid. This may be considered a compensatory mechanism, in which a new equilibrium of filtration and reabsorption is established by dilution of tissue fluid proteins. In the range of hypotonic plasma oncotic pressures (π_{PL} < 15 mm Hg), tissue fluid protein is diluted to a point where compensation is no longer possible. Under these circumstances, reabsorption decreases progressively, leading to an increased net flux of fluid into the tissues. The limiting factor for fluid transfer at this level shifts from one of dilution of proteins to the compliance of interstitial space, reflected in pronounced increases in tissue pressure and interstitial volume. Thus two separate mechanisms limiting the net transfer of fluid across the capillary wall appear to exist. At high plasma oncotic pressures (15–40 mm Hg), the limiting factor is mainly dilution of the tissue fluid protein. At lower oncotic pressures, the distensibility of the interstitial space is the major factor.

An essentially similar picture evolves in computer runs where the venous pressure was changed (Fig. 6). The venous pressure, in this instance considered to represent pressure in the smallest venous tributaries, was changed from 0 to 35 mm Hg. Corresponding venous capillary pressures are somewhat higher, as shown in the record (channel 8), as a result of the postcapillary resistance between the venous capillary and the small vein. Each incremental change in venous pressure is initially associated with relatively small changes in the interstitial volume. However, when the venous pressure is increased beyond 20–25 mm Hg, interstitial volume increases markedly. Tissue pressure shows a moderate increase from less than +1 mm Hg to a maximum of +5 mm Hg. Each incremental change in venous pressure is also associated with an almost identical decrease in the oncotic pressure of tissue fluid. At the highest venous pressure, dilution of the tissue fluid has progressed to a point where compensa-

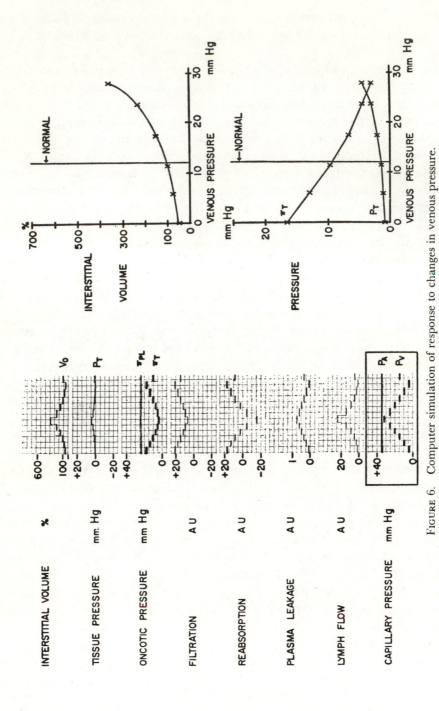

FIGURE 6.   Computer simulation of response to changes in venous pressure.

tion is no longer possible. Filtration shows a progressive decrease, associated in part with the decrease in tissue fluid oncotic pressure and in part with the increase in hydrostatic tissue pressures. Reabsorption, as would be expected, is profoundly affected by changes in the venous pressure, and is converted to filtration when the venous capillary pressure reaches 25 mm Hg. Plasma leakage progressively increases with increasing venous pressures, since bulk flow through the large-pore system is determined by the venous capillary pressure. Lymph flow also shows a progressive, but nonlinear, increase. When interstitial volume is plotted against venous pressure (Fig. 6, top right), the interstitial volume does not change significantly until venous pressure has been elevated by 10–15 mm Hg. Beyond this level, the interstitial volume increases rapidly to levels equivalent to edema. Tissue fluid oncotic pressure and tissue pressure plotted against venous pressure (Fig. 6, lower right) show the same basic features as when plasma oncotic pressure was changed. At low venous pressures, the tissue fluid oncotic pressure is high. Increasing venous pressures are counteracted to a large extent by equivalent changes in tissue fluid oncotic pressure. The limit of the compensatory range is reached at venous pressures of about 25 mm Hg, at which time tissue pressure begins to rise abruptly.

Effect of Changing Arterial Capillary Pressures

That edema is not a typical feature of hypertension until heart failure intervenes is well established clinically. Changes in arterial pressure have also been shown to have considerably less effect on capillary filtration rates than corresponding changes in venous pressure (30). Similar results have been obtained in computer runs in which the arterial capillary pressure was changed in steps from 40 to 15 mm Hg (Fig. 7). Over this pressure range, only insignificant changes were observed in interstitial volume and tissue pressure. Tissue fluid oncotic pressure increased from a normal of 10 mm Hg to 13 mm Hg, which may have been due to the reduction in filtration in the face of relatively constant plasma leakage. The reduction in filtration is a direct consequence of the reduced net filtration pressure in the arterial capillary. The reduction in reabsorption, in turn, reflects the increase in tissue oncotic pressure, which at its peak approaches the venous capillary hydrostatic pressure.

Computer Analysis of Tissue Pressure

It was pointed out in the first section of this report that measurements of tissue pressure by different techniques have yielded divergent results. Pressures recorded by hypodermic needle or ultramicroscopic glass micropipettes generally yield pressures ranging from 0 to +5 mm Hg, whereas hydrostatic pressures recorded in the free fluid space in subcutaneous capsules are normally negative. These divergent findings may be reconciled by considering the interface between the interstitial space and the free fluid within the capsule as a semipermeable membrane (Fig. 8). This figure illustrates diagrammatically the relationships between the blood vessels in the tissues surrounding the capsule and the free fluid within the capsule. The hydrostatic pressure within the capsule (P_c) is determined by the net flux of fluid from the inter-

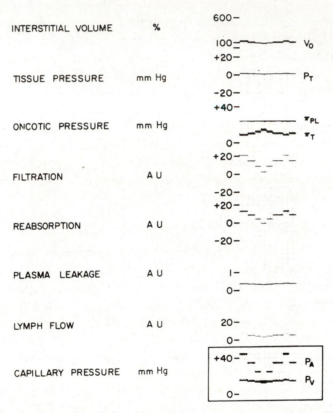

FIGURE 7.   Computer simulation of response to changes in arterial capillary pressure.

stitial space of surrounding tissues into the free fluid space ($\dot{V}_{fluid}$). The free intracapsular fluid has an average protein content of 1.9%, with a corresponding colloid osmotic pressure (π_c) of 4.3 mm Hg (28). In the interstitial space surrounding the capsule exists a hydrostatic pressure (P_T) and protein with a colloid osmotic pressure (π_T). If the interface between the free fluid and the interstitial space has the properties of a semipermeable membrane, the net fluid exchange may be defined by the following equation:

$$\dot{V}_{fluid} = K_6 (P_T - P_c - \pi_T + \pi_c) \tag{14}$$

where K_6 is a virtual permeability coefficient for the interface, and P_T and π_T denote the tissue pressure and tissue fluid oncotic pressure, respectively. P_C and π_C refer to hydrostatic and oncotic pressures of the free fluid in the capsule. The change in fluid volume within the capsule (ΔV_c) would then be an integral function of the fluid flux:

$$\Delta V_c = \int_0^t \dot{V}_{\text{fluid}}\, dt \tag{15}$$

The pressure in the capsule may be assumed to be a linear function of the volume change

$$P_C = K_7 \Delta V_c \tag{16}$$

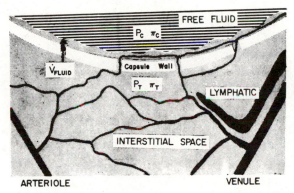

FIGURE 8. Fluid exchange between interstitial space and subcutaneous capsule. $\dot{V}_{\text{fluid}}$ = net fluid flux; P_C = hydrostatic pressure in capsule; π_C = oncotic pressure of free intracapsular fluid.

where K_7 represents the compliance of the capsule. In simulation of steady-state conditions, the steps described by equations 15 and 16 need not be performed; determining the capsule pressure for which the fluid flux is zero is sufficient. Three of the quantities describing the net driving pressure are known. P_T and π_T may be derived from the computer simulation program as described in previous sections, and π_c is 4.3 mm Hg (28). Thus the equation can be solved for P_c as the tissue pressure and tissue fluid oncotic pressure vary in response to changes in the input parameters. The results of a computer simulation run are shown in Fig. 9, in which the plasma oncotic pressure was changed and tissue fluid oncotic pressure, hydrostatic tissue pressure, intra-capsular hydrostatic pressure, and interstitial volume were recorded. The changes in tissue fluid oncotic pressure, tissue pressure, and interstitial volume are identical with those described previously, and need not be elaborated here. The computed hydrostatic pressure within the capsule is generally negative, however. When the plasma oncotic pressure is 40 mm Hg, the capsule pressure is about −19 mm Hg. As the oncotic pressure of plasma is reduced in 5 mm steps, the capsule pressure increases progressively. At the normal plasma oncotic pressure of 25 mm Hg, the intracapsular pressure is −5 mm Hg, which agrees well with Guyton's experimental measurements. A composite plot of the tissue hydrostatic, oncotic, and capsule pressures vs. plasma oncotic pressure is shown in Fig. 9, right. It is noteworthy that at normal plasma oncotic pressure the computed tissue pressure is about +1 mm

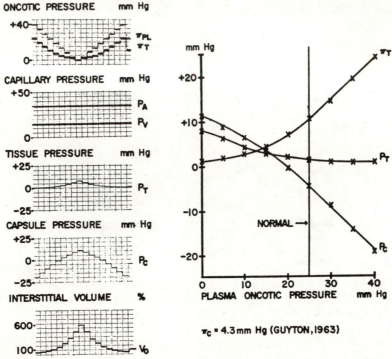

FIGURE 9. Computer simulation of equilibrium of fluid exchange between interstitial space and intracapsular fluid under conditions of changing plasma oncotic pressure.

Hg and the tissue fluid oncotic pressure about 10 mm Hg, whereas the computed intracapsular pressure is −5 mm Hg. As plasma oncotic pressures are increased from the normal level, correspondence between changes in tissue fluid oncotic pressure and capsular pressure is almost 1:1. As plasma oncotic pressures are reduced below 15 mm Hg, the capsule pressure approaches the tissue pressure. At the lowest values for plasma oncotic pressure, the capsule pressure parallels the tissue pressure with an offset corresponding to the oncotic pressure of the free fluid in the capsule (4.3 mm Hg). A basically similar response is seen when venous pressure is changed.

The data generated by the computer simulation yield a reasonable fit to

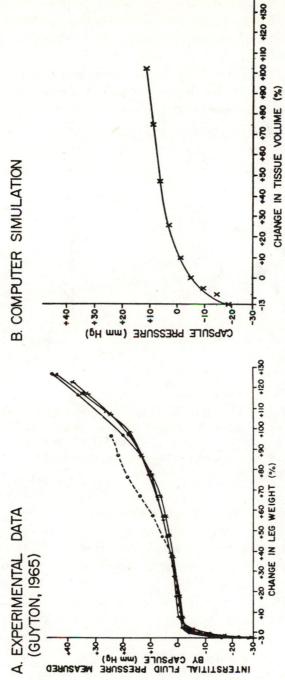

Figure 10. Comparison of experimental data of Guyton (31) with computed solution for intracapsular pressure. *Left-hand graph reprinted by permission from Dr. A. C. Guyton and The American Heart Association, Inc. and from Circulation Research (Interstitial fluid pressure: II. Pressure-volume curves of interstitial space, 1965, 16:452).*

Guyton's experimental data (28, 31). When computed intracapsular pressure is plotted against interstitial volume, expressed as a percentage change in total tissue volume, a fair fit is obtained over a relatively wide range (Fig. 10 *A* and *B*). The deviation in the lower range may be explained in part by the fact that the experimental data of Guyton were obtained in dehydrated preparations. Deviation in the high range may have been due to the simplifying assumption in the computer program that the interstitial volume is a linear function of tissue pressure. Deviations from linearity would be expected at large volume changes, however.

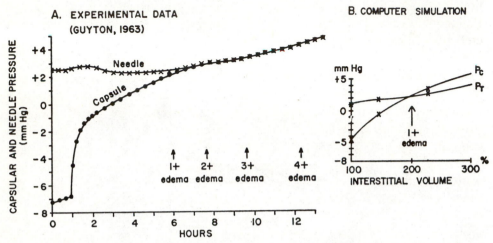

FIGURE 11.   Comparison of experimental data on intracapsular and needle pressures in animal experiments with computed values of tissue and intracapsular pressures. *Left-hand graph reprinted by permission from Dr. A. C. Guyton and The American Heart Association, Inc. and from Circulation Research (Concentration of negative interstitial pressure based on pressures in implanted perforated capsules, 1963, 12:399).*

A second comparison of computer-generated data with experimental data is shown in Fig. 11. Guyton plotted intracapsular pressure and tissue pressure, recorded by needle, during development of edema (Fig. 11 *A*) (31). Computed values of tissue pressure and intracapsular pressures show a similar divergence, which initially amounts to 6.5 mm Hg. After 1 + edema has developed, the pressure recorded within the capsule and by the needle coincide in Guyton's experiments. In the computer simulation, tissue and capsule pressures cross over when the interstitial volume is increased by 100%, corresponding to 1 + edema (Fig. 11 *B*). In the animal experiments, needle and capsule pressures were identical as edema increased. In the computer simulation, however, capsule pressure slightly exceeded tissue pressure.

COMPARISON OF COMPUTER SIMULATION DATA
WITH EXPERIMENTAL DATA

Normal Values

Despite its relative simplicity, the computer model has agreed surprisingly well with experimental data in the literature. Normal tissue pressure in the range of +1 mm Hg is in line with McMaster's (26) measurements and also with independent measurements in our laboratory. The relative magnitude of filtration, reabsorption, and lymph flow is somewhat higher than estimated by Landis and Pappenheimer (3). Computer analysis indicated that lymph flow normally amounts to 30% of filtration; the estimate of Landis and Pappenheimer ranged from 10 to 20%. Adjustment of some computer parameters may bring these results closer in line. The most striking divergence from previously published normal values were obtained for oncotic pressure of tissue fluid, since computer runs averaged 10 mm Hg, which corresponds to a tissue fluid protein concentration of 3.5%. Whereas the protein content of lymph derived from cardiac muscle, lungs, or gastrointestinal tract may exceed this value, lymph from skin and skeletal muscle usually has a lower protein content. This unexpectedly high value can be explained, however, on the basis of physical chemical properties of the ground substance, which occupies a substantial fraction of the interstitial space. The ground substance in the connective tissue of skin is composed mainly of hyaluronic acid and chondroitin sulfate (32). Characteristically the macromolecules of these mucopolysaccharides form an intertwining meshwork, in which the mesh diameter is sufficiently small to exclude the protein but is freely permeable to smaller molecules such as water, electrolytes, and glucose. The fluid bound in the ground substance thus is not available to the protein; i.e. the plasma protein space is not identical with the total interstitial space.

Biochemical assay of human skin shows an average content of 0.2% mucopolysaccharides (32). Since the interstitial space occupies approximately 20% of the total skin volume, the concentration of mucopolysaccharides within the interstitial space could be as high as 1%. The osmotic pressure of a 1% solution of hyaluronic acid has been estimated to be 4.5 mm Hg (33). 1 g of hyaluronic acid may bind as much as 100 ml of water in the absence of other sterically excluded macromolecules, such as plasma albumin. In the presence of albumin, however, water will be extracted from the meshwork of the ground substance, and free fluid spaces will exist within the ground substance. The water bound in the ground substance thus is in a dynamic equilibrium with the free fluid phase. The syneresis is associated with a pronounced nonlinear increase in osmotic pressure. For instance, a 2% solution of hyaluronic acid exerts an osmotic pressure of 18 mm Hg (33).

The basic concept of the interstitial space as a two-phase structure has been supported by a number of physiological and morphological studies, as summarized in a previous publication (34). Of particular interest is a study by Gersh and Catchpole (35), in which Evans blue was used as a vital dye. The Evans blue, which presumably was bound to plasma albumin, was found to be distributed in discrete areas within the ground substance. In these same

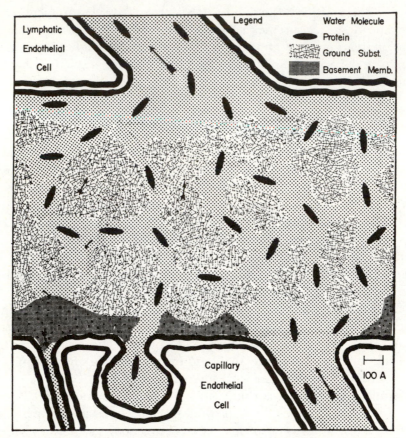

FIGURE 12.   Interrelationship of ground substance, free fluid, and fluid and protein exchange in interstitial space. The large pore and the tight junction between capillary endothelial cells and protein molecules are drawn approximately to scale.

areas soluble mucopolysaccharides were found, corresponding to free fluid space. The combined effect of the osmotic pressure of the mucopolysaccharides in the ground substance and exclusion of protein may account for the unexpectedly high values for tissue fluid oncotic pressure required for an equilibrium of fluid fluxes.

The interrelationship of ground substance, free fluid, and fluid and protein exchange in the interstitial space is outlined diagrammatically in Fig. 12.

The figure represents the interstitial space between a venous capillary (bottom) and a lymphatic capillary (top). The capillary endothelium shows a 250 A large pore, through which plasma, containing water and protein, is filtered. On the left side is shown a tight junction 40 A wide, through which reabsorption occurs. Protein molecules are restricted to the free fluid phase in the interstitial space, whereas water freely permeates the meshwork of the ground substance. The arrows indicate the net drift of the solvent through the free fluid spaces as well as through the basement membrane and ground substance. Since the protein molecules are restricted to the free fluid phase, they will exert a higher osmotic pressure than if the bound fluid were available for dilution. The protein concentration in the free fluid of the interstitial space may thus be considerably higher than the concentration in either lymph or capillary filtrate, and thus exert a correspondingly higher oncotic pressure. A quantitative evaluation of the role of the ground substance is not possible at this stage, however, since information on fluid fluxes in gels is scanty.

In the studies of Pappenheimer and Soto-Rivera on the isogravimetric hind limb preparation, the average protein osmotic pressure in interstitial fluid was estimated to be 1.4 mm Hg (30). This value is considerably lower than those predicted either from estimates of interstitial protein concentration by tracer studies or by the computer analysis. Pappenheimer and Soto-Rivera's data, however, can be fitted to the computer simulation data if one considers the fact that the blood used in the majority of their experiments had colloid osmotic pressures lower than normal. In 18 out of 20 experiments, the osmotic pressure of the plasma used in the perfusion procedure ranged between 8 and 20 mm Hg, with an average of 15 mm Hg. This low value was believed to result from dilution of the plasma with tissue fluid during the bleeding of the donor animals. It is noteworthy that, when the plasma oncotic pressure is reduced to 15 mm Hg in the computer analysis, the corresponding oncotic pressure of tissue fluid is +3 mm Hg (Fig. 5). Since the tissue pressure at this plasma protein concentration is almost identical with the oncotic pressure of the tissue fluid, their effects cancel out. The isogravimetric pressure under these conditions accurately represents the oncotic pressure of plasma. That Pappenheimer's experiments were carried out under these conditions is perhaps fortuitous, since the validity of the computations of capillary filtration coefficient as well as of changes in pre- and postcapillary resistance depends critically on the assumption of negligible tissue hydrostatic and oncotic pressures. Results obtained by Pappenheimer and Soto-Rivera after periods of prolonged filtration or absorption can also be duplicated qualitatively in the computer simulation. The tissue fluid in the isolated hind limb was first concentrated by allowing net absorption to occur. At minimum limb weight the isogravimetric pressure amounted to only two-thirds of the plasma protein pressure, which was attributed to increased concentration of protein in the tissue fluid. Capillary pressure was then increased above the isogravimetric value, leading to filtration throughout the capillary network. Filtration of 15 ml of fluid into the interstitial space diluted the tissue fluid protein sufficiently to increase the isogravimetric pressure to 92% of the plasma oncotic pressure. Further filtration did not increase the isogravimetric pressure significantly. It is noteworthy that in the computer analysis the crossover of tissue hydrostatic and oncotic pressures occurs when venous pressure is elevated to levels between 25 and 30 mm Hg. In other experiments, the isolated hind limb preparation was initially perfused with plasma having an oncotic pressure of 17.2 mm Hg for $2\frac{3}{4}$ hr. Subsequently plasma rendered hypertonic by addition of bovine albumin ($\pi_{PL} = 39.5$ mm Hg) was substituted. The first measurements of isogravimetric pressure, 10–15 min after the perfusion of hypertonic plasma was begun, show isogravimetric pressures averaging 60% of the plasma oncotic pressure. During the perfusion period of $5\frac{1}{2}$ hr, the isogravimetric pressure decreased to a level of approximately 25% of the plasma protein pressure without a change in the filtration coefficient. This decrease was attributed to an abnormal permeability of the capillary membranes to crystalline bovine albumin. The alternative should be considered, however, namely that the initial perfusion of the experimental preparation with hypotonic plasma would wash out protein from the interstitial space into the normally collapsed lymphatics. A new equilibrium would be restored over a prolonged time interval, since the amount of protein moving through the large pore system is small compared to the interstitial fluid volume. In comparison, when oncotic pressure is elevated to 40 mm Hg in the computer simulation, tissue fluid oncotic pressure rises to a level of 23 mm Hg. The effective osmotic pressure ($\pi_{PL} - \pi_T$) is approximately 40% of the total plasma osmotic pressure, as compared with Pappenheimer's experimental determination of 25%. Since removal of protein by lymphatic drainage is prevented in the isogravimetric hind limb preparation, the lower values at equilibrium are not unexpected. In the computer simulation of lymphedema, the corresponding effective oncotic pressure is 15% of the plasma oncotic pressure (Fig. 4).

Pappenheimer and Soto-Rivera pointed out that diffusion coefficients of plasma protein are such that relatively large concentration gradients are possible between tissue fluid undergoing reabsorption at the venous end and freshly formed capillary filtrate at the arterial end. Even if all filtration and absorption processes were stopped, some 20 min would be required to reach 90% of equilibration of the protein concentration over a distance of 50 μ. However, significant osmotic gradients associated with unequal distribution of protein are unlikely in the interstitial space, since osmotic attraction of water into areas of high concentration would lead to rapid equilibration. In contrast with the relatively slow diffusion rates of plasma proteins, only 30 sec would be required to reach 66% equilibration of protein concentration over a distance of 50 μ by redistribution of water (34). Thus, large gradients in osmotic pressure are unlikely within the interstitial space, except on a molecular scale such as represented in Fig. 12.

Effect of Changing Plasma Oncotic Pressure

Data obtained from the computer analysis also agree reasonably with experimental studies in which plasma oncotic pressure was altered by continuous infusion of Ringer's solution. A compensatory change in tissue fluid protein concentration, as plasma oncotic pressure is altered, has been demonstrated experimentally by Morris (36). In his experiments, hemodilution was induced by infusing Ringer's solution at a rate of 100 ml/kg/5 hr. Concentrations of protein in plasma and intestinal lymph were measured. Prior to the Ringer's infusion, the difference in colloid osmotic pressure between plasma and lymph was 8 mm Hg; at the end of the experiment, 5 hr later, this difference was 9 mm Hg. The reduction in plasma oncotic pressure was thus compensated by an almost identical reduction of tissue fluid oncotic pressure. Infusion of Ringer's solution also led to a 4-fold increase in lymph flow from the intestinal lymphatics. In the computer simulation, lymph flow increases by a factor of 3 for a similar change in plasma protein concentration. Similarly, Földi, Rusznyák, and Szabó (37) found a 4-fold increase in thoracic duct lymph flow in animals rendered hypoproteinemic by plasmapheresis.

Qualitative agreement has also been obtained by comparing data from the computer analysis with experimental studies on hypoproteinemia. It was pointed out that in the computer simulation plasma oncotic pressure has to be lowered to 10–15 mm Hg before changes in the interstitial volume occur which correspond to 1+ edema. A number of studies (4–6) indicated that edema occurs after plasmapheresis only if the protein level of the plasma drops below 3–3.5%, corresponding to a colloid osmotic pressure of 10–12 mm Hg. Similar observations have been made in clinical studies on nephrotic patients.

Hypoproteinemic conditions are associated with large increases in flow of lymph with low protein concentration. The leakage of protein through the large-pore system would be expected to be decreased in hypoproteinemia, both as a consequence of the decreased protein content of plasma, and also because of the reduced pressure gradient across the venous capillary wall. This is in contrast with edema induced by elevation of venous pressure, in which the pressure gradient across the large-pore system is actually elevated. One would thus predict that the protein content of edema fluid associated with cardiac failure should be higher than that associated with hypoproteinemic conditions. This prediction is supported by data summarized by Landis and Pappenheimer (3), which indicate that in hypoproteinemic states in most instances the protein content of edema fluid ranges between 0.1 and 0.27%, whereas in cardiac failure edema fluids contain from 0.1 to 1% protein, with an average of 0.4%.

Effects of Changes in Venous Pressure

Many features of the changes in capillary fluid exchange which occur when venous pressure is altered are also duplicated in the computer analysis. In the previously quoted study of Morris (36), changes in intestinal lymph flow and protein concentration in response to an increase in portal venous pressure were measured. Portal pressure was elevated from the control level of 8 mm Hg to 16 mm Hg by partial occlusion of the vena cava between the liver and the diaphragm. The elevation in venous pressure produced a 2-fold increase in intestinal lymph flow, and a reduction in lymphatic protein content from 4.2 to 3.4%, corresponding to a change in colloid osmotic pressure from 12 to 7.5 mm Hg. For corresponding venous pressure values in the computer analysis, lymph flow increases by a factor of 2.2, and the tissue fluid oncotic pressure decreases by 6 mm Hg.

In similar experiments, carried out by White et al. (38), protein concentration and lymph flow were measured in the forepaws of unanesthetized dogs. Spontaneous activity during the experimental period produced some variability in the data, and only average values are presented here. When the venous pressure in the forepaw was elevated from 14 to 26 mm Hg by inflation of a cuff, lymph flow increased by a factor of 2.1. A further increase of venous pressure to 34 mm Hg increased the lymph flow to a value 4.1 times the control flow. Data obtained from the computer analysis show a 3-fold and a 4.8-fold increase in lymph flow for corresponding changes in venous pressure. The absolute magnitudes of the protein concentration differ markedly in the experiment and in the computer simulation. The percentage changes are quite similar, however. In the experiments of White et al., elevation of the venous pressure to 26 mm Hg reduced lymph protein concentration to 42% of the control value. Further elevation of the venous pressure to 34 mm Hg reduced the protein concentration to 27% of the control value. In comparison, the computer analysis yielded a reduction of the oncotic pressure of tissue fluid to 50% and 33% of the control value for the corresponding changes in venous pressure.

By drastic elevation of venous pressure, excessive filtration into the interstitial space can be induced, thus elevating the tissue pressure as reported by McMaster (39). In his experiments a cuff was inflated around the forearm or thigh of human subjects, and tissue pressure was recorded by inserting fine hypodermic needles into the connective tissue of the skin of the arm or ankle. After the cuff had been inflated to a pressure of 80–87 mm Hg, the interstitial pressure reached an equilibrium ranging from 13 to 17 mm Hg after 20–30 min. Computer simulation of this experiment yielded an equilibrium value for tissue pressure of 25 mm Hg.

Pressure in Subcutaneous Capsules

The basic question whether pressures recorded in subcutaneous capsules represent hydrostatic pressures in tissues must be regarded as unresolved. The fit of the computer data to Guyton's experimental data indicates at least that alternative possibilities may exist. The consistency with which the negative pressures in the subcutaneous capsules is reproduced in different laboratories serves as a strong indication that the observations are not artifactual The validity of the assumed identity of tissue pressures and capsule pressures, however, rests on the assumption of free communication between fluid in the capsule and the free fluid in the interstitial space. Guyton's observation that Evans blue injected into the capsule appears in the tissue surrounding the capsule seems to support this assumption. These experiments were conducted, however, with hydrostatic pressures of $+10$ mm Hg within the capsule, which may have been sufficient to violate the integrity of the surrounding tissues. With capsules of the dimensions used by Guyton, a pressure of 10 mm Hg would give rise to a total wall tension of 0.5–1 g/cm. In comparison, the total tension at the tip of the 30 gauge needle would only amount to 0.01 g/cm for comparative pressures.

When native capsule fluid is replaced by hypertonic protein solutions, the composition of the capsule fluid retains its hypertonicity for prolonged periods. Thus, in one instance when the capsule fluid was replaced by a 5% protein solution, concentration 1 month later was still 4.1%. This extremely slow disappearance of protein from the capsules is consistent with the concept that the interface between tissue and capsule is relatively impermeable to protein. The protein composition of the intracapsular fluid may represent an average of the composition of the free fluid phase in the interstitial space, but the time course of equilibration may be prolonged to an extent where it has not yet been measured. It is noteworthy that the computed normal protein concentration of tissue fluid, amounting to 3.5%, falls between the values of 4.1%, observed 1 month after injection of hypertonic protein solution, and 1.96%, obtained about 4 wk after implantation of the capsule. However, Guyton's observation that changes in the protein concentration in the capsule do not alter the recorded capsule pressure is difficult to explain. The volume of fluid contained within the capsule is large compared to the free fluid volume within the interstitial space, and thus the tissue immediately surrounding the capsule may be in a state of relative dehydration, which would account for the maintained negative pressures.

The fact that the intracapsular pressures reflect changes in hydrostatic tissue pressures cannot be disputed. The converse, however, is not necessarily true, namely that the capsule pressures are independent of changes in tissue fluid oncotic pressure. The latter possibility might be excluded by experiments supplementing Guyton's studies, in which local injection of saline produced edema, resulting in a rise in capsule pressure into the positive range. Injection of an identical volume of native blood plasma should give identical results, if free communication exists between the tissue fluids and the capsule. If, on the other hand, the interface between tissues and the free fluid in the capsule has the properties of a semipermeable membrane, the elevated tissue fluid oncotic pressure should drive the intracapsular pressure to more negative levels. This experiment has not been performed.

SUMMARY AND CONCLUSIONS

Fluid balance at the capillary level has been simulated with an analogue computer program, based on experimental data on regional differences in capillary permeability, surface area, and hydrostatic pressures. The program takes into account four fluid fluxes into and out of the interstitial space: filtration, reabsorption, plasma leakage through the large-pore system in capillaries, and removal of tissue fluid by lymphatics. The program also takes into account changes in tissue fluid protein concentration, as determined by differences in protein fluxes into the interstitial space through the large-pore system in capillaries, and protein removal by the lymphatics. Solutions are obtained for tissue hydrostatic pressure, tissue fluid osmotic pressure, interstitial space volume, and lymph flow. Simulation of these processes yields qualitative agreement with clinical data. Changes in input parameters, e.g. plasma oncotic pressure, venous pressure, or arterial capillary pressure, yield results which agree well with physiological data obtained in many experimental studies. The computer analysis has shed light on the mechanism whereby edema formation is prevented when plasma oncotic pressures are reduced by 10–15 mm Hg, or, alternatively, venous pressures are elevated by a similar amount. Dilution of the interstitial plasma protein pool with a consequent reduction of its oncotic pressures appears to be the major factor, as originally surmised by Starling. When the plasma oncotic pressure is reduced below 15 mm Hg, or venous pressure elevated by more than 10 mm Hg, excessive dilution of tissue fluid protein occurs. The increased filtration leads to edema, the extent of which is limited only by lymphatic removal of tissue fluid and the compliance of the interstitial space. The computer analysis in all instances gives positive values for tissue pressure, in agreement with experimental data obtained by needle puncture. The negative tissue pressures observed in subcutaneous capsules can be reproduced in the simulation program, however, if the interface between the capsule and the surrounding interstitial space is assumed to have the properties of a semipermeable membrane.

This work was supported by grants 2-K3-HE-22,465 and HE 10861 from the National Institutes of Health.

The author wishes to express his gratitude to Mr. Burton Weston, who participated actively and enthusiastically in all phases of these studies, ranging from data acquisition to preparation of illustrations. The valuable contributions by Dr. Don Stromberg, Mr. Dennis Lee, and Mrs. Coralee Huynh are also acknowledged with deep appreciation.

REFERENCES

1. STARLING, E. H. 1896. On the absorption of fluids from the connective tissue spaces. *J. Physiol., (London)*. **19**:312.
2. LANDIS, E. M. 1930. Microinjection studies of capillary blood pressure in human skin. *Heart*. **15**:209.
3. LANDIS, E. M., and J. R. PAPPENHEIMER. 1963. Exchange of substances through the capillary walls. *In Handbook of Physiology, Section II; Circulation*. W. F. Hamilton and P. Dow, editors. American Physiological Society, Washington, D.C. **2**:961.
4. BARKER, M. H., and E. J. KIRK. 1930. Experimental edema (nephrosis) in dogs in relation to edema of renal origin in patient. *A.M.A. Arch. Internal Med.* **45**:319.
5. LEITER, L. 1931. Experimental nephrotic edema. *A.M.A. Arch. Internal Med.* **48**:1.
6. DARROW, D. C., E. G. HOPPER, and M. K. CARRY. 1932. Plasmapheresis edema. I. The relation of reduction of serum proteins to edema and the pathological anatomy accompanying plasmapheresis. *J. Clin. Invest.* **11**:683.
7. FÖLDI, M., I. RUSZNYÁK, and G. SZABÓ. 1949. Role of lymph circulation in the origin of phlebohypertonic oedemas. (Hungarian.) *Quoted in* RUSZNYÁK, I., M. FÖLDI, and G. SZABÓ. 1960. Lymphatics and Lymph Circulation. Pergamon Press, New York. 235.
8. BEECHER, H. K. 1937. Adjustment of the flow of tissue fluid in the presence of localized, sustained high venous pressure as found with varices of the great saphenous system during walking. *J. Clin. Invest.* **16**:733.
9. GUYTON, A. C., and A. W. LINDSAY. 1959. Effect of elevated left atrial pressure and decreased plasma protein concentration on the development of pulmonary edema. *Circulation Res.* **7**:649.
10. ROUS, P., H. P. GILDING, and F. SMITH. 1930. The gradient of vascular permeability. *J. Exptl. Med.* **51**:807.
11. MORI, K., S. YAMADA, R. OHORI, M. TAKADA, and T. NAITO. 1963. Observations *in vivo* on the extravasation of various dye fluids from blood vessels into the connective tissue. *Okajima's Folia Anat. Japon.* **39**:277.
12. LANDIS, E. M. 1964. Heteroporosity of the capillary wall as indicated by cinematographic analysis of the passage of dyes. *Ann. N.Y. Acad. Sci.* **116**:765.
13. WIEDERHIELM, C. A. 1967. Analysis of small vessel function. *In Physical Bases of Circulatory Transport: Regulation and Exchange*. E. B. Reeve and A. C. Guyton, editors. W. B. Saunders Company, Philadelphia. 313.
14. INTAGLIETTA, M. 1967. Evidence for a gradient of permeability in frog mesenteric capillaries. *Bibliotheca Anat.* **9**:465.
15. DAVIS, M. J., AND J. C. LAWLER. 1958. The capillary circulation of the skin. *A.M.A. Arch. Dermatol.* **77**:690.
16. WETZEL, N. C., and Y. ZOTTERMAN. 1926. On differences in the vascular colouration of various regions of the normal human skin. *Heart*. **13**:357.
17. WIEDEMAN, M. P. 1963. Dimensions of blood vessels from distributing artery to collecting vein. *Circulation Res.* **12**:375.
18. GROTTE, G. 1956. Passage of dextran molecules across the blood-lymph barrier. *Acta Chir. Scand.* **211**:1.
19. WASSERMAN, K., and H. S. MAYERSON. 1951. Exchange of albumin between plasma and lymph. *Am. J. Physiol.* **165**:15.
20. OEFF, K. 1954. Umsatz von radioaktiven Sermeiweissfraktionen. III. Versuche an normalen Kaninchen. *Z. Ges. Exptl. Med.* **123**:434.

21. ABDOU, I. A., W. O. REINHARDT, and H. TARVER. 1952. Plasma protein. III. The equilibrium between the blood and lymph protein. *J. Biol. Chem.* **194**:15.
22. TAKEDA, Y. 1964. Metabolism and distribution of autologous and homologous albumin-I^{131} in the dog. *Am. J. Physiol.* **206**:1223.
23. FIELD, M. E., O. C. LEIGH, JR., J. W. HEIM, and C. K. DRINKER. 1934. The protein content and osmotic pressure of blood serum and lymph from various sources in the dog. *Am. J. Physiol.* **110**:174.
24. RÉNYI-VÁMOS, F. 1954. New investigations of the lymphatic system of certain organs. Doctorate Thesis. Budapest. (Hungarian.) *Quoted in* RUSZNYÁK, I., M. FÖLDI, and G. SZABÓ. 1960. Lymphatics and Lymph Circulation. Pergamon Press, New York. 547.
25. SZABÓ, G. 1954. Factors influencing lymphogenesis and lymph flow. Doctorate Thesis. Budapest. (Hungarian.) *Quoted in* RUSZNYÁK, I., M. FÖLDI, and G. SZABÓ. 1960. Lymphatics and Lymph Circulation. Pergamon Press, New York. 547.
26. McMASTER, P. D. 1946. The pressure and interstitial resistance prevailing in the normal and edematous skin of animals and man. *J. Exptl. Med.* **84**:473.
27. WIEDERHIELM, C. A., J. W. WOODBURY, S. KIRK, and R. F. RUSHMER. 1964. Pulsatile pressures in the microcirculation of frog's mesentery. *Am. J. Physiol.* **207**:173.
28. GUYTON, A. C. 1963. A concept of negative interstitial pressure based on pressures in implanted perforated capsules. *Circulation Res.* **12**:399.
29. KATO, F. 1966. The fine structure of the lymphatics and the passage of China ink particles through their walls. *Nagoya Med. J.* **12**:221.
30. PAPPENHEIMER, J. R., and A. SOTO-RIVERA. 1948. Effective osmotic pressure of the plasma proteins and other quantities associated with the capillary circulation in the hindlimbs of cats and dogs. *Am. J. Physiol.* **152**:471.
31. GUYTON, A. C. 1965. Interstitial fluid pressure. II. Pressure-volume curves of interstitial space. *Circulation Res.* **16**:452.
32. LOEWI, G. 1961. The acid mucopolysaccharides of human skin. *Biochim. Biophys. Acta.* **52**:435.
33. OGSTON, A. G. 1966. On water binding. *Federation Proc.* **25**:986.
34. WIEDERHIELM, C. A. 1966. Transcapillary and interstitial transport phenoma in the mesentery. *Federation Proc.* **25**:1789.
35. GERSH, I., and H. R. CATCHPOLE. 1949. The organization of ground substance and basement membrane and its significance in tissue injury disease and growth. *Am. J. Anat.* **85**:457.
36. MORRIS, B. 1956. The exchange of protein between the plasma and the liver and intestinal lymph. *Quart. J. Exptl. Physiol.* **41**:326.
37. FÖLDI, M., I. RUSZNYÁK, and G. SZABÓ. 1951. Role of lymph circulation in the formation of hypalbuminaemic oedemas. (Hungarian.) *Quoted in* RUSZNYÁK, I., M. FÖLDI, and G. SZABÓ. 1960. Lymphatics and Lymph Circulation. Pergamon Press, New York. 253.
38. WHITE, J. C., M. E. FIELD, and C. K. DRINKER. 1933. On the protein content and normal flow of lymph from the foot of the dog. *Am. J. Physiol.* **103**:34.
39. McMASTER, P. D. 1946. The effect of venous obstruction upon interstitial pressure in animal and human skin. *J. Exptl. Med.* **84**:495.

Author Citation Index

Subject Index